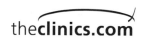

HEMATOLOGY/ ONCOLOGY CLINICS OF NORTH AMERICA

Mesothelioma

GUEST EDITOR
Hedy Lee Kindler, MD

December 2005 • Volume 19 • Number 6

SAUNDERS
An Imprint of Elsevier, Inc.
PHILADELPHIA   LONDON   TORONTO   MONTREAL   SYDNEY   TOKYO

W.B. SAUNDERS COMPANY
A Division of Elsevier Inc.

Elsevier, Inc. · 1600 John F. Kennedy Boulevard · Suite 1800 · Philadelphia, Pennsylvania 19103-2899

http:/www.hemonc.theclinics.com

HEMATOLOGY/ONCOLOGY CLINICS OF NORTH AMERICA
December 2005
Editor: Kerry Holland

Volume 19, Number 6
ISSN 0889-8588
ISBN 1-4160-2776-9

The ideas and opinions expressed in *Hematology/Oncology Clinics of North America* do not necessarily reflect those of the Publisher. The Publisher does not assume any responsibility for any injury and/or damage to persons or property arising out of or related to any use of the material contained in this periodical. The reader is advised to check the appropriate medical literature and the product information currently provided by the manufacturer of each drug to be administered to verify the dosage, the method and duration of administration, or contraindications. It is the responsibility of the treating physician or other health care professional, relying on independent experience and knowledge of the patient, to determine drug dosages and the best treatment for the patient. Mention of any product in this issue should not be construed as endorsement by the contributors, editors, or the Publisher of the product or manufacturers' claims.

Hematology/Oncology Clinics of North America (ISSN 0889-8588) is published bi-monthly by W.B. Saunders Company. Corporate and editorial offices: Elsevier, Inc., 1600 John F. Kennedy Boulevard, Suite 1800, Philadelphia, PA 19103-2899. Accounting and circulation offices: 6277 Sea Harbor Drive, Orlando, FL 32887-4800. Periodicals postage paid at Orlando, FL 32862, and additional mailing offices. Subscription prices are $220.00 per year (US individuals), $110.00 per year (US students), $330.00 per year (US institutions), $280.00 per year (foreign individuals), $140.00 per year (foreign and Canadian students), $395.00 per year (foreign and Canadian institutions), $250.00 per year (Canadian individuals). Foreign air speed delivery is included in all *Clinics* subscription prices. All prices are subject to change without notice. POSTMASTER: Send address changes to *Hematology/ Oncology Clinics of North America*, W.B. Saunders Company, Periodicals Fulfillment, Orlando, FL 32887-4800. **Customer Service: 1-800-654-2452 (US). From outside the US, call 407-345-4000.** E-mail: hhspcs@harcourt.com

Hematology/Oncology Clinics of North America is covered in *Index Medicus, EMBASE/Excerpta Medica, and BIOSIS.*

Printed in the United States of America.

HEMATOLOGY/ONCOLOGY CLINICS
OF NORTH AMERICA

ELSEVIER
SAUNDERS

Mesothelioma

GUEST EDITOR

HEDY LEE KINDLER, MD, Associate Professor of Medicine, Section of
Hematology/Oncology, University of Chicago, Chicago, Illinois

CONTRIBUTORS

RICHARD ALEXANDER, MD, Deputy Director, Center for Cancer Research; and
Head, Surgical Metabolism Section, Surgery Branch, National Cancer Institute,
National Institutes of Health, Bethesda, Maryland

SAMUEL G. ARMATO III, PhD, Assistant Professor of Radiology and the Committee
on Medical Physics, Department of Radiology, University of Chicago,
Chicago, Illinois

RAPHAEL BUENO, MD, Associate Chief, Division of Thoracic Surgery, Brigham and
Women's Hospital; and Associate Professor of Surgery, Department of Surgery,
Harvard Medical School, Boston, Massachusetts

HELEN CLAYSON, MBBS, FRCP, FRCGP, Medical Director, Hospice of St. Mary of
Furness, Cumbria; and Honorary Research Fellow, University of Sheffield,
Sheffield, United Kingdom

JENETTE CREANEY, PhD, Senior Research Officer, School of Medicine and
Pharmacology, University of Western Australia, Nedlands,
Western Australia, Australia

JONATHAN E. DOWELL, MD, Assistant Professor of Internal Medicine, University of
Texas–Southwestern Medical Center; and Chief, Division of Hematology &
Oncology, Dallas Veterans Affairs Medical Center, Dallas, Texas

KENNETH M. FORSTER, PhD, Department of Radiation Oncology, University of
Texas Southwestern Medical Center, Dallas, Texas

RAFFIT HASSAN, MD, Principal Investigator, Laboratory of Molecular Biology,
Center for Cancer Research, National Cancer Institute, National Institutes of
Health, Bethesda, Maryland

HEDY LEE KINDLER, MD, Associate Professor of Medicine, Section of
Hematology/Oncology, University of Chicago, Chicago, Illinois

LEE M. KRUG, MD, Thoracic Oncology Service, Department of Medicine, Memorial
Sloan-Kettering Cancer Center, New York, New York

BILL NOBLE, MB ChB, MRCGP, MD, Macmillan Senior Lecturer in Palliative Medicine, Academic Unit of Supportive Care, University of Sheffield, Sheffield, United Kingdom

GEOFFREY R. OXNARD, MD, Department of Medicine, Massachusetts General Hospital, Boston, Massachusetts

EVAN PISICK, MD, Department of Medicine, Section of Hematology/Oncology, Tufts–New England Medical Center, Boston, Massachusetts

DAVID RICE, Department of Thoracic Surgery, University of Texas M.D. Anderson Cancer Center, Houston, Texas

BRUCE W.S. ROBINSON, MBBS, MD, Professor of Medicine, School of Medicine and Pharmacology, University of Western Australia; and Western Australian Institute of Medical Research, Nedlands, Western Australia, Australia

RAVI SALGIA, MD, PhD, Department of Medicine, Section of Hematology/Oncology, University of Chicago Medical Center, University of Chicago Cancer Research Center, Pritzker School of Medicine, Chicago, Illinois

JANE SEYMOUR, RGN, BA (hons), MA, PhD, Sue Ryder Care Professor in Palliative and End-of-Life Studies, School of Nursing, University of Nottingham, Nottingham, United Kingdom

W. ROY SMYTHE, MD, Department of Surgery, Texas A&M University Medical School, College Station, Texas

JEREMY P.C. STEELE, MD, Consultant in Medical Oncology, Bart's Mesothelioma Research Group, St. Bartholomew's Hospital and Medical College, London, United Kingdom

DANIEL H. STERMAN, MD, Associate Professor of Medicine, Thoracic Oncology Research Laboratory, Pulmonary, Allergy, and Critical Care Division, Department of Medicine, University of Pennsylvania Medical Center, Philadelphia, Pennsylvania

CRAIG W. STEVENS, MD, PhD, Division of Radiation Oncology, H. Lee Moffitt Cancer Center, Tampa, Florida

HEMATOLOGY/ONCOLOGY CLINICS
OF NORTH AMERICA

Mesothelioma

CONTENTS

VOLUME 19 · NUMBER 6 · DECEMBER 2005

Preface xi

Hedy Lee Kindler

**Molecular Biology of Malignant Mesothelioma:
A Review** 997

Evan Pisick and Ravi Salgia

Malignant mesothelioma (MM) is an uncommon tumor with high mortality and morbidity rates. It arises from mesothelial cells that line the pleural, pericardial, peritoneal, and testicular cavities. This is a disease with an indolent course because tumors arise 20 to 40 years after exposure to an inciting agent. Extensive research has shown that mesothelial cells are transformed into MM cells through various chromosomal and cellular pathway defects. These changes alter the normal cells' ability to survive, proliferate, and metastasize. This article discusses the alterations that occur in transforming normal mesothelial cells into MM. It also details some of the signal transduction pathways that seem to be important in MM with the potential for novel targeted therapeutics.

**Detection of Malignant Mesothelioma in
Asbestos-Exposed Individuals: The Potential Role
of Soluble Mesothelin-Related Protein** 1025

Jenette Creaney and Bruce W.S. Robinson

Malignant mesothelioma (MM) is strongly associated with asbestos exposure. Measurement of soluble mesothelin-related protein (SMRP) levels in the serum may prove valuable as an adjunct to current tests for the diagnosis of MM and for monitoring MM patients for the early detection of disease recurrence. SMRP measures also may be useful in an overall screening program for MM because early results show that some individuals have elevated levels 1 to 4 years before symptom development. Although individuals with occupational and nonoccupational asbestos exposure are justifiably concerned about their risk of developing MM, consideration must be given to the complex issues surrounding screening for this disease, and a more substantial evaluation of the SMRP marker must be undertaken before deciding to promote a screening program.

Prognostic Factors for Mesothelioma   1041
Jeremy P.C. Steele

Our understanding of malignant mesothelioma has increased rapidly in the last 5 years. The prognosis remains poor for most patients, however. Radical surgery is inappropriate for most, and palliative chemotherapy can be toxic if used without care. Patient selection is crucial, and prognostic factors allow us to predict which patients are likely to benefit from intensive treatment. Longer survival is associated with epithelioid histology, earlier stage, female gender, left-sided primary, nonexposure to asbestos, no history of smoking, and a lack of symptoms at presentation. Numerous genes of significance are identified and many have been shown to correlate with clinical outcome. Molecular data will provide prognostication of exceptional accuracy, biologic insights, and targets for improved treatment.

The Radiologic Measurement of Mesothelioma   1053
Samuel G. Armato III and Geoffrey R. Oxnard

The radiologic evaluation of disease, which now includes the quantification of disease, has become an essential part of clinical medicine. The unique circumferential and often scalloped morphology of mesothelioma, however, distinguishes it from other thoracic neoplasms. The challenges of measuring mesothelioma are many. In this article, the authors explore the demands, the current standard of clinical practice, and the opportunities associated with the radiologic measurement of mesothelioma.

Nonpleural Mesotheliomas: Mesothelioma of the Peritoneum, Tunica Vaginalis, and Pericardium   1067
Raffit Hassan and Richard Alexander

Mesotheliomas are tumors that arise from the mesothelial cells of the pleura, peritoneum, pericardium, or tunica vaginalis. Although the number of new mesothelioma cases diagnosed each year in the United States seems to be leveling off or decreasing, several other countries are projected to have continued increased incidence of mesothelioma over the next several years. Of the approximately 2500 new cases of mesothelioma in the United States each year, most are pleural mesotheliomas. The peritoneum is the second most common site of mesothelioma development and accounts for approximately 10% to 20% of all mesotheliomas. Mesotheliomas that involve the pericardium or originate from the tunica vaginalis are rare tumors. Given the rarity of these tumors, it is difficult to obtain precise information regarding their incidence, natural history, and optimal management.

Multimodality Treatments in the Management of Malignant Pleural Mesothelioma: An Update   1089
Raphael Bueno

> Malignant pleural mesothelioma (MPM) is relatively unique among cancers, since the local and regional disease rather than the systemic disease usually contributes to death. Because of its multifocal distribution in the chest, MPM progresses locally by compressing the lung, heart, and major vessels, and causes death by cardiac tamponade and lung collapse physiology. The therapy for this aggressive local malignancy is currently inadequate. In most cases there is insufficient time for systemic disease to develop or contribute to mortality. The first order of therapy in MPM is currently, as it has been for decades, to control effectively the tumor's locoregional spread and then deal with controlling the distant disease.

Radiotherapy for Mesothelioma   1099
Craig W. Stevens, Kenneth M. Forster, W. Roy Smythe, and David Rice

> Three to four thousand cases of malignant pleural mesothelioma will occur in the United States this year. Single-modality therapy with radiation plays a role for palliation. Radiation can prevent tumor recurrence at drain/instrumentation sites and provide symptomatic relief of pain and other complaints. Combinations of surgery and radiation also have been attempted with curative intent. The best local control has been found—EPP followed by radiotherapy. Locoregional tumor recurrence can be dramatically reduced with combinations of extrapleural pneumonectomy and radiation therapy. Survival in aggressively treated early-stage patients is excellent. However, the preponderance of death from distant metastases makes the development of better systemic therapy essential. Better therapy also must be developed for patients who are not candidates for extrapleural pneumonectomy.

An Overview of Chemotherapy for Mesothelioma   1117
Lee M. Krug

> Mesothelioma is an extraordinarily challenging disease to treat. While numerous clinical trials testing various chemotherapeutic agents have been conducted over the last several decades, only recently have larger studies proven the efficacy of newer chemotherapy regimens. This article reviews the data regarding specific classes of chemotherapeutic agents. The role of treatment in various disease settings and the difficulty in assessing the benefit of that therapy is discussed. Finally, an update is provided on novel therapeutics being testing in mesothelioma.

Antiangiogenic Therapies for Mesothelioma 1137
Jonathan E. Dowell and Hedy Lee Kindler

A large body of preclinical evidence suggests that angiogenesis plays a key role in the pathogenesis of malignant mesothelioma. Several mediators of angiogenesis seem to be autocrine growth factors in mesothelioma, and in preclinical models, agents that target angiogenesis produce tumor regression. Several clinical trials are currently evaluating the efficacy of inhibitors of angiogenesis in mesothelioma. This article details the preliminary results of these trials and future directions.

Gene Therapy for Malignant Pleural Mesothelioma 1147
Daniel H. Sterman

Gene therapy for mesothelioma is currently in its adolescence. The expansion of knowledge regarding molecular aspects of mesothelioma carcinogenesis has facilitated the development of promising gene therapy modalities that target specific oncoproteins and mutant tumor suppressor genes. Although implementation of any of these gene therapy approaches as part of standard medical care for patients who have mesothelioma remains years in the future, the field is finally progressing toward more definitive phase II/III efficacy studies. Unfortunately, the marginal benefits garnered from standard anticancer treatments in mesothelioma argue strongly for continued participation in clinical studies of various experimental approaches, particularly gene therapy. These trials serve multiple purposes: to establish safety, determine proper dosing, evaluate for efficacy, and, in an iterative fashion, guide future avenues of laboratory investigation.

Mesothelioma from the Patient's Perspective 1175
Helen Clayson, Jane Seymour, and Bill Noble

This study reports findings from qualitative semi-structured interviews with 15 patients who suffered from mesothelioma. The results are described under four headings that reflect the main themes that arose from the data: coping with symptoms (particularly breathlessness and pain), finding out about mesothelioma and its implications, the trauma of medical interventions, and psychosocial issues. The results illustrate the severe disease burden that is borne by people who have mesothelioma. It is hoped that a greater understanding of mesothelioma from a patient's perspective could inform the response of health care professionals.

Cumulative Index 2005 1191

HEMATOLOGY/ONCOLOGY CLINICS
OF NORTH AMERICA

ELSEVIER
SAUNDERS

FORTHCOMING ISSUES

February 2006

> **Radiation Medicine for the Practicing Oncologist, Part I**
> Charles Thomas, MD, and Lisa Kachnic, MD
> *Guest Editors*

April 2006

> **Radiation Medicine for the Practicing Oncologist, Part II**
> Charles Thomas, MD, and Lisa Kachnic, MD
> *Guest Editors*

June 2006

> **Prostate Cancer**
> William Oh, MD
> *Guest Editor*

RECENT ISSUES

October 2005

> **Sickle Cell Disease**
> Cage S. Johnson, MD
> *Guest Editor*

August 2005

> **Central Nervous System Lymphomas**
> Lisa M. DeAngelis, MD, and Lauren E. Abrey, MD
> *Guest Editors*

June 2005

> **Sarcomas**
> Robert G. Maki, MD, PhD
> *Guest Editor*

PREFACE

Mesothelioma

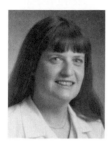

Hedy Lee Kindler, MD

Guest Editor

I t is with great pleasure that I introduce this issue on malignant mesothelioma for *Hematology/Oncology Clinics of North America*. International experts have been invited to share their expertise on a comprehensive range of topics, and we hope that you will appreciate their insights.

Drs. Pisick and Salgia summarize recent advances in our understanding of the complex molecular biology of this cancer, which may yield rational targets for future therapeutic interventions. Individuals exposed to asbestos often have significant concerns regarding their risk of mesothelioma. Drs. Creaney and Robinson discuss their exciting data on the use of soluble mesothelin-related protein for the early detection and monitoring of mesothelioma, in the context of the complex issues surrounding screening for this cancer.

In a disease as heterogenous as mesothelioma, in which anatomic stage is often difficult to discern before resection, an understanding of relevant prognostic factors is essential for selecting the right treatment approach, as Dr. Steele describes in his review. Drs. Armato and Oxnard discuss the challenges underlying accurate radiologic measurement and response assessment that results from the scalloped morphology and circumferential growth pattern of mesothelioma.

The pleura is the most common anatomic site of origin of mesothelioma. Drs. Hassan and Alexander provide a comprehensive overview of the natural history and treatment options for the less common mesotheliomas of the peritoneum, tunica vaginalis, and pericardium. Although pleural mesothelioma is principally a loco-regional disease, surgery as a single modality is rarely curative. Dr. Bueno discusses current strategies for multi-modality treatment.

0889-8588/05/$ – see front matter
doi:10.1016/j.hoc.2005.11.001

Radiation, a key component of multimodality therapy, is comprehensively reviewed by Dr. Stevens.

Pemetrexed, a multi-targeted antifolate which improves response, survival, and quality of life in mesothelioma patients, is the first FDA-approved drug for this cancer. As Dr. Krug describes, several other drugs have demonstrated activity, and many new agents are being evaluated. Angiogenesis may be a critical step in the pathogenesis of mesothelioma. Dr. Dowell and I delineate the biology of vascular endothelial growth factor (VEGF) in this disease, and discuss ongoing clinical trials of VEGF inhibitors. The localized nature of mesothelioma and the accessibility of the pleural space for the delivery of experimental agents has facilitated the evaluation of gene therapy, as Dr. Sterman details in his overview.

In 2005, about 2500 Americans will be faced with a new diagnosis of mesothelioma. Using qualitative patient interviews, Dr. Clayson and her colleagues share their insights about the experience of mesothelioma and its meaning for the patient. I would like to dedicate this issue of *Hematology/Oncology Clinics of North America* to those individuals who cope daily with the challenges of living with mesothelioma, and to the memory of those patients, including my father, who have lost their battle with this deadly disease.

Hedy Lee Kindler, MD
Section of Hematology/Oncology
University of Chicago
5841 South Maryland Avenue
MC 2115
Chicago, IL 60637, USA
E-mail address: hkindler@medicine.bsd.uchicago.edu

Hematol Oncol Clin N Am 19 (2005) 997–1023

Molecular Biology of Malignant Mesothelioma: A Review

Evan Pisick, MD[a], Ravi Salgia, MD, PhD[b],*

[a]Department of Medicine, Section of Hematology/Oncology, Tufts–New England Medical Center, Boston, MA, USA
[b]Department of Medicine, Section of Hematology/Oncology, University of Chicago Medical Center, University of Chicago Cancer Research Center, and Pritzker School of Medicine, 5841 South Maryland Avenue, M 255A, MC2115, Chicago, IL 60637, USA

M alignant mesothelioma (MM) is an uncommon tumor that arises from mesothelial cells that line the pleural cavity and, less commonly, the pericardium, peritoneum, and testicular cavities [1]. Approximately 2000 new cases are diagnosed each year in the United States, with an even higher number worldwide [2]. More than 80% of cases can be attributed to asbestos fiber exposure, but approximately 20% of cases may be related to alternative factors, including exposure to simian virus 40 (SV40), radiation, and thorotrast [3]. Asbestos exposure also can lead to the formation of other tumors, such as lung cancer, when combined with smoking and can cause noncancerous lung diseases, such as asbestosis. Most cases of MM diagnosed each year arise from the pleura, with approximately 10% of cases affecting the peritoneum and rarer cases including the pericardium and tunica vaginalis of the testes.

MM is a disease of different subtypes, genetic alterations, and signal pathway disruptions. Although these tumors can arise in different cavities of the human body, they all arise from mesothelial cells and have similar cellular dysfunction. There are three main histologic subtypes, including epithelial sarcomatoid and biphasic forms.

ETIOLOGY

MM was first shown to be associated with occupational and environmental exposure to crocidolite fibers by Wagner and colleagues [4] in 1960 in the northwest Cape Province of South Africa. They described a 30- to 40-year lag

This article was supported in part by the Mesothelioma Applied Research Foundation, American Cancer Society Research Scholar grant RSG-02-244-03-CCE, National Cancer Institute grant R01-CA100750-02, and institutional support from the University of Chicago Cancer Research Center (to R. Salgia).
* Corresponding author. E-mail address: rsalgia@medicine.bsd.uchicago.edu (R. Salgia).

0889-8588/05/$ – see front matter
doi:10.1016/j.hoc.2005.09.012

between exposure and the formation of malignant pleural mesotheliomas (MPMs) [5]. As the number of reported cases increases, it has been predicted that there will be a 5% to 10% increase in mortality per annum over the 10,000 deaths per year reported worldwide at least until the year 2020 [6]. These numbers reflect the continued mining and use of these fibers worldwide. Although the use of crocidolite fibers was discontinued in the United Kingdom in 1970 and most of Western Europe by 1980, many regions throughout the world continue to use these fibers [7]. In the 1960s, malignant peritoneal mesotheliomas comprised up to 30% of cases of this disease, but that number has decreased to less than 10% as the number of pleural tumors has risen [8,9]. Rarer cases involve the pericardium and tunica vaginalis of the testes.

Asbestos is a generic term that encompasses many different types of naturally occurring fibers, some of which are linked to the formation of MM [10]. There are two major groups of asbestos fibers: the serpentine fibers, of which chrysolite is the only form, and the amphibole fibers, which include crocidolite, the most oncogenic form, amosite, anthophyllite, and tremolite [10–14]. In the 1960s and 1970s, many case-controlled studies of MPM were conducted, all of which demonstrated an association between occupational exposure to asbestos and formation of tumors, with relative risks ranging from 2.3 to 7 [15–20]. Recently, 43 separate cohort studies were summarized by McDonald [21] in 2000, in which he showed a proportional mortality rate ranging from 2.5 to 102.3, with the highest numbers seen in individuals exposed to crocidolite fibers.

Other fibers, including amosite, chrysolite, tremolite, and anthophyllite, have less convincing data linking exposure to formation of MM [21–25]. The latter two fibers are rarely used commercially, so few data exist to link them to tumor formation. Less compelling evidence links amosite and chrysolite to MM formation, but cases have been reported in factories that use this material in the production of insulation.

Nonoccupational exposure to asbestos particles occurs in parts of the world in which these fibers are mined and then used in construction of local villages. In Turkey, cases of MM are being reported in towns characterized by volcanic tuffs and natural caves. In the villages of Karain and Tuzkoy in Cappadocia, it has been documented that more than 50% of deaths can be attributed to MM [26]. Buildings in Cappadocia were built from stone mined from the nearby natural caves, which contained a large amount of asbestos fibers, whereas in Karain only some asbestos was found in the buildings [26–28]. The asbestos fiber that was discovered was tremolite and another highly carcinogenic fiber known as erionite. The latter fiber is widespread in both of these villages and was shown to cause MM when injected intrapleurally into animals, and it is believed to be the causative agent [26].

Even with the high level of MM formation, not all residents of these towns were affected equally. It was noted that in some homes, entire families were afflicted with this disease, whereas nearby houses had no reported cases [26]. All the homes were built from stones from the same caves, and researchers believed that there might be a genetic predisposition to the formation in MM. This hypothesis was strengthened when researchers discovered that there was only one case of MM in the nearby town of Karlik, which also was built with stone from the same caves that produced stone for Karain and Tuzkoy. The tumor was found in a woman from Karain who was living Karlik.

To strengthen their argument for a genetically transmitted predilection for MM, a researcher lived in the village of Karain for almost 3 years [29]. Pedigrees of several families with a large amount of MM cases were constructed. The researcher demonstrated that approximately 50% of descendants of affected parents developed this disease and that when a person from an unaffected family married into an affected family, their descendants developed MM. These findings strengthened the hypothesis of a genetically transmitted susceptibility to the formation of MM that may be passed on in an autosomal dominant pattern.

A few cases have been reported of MM forming in patients with no known exposure to asbestos fibers. Some researchers hypothesize a role for SV40, which is discussed in detail later. Other etiologic factors include previous radiation exposure for treatment of other cancers and thorium dioxide [3].

CHROMOSOMAL ABERRATIONS

Through genomic hybridization analysis, several genetic alterations have been discovered in mesothelioma cells. Loss of genetic material is common in this disease and it is believed that loss of tumor suppressor genes and function facilitates in the oncogenesis of mesothelial cells. Chromosomal damage may occur when asbestos fibers interact directly with the mitotic spindle apparatus or may act on cellular proliferation, which allows spontaneous genetic mutations to occur unchecked over time. There has been documentation of loss of genetic material on the short (p) arms of chromosomes 1, 3, and 9 and the long (q) arms of chromosomes 6, 15, and 22 [30]. The observed deletions varied from study to study and even country to country. It has been suggested that studies that use tumor samples may have been contaminated from normal stromal cells, thus the number of true chromosomal abnormalities is lower than has been reported.

A common chromosomal abnormality detected in MM is the loss of genetic material at 3p21, with the highest percentage of loss at 3p21.3 [31]. This region has known tumor suppressor candidate genes and is seen in other malignancies, including lung cancer, nonpapillary renal cell cancer, uterine cancer, follicular thyroid cancer, and breast cancer [32]. Of note, the β-catenin gene (CTNNB1) is located at 3p21.3. The protein product of this gene is important in Wnt signaling seen in MM cells and cell lines. It is also important to note that this region has been shown to be unaffected in nine of ten MM cells and cell lines tested [33].

On chromosome 1, 70% of cases have been noted to have deletions at 1p21-p22 [34]. Potential tumor suppressor gene candidates are being mapped to this region. Several different regions are affected on chromosome 6, including 6q14-q21, 6q16.6-q21, 6q21-q23.2, and 6q25. Deletions of similar regions have been detected in other forms of cancer, including breast cancer, ovarian cancer, and non-Hodgkin's lymphoma [35–37]. The short arm of chromosome 9 has two tumor suppressor genes that can be deleted in this disease, including p16/

CDKN2A and $p14^{ARF}$. The long arm of chromosome 15 has loss of genetic material in the region 15q11.1-q15. Loss of this region is also seen in other diseases, including prostate cancer, ovarian cancer, parathyroid adenomas, and metastatic tumors of breast, lung, and colon [38–41]. Several of these genetic aberrations are discussed in detail.

NORMAL CELL CYCLE

The cell cycle is a tightly controlled process with greatest regulation occurring during the G1 phase. During this phase, there is a restriction point at which time the cell becomes dedicated to dividing. If the cell is under stress or there is DNA damage, regulatory processes signal the cell to repair the damage or die. This process occurs because the S, G2, and M phases of the cycle are autonomous and any damage at these points leads to nonviable cells. These latter phases, which are not discussed in detail in this article, are primarily for replication and segregation of chromosomal DNA into two daughter cells [42,43].

Most mammalian cells generally remain in the quiescent (G0) phase. They proliferate in response to mitogenic signals, such as hormones, cytokines, growth factors, and cell-cell contact. Once the signal to divide is received by a cell, a process is started that moves the cell from the G0 to the G1 phase. In the G1 phase, many processes act to ensure that only intact chromosomal DNA is replicated. Once these criteria are met, the cells move toward a restriction point, at which time the process is either aborted for repairs or apoptosis or the cell moves toward division.

Restriction point control is believed to be regulated by cyclin-dependent protein kinases (CDKs), which are regulated by cyclins D, E, and A. Cyclin D is a family of three, including cyclins D1-3 [44–49]. They are not only the earliest cyclins to be synthesized in the cell but they also occur in direct response to growth stimuli. Withdrawal of a growth stimulus leads to decreased cyclin D expression; these proteins are labile. Cyclin D has two binding partners, including CDK4 and CDK6 [50]. The complexes that are formed are first seen in the mid-G1 phase, with maximum levels being attained at the G1-S transition. The importance of the cyclin D-CDK complex in restriction point control has been shown by several groups. G1 phase arrest occurs when CDK inhibitors, the INK4 proteins, or neutralizing antibodies are introduced to cells before the restriction point [51–57].

The cyclin D-CDK4 and CDK6 complexes exert their effect by phosphorylating the retinoblastoma gene product (pRb) [58–60]. In its hypophosphorylated state, pRb binds to a family of transcription factors known as E2F-1, -2, and -3 and renders them inactive [61–65]. Once phosphorylated, pRb disengages the E2Fs, a process required for expression of S phase genes. The initial phosphorylation of pRb is caused by the cyclin D-CDK and CDK6 complexes and depends on mitogen [50,58–60,66–71]. pRb is sustained in a phosphorylated state by another cyclin, cyclin E [72–75]. This protein partners with CDK2 and acts to further accelerate phosphorylation of pRb and release of E2Fs. The cyclin E gene is a target of E2Fs and acts as a positive feedback, with its highest levels being expressed at the G1-S phase transition [75–82]. At this point, pRb phosphorylation becomes mitogen independent through the cyclin E-CDK2 complex.

Cyclin A- and B-dependent kinases maintain pRb phosphorylation throughout the cell cycle until the cell has divided and re-entered the G1 or G0 phase [44–48]. Once the cell enters S phase, cyclin E levels start to drop as CDK2 phosphorylates it, which leads to ubiquitin-dependent proteolysis [83,84]. Simultaneously, cyclin A-CDK2 complexes accumulate and bind to and phosphorylate pRb-regulated E2Fs. This phosphorylation leads to an inability of E2Fs to bind DNA, a function lacking in the cyclin E-CDK2 complex [85–87].

Inhibition of cyclin D-, A-, and E-dependent kinases are regulated by the CDK inhibitors $p21^{CIP1}$, $p27^{KIP1}$, and $p57^{KIP2}$ [88–97]. Cells that are quiescent express high levels of $p27^{KIP1}$, but these levels drop once cells enter the cell cycle [98,99]. As cells progress through the cycle, residual $p27^{KIP1}$ is sequestered with cyclin D-CDK complexes, which leads to increased cyclin E-CDK2 and cyclin A-CDK2 activities [94–96,98,99]. $P27^{KIP1}$ levels and function are controlled by translational and posttranslation mechanisms and phosphorylation by cyclin E-CDK2 complexes [100–102].

INK4 FAMILY

The CDK inhibitors known as the INK4 family consist of multiple proteins, including $p16^{INK4a}$/MTS1/CDKN2A, $p15^{INK4b}$, $P18^{INK4c}$, and $p19^{INK4d}$. Xiong and colleagues [103] first discovered $p16^{INK4a}$ while studying the cyclin-CDK complexes in SV40-transformed cells. Serrano and colleagues [51] sequenced the human $p16^{INK4a}$ cDNA. The $p16^{INK4a}$ gene is located on chromosome 9p21 along with other members in the INK4 family.

Kamb and colleagues [54] noted that within the genomic DNA for $p16^{INK4a}$, an additional segment was found and designated MTS2. This sequence proved to be the second exon for $p15^{INK4b}$. The first exon for $p15^{INK4b}$ was not found in this region but was located 30 base pairs away. These two tandomly linked genes are presumed to have occurred because of gene duplication. Although $p16^{INK4a}$ is encoded by three exons, $p15^{INK4b}$ is encoded by only two [104,105]. Two other INK4 family members, $p18^{INK4c}$ and $p19^{INK4d}$, were cloned after CDK4 immunoprecipitates were noted to bring down additional low molecular weight proteins [53,55]. These proteins were cloned from cDNAs isolated by a two-hybrid screening process using CDK4 and CDK6 [55–57,106]. The $p18^{INK4c}$ and $p19^{INK4d}$ genes are located on chromosomes 1p32 and 19p13, respectively [55,57,106,107].

The INK4 family story gets more complicated because an additional exon has been noted between the INK4a and INK4b genes and was designated exon 1β [108–112]. This exon is transcribed from a different promoter than the one used for $p16^{INK4a}$ but becomes spliced to the second and third exons of $p16^{INK4a}$. This different transcript, known as the β transcript, encodes a smaller alternative reading frame (ARF) protein known as $p14^{ARF}$ and $p19^{ARF}$ in humans and mice, respectively [108,113].

The INK4 family proteins function as CDK inhibitors. All four proteins in this family interact with CDK4 and CDK6 exclusively and act as competitive inhibitors [51,53,55–57,106,111]. Using in vitro translation or recombinant proteins, several groups have shown that INK4 proteins and CDK4 and CDK6 bind directly in the absence of cyclins [51,53,56,57,104,106,114]. When cyclin D is added, the interaction between INK4 proteins and CDK4 and CDK6 is not affected and the interaction between cyclin D and CDK4 or CDK6 is prevented [67,106,114–116]. These interactions do not displace cyclin D but inhibit the action of the whole complex. This process has not yet been shown to occur in vivo in mammalian cells. Cyclin D has a half-life measured in minutes, whereas the half-life of INK4 proteins is measured in hours [117–119]. It is believed that cyclin D in vivo is degraded rapidly and that currently INK4 proteins can bind to and inhibit CDK4 and CDK6 [120]. This finding is in contrast to the CIP/KIP family of CDK inhibitors, which can bind CDKs and cyclins to make an active or inactive complex [121].

High levels of p16^{INK4a} were noted in pRb-negative cells and in cells with nonfunctioning pRb [51]. There seems to be an inverse relationship between p16^{INK4a} and pRb levels, which is seen in many tumor cell lines. For example, small cell lung cancer cell lines have pRb defects and high p16INK4a levels, whereas non–small cell lung cancer cell lines have wild-type pRb and defective p16INK4a [122–127]. This inverse relationship between p16^{INK4a} and pRb demonstrates that p16^{INK4a} is important in the cell cycle, especially in the G1 phase.

The INK4a gene alternative reading frame protein, p14^{ARF}, is also important in the cell cycle but acts through the tumor suppressor p53 [128–130]. p14^{ARF} does not bind or inhibit CDKs, but ectopic expression of this gene causes cell cycle arrest [113,130–133]. p14^{ARF} protects p53 from degradation by binding to inhibiting MDM2, which targets p53 for ubiquitin-mediated degradation [129,130,134]. p14^{ARF} also has been shown to upregulate p21^{CIP1}, which is a CDK inhibitor and can contribute to cell cycle arrest [128,130]. The inverse relationship noted between p16^{INK4a} and pRb also has been observed between p14^{ARF} and p53 [113,128,130,133]. Elevated levels of p14^{ARF} have been noted in p53 negative cells, with decreased p14^{ARF} levels noted in cells as the level of p53 increases.

p16^{INK4a}/p14^{ARF} ALTERATIONS

In MM cells, chromosomal damage occurs either as a direct result of asbestos exposure or because of replication of cells with damaged genomic DNA. One site commonly affected is the short arm of chromosome 9p21, which is the location of the INK4a gene and transcribes for the p16^{INK4a} and p14^{ARF} proteins. Murthy and Testa [30] demonstrated this homozygous deletion in 40 MM cell lines and 23 of 42 MM primary tumors. Other groups also have shown deletion of this region of chromosome 9 in 85% and 22% of MPM cell lines and primary MM tumors, respectively [135]. Along with homozygous deletion, decreased levels of these two proteins may occur because of point mutation in the genes or hypermethylation of 5' CpG islands [123]. Hirao and colleagues [136] demonstrated that 8.8% of their primary MM tumors had a methylated p16^{INK4a} promoter, 22.2% had a p16^{INK4a} deletion, and 2% had a point mutation within the p16^{INK4a} gene. No hypermethylation of the p14^{ARF} promoter was noted.

The absence or alteration of p16^{INK4a} and p14^{ARF} may be important in transformation and proliferation of MM cells. This occurrence has been shown by several groups that have demonstrated cell cycle arrest in MM cells that were transfected with either p16^{INK4a} or p14^{ARF} constructs. Frizelle and colleagues [137] observed cell cycle arrest, inhibition of pRb phosphorylation, diminished cell growth, and increased apoptosis in MM cells transfected with a p16^{INK4a}-containing adenovirus. Similar results were seen in MM cells transfected with p14^{ARF}, as long as wild-type p53 was present [138].

RECEPTOR TYROSINE KINASES

Several receptor tyrosine kinases (RTKs) are expressed on the surface of MM cells, including c-Met, epidermal growth factor receptor, c-erbB-2 (HER2/Neu), vascular endothelial growth factor receptor (VEGF-R), c-kit, insulin-like growth factor receptor-I and -II, and fibroblast growth factor receptor. Like many other cancers, RTKs may play an important role in cell survival, proliferation, and motility. Epidermal growth factor, insulin-like growth factor-I, transforming growth factor-β, β-fibroblast growth factor, and platelet-derived growth factor stimulate the synthesis of hyaluronan and proteoglycans by MM cells.

c-MET

c-Met is an RTK expressed on the surface of normal and malignant cells [139–141]. This receptor is activated by the ligand hepatocyte growth factor (HGF), also known as scatter factor. c-Met is a disulfide-linked α−β heterodimer that has been identified as a proto-oncogene. The gene is located on chromosome 7 band 7q21-q31 [142,143]. The gene for the ligand, HGF, is also located on chromosome 7 band 7q21.1 [144].

The primary transcript for c-Met is a 150-kDa fragment that is glycosylated to a precursor protein that is 170 kDa. This protein is further glycosylated and subsequently cleaved into a 50-kDa α -chain and a 140-kDa β-chain. The α-subunit of this heterodimer is completely extracellular, whereas the β-subunit traverses the cell membrane and contains an intracellular portion at the C-terminus that contains a tyrosine kinase (TK) domain. The β-subunit contains several other domains, including (1) an N-terminus Sema domain embodied with the MRS cysteine-rich region, (2) a PSI domain found in plexins, semaphorins, and integrins, (3) IPT repeats, known as TIG domains, which are also found within immunoglobulins, plexins, and transcription factors, (4) a transmembrane domain, and (5) a juxtamembrane (JM) domain located next to the TK domain. The TK domain of Met shares homology with Ron and Sea, which belong to the same family of RTKs [145].

The Met subfamily of RTKs shares homology with semaphorins and semaphorin receptors, which are important in mediating cell scattering [146–150].

The Met subfamily also mediates cell scattering. The extracellular portions of Met, Ron, and Sea contain regions of homology with semaphorins, including the Sema domain and the MRS [151]. Semaphorin receptors (plexins) do not possess any homology to the intracellular kinase domain of the Met subfamily.

The function of c-Met is in cell motility. It is activated by HGF, which is released in a paracrine fashion [152–158]. Upon binding of HGF to the extracellular portion of c-Met, intracellular tyrosine residues on the β-subunit are autophosphorylated by its TK domain. Several tyrosine residues are tyrosine phosphorylated, including Y1003, Y1230, Y1234, Y1235, Y1313, Y1349, and Y1356. Residue Y1313 is important in binding to phosphpatidylinositol-3 kinase (PI3-K), which also can be phosphorylated in response to HGF binding to c-Met. Phosphorylation of residues Y1349 and Y1356 activates the multisubstrate signal transducer docking site, which interacts with such proteins as SHC, Src, Gab1, GRB2, PI3-K, PLC-γ, and SHP2. The Y1003 residue, located within the JM domain, is important for binding to c-Cbl. This interaction plays a role in ubiquination and internalization of the c-Met receptor and regulates its activity [159,160].

c-Met is expressed in various cell types and tissues. With increased amplification and expression comes the possibility of mutations, especially within the JM or TK domains. Thus far, at least 17 different JM domain and TK domain mutations have been described in different malignant tissues and cell lines [161–165]. c-Cbl regulates c-Met activity by ubiquinating the receptor after binding to tyrosine residue Y1003 within the JM domain. This process causes internalization and subsequent degradation. In gastric carcinoma, deletion of this site has been described. Peschard and colleagues [166] described transforming activity in epithelial cells and fibroblasts when the tyrosine residue at Y1003 is changed to phenylalanine. These mutations may lead to increased activity of the TK domain and cause aberrant and unregulated cell proliferation, survival, and motility. These mutations have yet to be described in MM.

Tolnay and colleagues [167] demonstrated that paraffin-embedded MM tumor samples showed an overexpression of c-Met and its ligand HGF. Increased production of HGF was found in 33 of 39 samples with a corresponding overexpression of c-Met in 29 of 39 samples. This coexpression suggests a possible self-stimulation of tumor cells. The HGF-positive MM also had a significantly higher microvessel density compared with its HGF-negative counterpart.

Knowing that c-Met and HGF overexpression occurs in MM, what does this mean in the disease process? Harvey and colleagues [168] demonstrated that HGF acts as a strong chemoattractant for MPM cell lines and caused enhanced cell adhesion and invasion into Matrigel. This invasion could have occurred because of increased expression of matrix metalloproteinases, which enhance degradation of extracellular stroma. This group identified three metalloproteinases that had increased expression in MM cell lines when exposed to HGF: metalloproteinase-1, 9, and membrane-bound MT1-metalloproteinase. There was minimal effect on metalloproteinase inhibitor tissue inhibitors of metalloproteinase-1 and no effect on tissue inhibitor of metalloproteinase-2 expression.

Serine proteases also were overexpressed in these cell lines after exposure to HGF and were involved in HGF-induced invasion.

Similar findings were described by Klominek and colleagues [169] when they demonstrated HGF production in 3 of 11 MM cell lines, c-Met expression in 11 of 11 MM cell lines, and 6 of 6 tumor samples. Mesothelial cell lines and mesothelial samples from patients who did not have MM failed to express HGF or c-Met. When MM cell lines were exposed to recombinant human HGF, directional and random motility occurred. When the cells were exposed to an anti-HGF monoclonal antibody, cellular motility was inhibited.

c-Met does not need to be activated by HGF to affect MM cells. Cacciotti and colleagues [170] demonstrated activation of c-Met in human mesothelial cells transfected with full-length SV40 DNA (SV40-HMC). The activation of this RTK was associated with S-phase entry, acquisition of a fibroblastoid morphology, and assembly of viral particles. When cells were treated with suramin or HGF-blocking antibodies, large T antigen–positive cells reverted back to their spindle-shaped morphology. These data suggest that HGF and c-Met play an important role in mesothelioma cell motility and invasion into extracellular stroma.

Inhibitors that target c-Met or HGF are being developed. Several strategies include antibodies, small molecule TK inhibitors, and downstream signal transduction inhibitors.

c-KIT

c-Kit and its ligand, stem cell factor, are important in the maturation of hematopoietic and germ cells. The expression of this RTK has been linked to drug resistance in MM cells. Catalano and colleagues [171] identified a pathway within MM cell lines that involved c-Kit, stem cell factor, and the Slug protein. They created a multidrug-resistant cell line from parental MM cell lines. These cells expressed c-Kit and stem cell factor and higher levels of Slug. When Slug or c-Kit was downregulated using iRNA technology, the MM cell line became sensitized to apoptosis by several different chemotherapeutic agents. When c-Kit was transfected into the parental cell line, Slug levels rose and the cells became resistant to chemotherapy.

A recent study using the c-Kit and platelet-derived growth factor-R inhibitor imatinib mesylate demonstrated no activity in patients who had MM. Seventeen patients who had unresectable MPM were dosed with 600 mg daily of imatinib mesylate in 28-day cycles. Results showed no objective responses with a progression-free survival of 7.4 weeks (range, 2–24 weeks) and a 1-year survival rate of 62% [172].

VASCULAR ENDOTHELIAL GROWTH FACTOR RECEPTOR

VEGF and VEGF-R may play a role in MM angiogenesis and lymphangiogenesis. VEGF-R is a family of RTKs that include fms-like TK (flt)-1, kinase domain-containing receptor, and flt-4. Expression levels of VEGF, VEGF-C, and VEGF-R are all increased in MM cell lines. A strong correlation between

VEGF-C expression levels and microlymphatic vessel density has been demonstrated. A significant correlation also was observed between microlymphatic vessel density and flt-4 and microvessel density and VEGF [173]. MM cells infected with SV40 showed an increase in VEGF expression and led to enhanced proliferation [174]. This process is accomplished via an autocrine loop, which was demonstrated when proliferation of human MM cells were inhibited when the cells were exposed to soluble flt-1. Experiments revealed that the SV40-T antigen protein is involved in VEGF promoter activation. The anti-VEGF monoclonal antibody bevacizumab is currently being tested in a randomized phase II trial in combination with gemcitabine and cisplatin in MM.

SIGNAL PATHWAYS
In MM, cellular pathways are altered, which causes disruption of the normal cell cycle, including inhibiting apoptosis. These changes can be caused by the effect of asbestos fibers directly on mesothelial cells, hormones, and cytokines released by the surrounding tissues in response to damage, virally encoded proteins, and loss of normal protein function because of DNA damage. Many researchers have demonstrated that one, if not multiple, alterations can occur and are present in MM cells and cell lines.

Wnt PATHWAY
The first pathway, and most studied, is the Wnt-1 pathway. The Wnt family is a group of glycoproteins that are excreted from the cell and interact with its receptor Frizzled (Fz). This group of proteins is important in embryogenesis, cell proliferation, and determining cell fate. The Wnt-Fz interaction activates canonical and noncanonical pathways.

The canonical pathway signals through a protein called Dishevelled (Dvl) and leads to accumulation and stabilization of β-catenin [175–179]. This process results in translocation of β-catenin to the nucleus, where it binds to and activates T-cell factor/lymphocyte enhancer factor transcription factors, which then activate transcription of Wnt target genes [180,181]. These genes include c-myc, c-jun, and cyclin D1 [182–185]. The activation of this pathway inhibits apoptosis and promotes cell survival. β-Catenin levels are regulated negatively by glycogen synthase kinase β [186]. A complex that includes β-catenin, glycogen synthase kinase β, axin, adenomatous polyposis coli, and casein kinase 1 leads to the phosphorylation of β-catenin, which then leads to ubiquitin proteosome degradation of β-catenin [180,181].

Uematsu and colleagues [187] demonstrated that Dvl and β-catenin are overexpressed in MM cells and cell lines. Dvl, which consists of several membrane-proximal signaling intermediates, is part of the Wnt pathway. Dvl proteins contain three domains: a dix domain, a PDZ domain involved in protein-protein interaction, and a DEP domain [188]. Downstream of these proteins is glycogen synthase kinase β. MPM cells and cell lines were transfected with a PDZ domain deletion mutant. In these cells, the mutant caused inhibition of Dvl and subsequently led to a decrease in β-catenin levels, which also led to a decrease in

T-cell factor–mediated transcription and suppressed tumorigenesis in vitro and in vivo. Decreases in c-myc and cyclo-oxygenase-2 levels also were observed in two different cell lines, respectively [187].

Aberrant Wnt signaling also can occur because of loss of a group of glyco-proteins that normally antagonize Wnt signaling. Secreted Frizzle-related proteins are a family of five glycoproteins that share similar sequence with the Fz receptor extracellular domain [189–191]. The main difference is that secreted Frizzle-related proteins lack a transmembrane domain and are unable to trans-duce signals upon binding ligand [189]. Lee and colleagues [192] demonstrated that downregulation of secreted Frizzle-related proteins occurs in MM cells and cell lines and is caused by hypermethylation of the secreted Frizzle-related protein gene promoters. By transfecting secreted Frizzle-related protein gene constructs into MM cell lines, they were able to induce apoptosis and suppress cell growth.

Dickkopf-1 is also an antagonist of the Wnt signaling pathway that binds to the LDL receptor-related protein 5/6, which is a Wnt coreceptor [193,194]. This essential interaction is blocked and signaling ceases. Kremen, a membrane-anchored protein, binds to Dickkopf-1 and leads to endocytosis of the LDL receptor-related protein 5/6 receptor [195]. Dickkopf-1 levels are downregulated in various cancers; restoring its function may lead to apoptosis [192,196–200].

Noncanonical signaling occurs in the absence of β-catenin and may occur through calcium flux, c-Jun NH2-terminal kinase, and G proteins [201]. Using β-catenin–deficient MM cell lines, You and colleagues [202] were able to demonstrate restoration of apoptosis and growth suppression when inhibit-ing Wnt-1 or Dvl. This effect was negated when c-Jun NH2-terminal kinase was inhibited using a small molecule inhibitor. Using the same cell lines, Lee and colleagues [196] demonstrated apoptosis and growth suppression once Dickkopf-1 levels were restored. When a c-Jun NH2-terminal kinase small mole-cule inhibitor was introduced to the Dickkopf-1 restored β-catenin–deficient MM cell lines, apoptosis ceased and growth was no longer suppressed. These two observations revealed that c-Jun NH2-terminal kinase is important in WNT signaling in β-catenin–deficient MM cell lines.

mTOR PATHWAY

Another important protein in cell signaling is mammalian target of rapamycin (mTOR), which plays a central role in transcription and translation in response to growth factors and nutrients. mTOR, also known as FRAP, RAPT, and RAFT, was discovered because of its FK506 binding protein (FKBP)-rapamycin binding properties after its counterpart TOR was originally discovered in yeast [203–206]. mTOR contains a C-terminus Ser/Thr protein kinase domain that shares homology with the PI3-K catalytic domain [206–209]. Several other proteins, including RAD3, DNA-PKc, ATM, and TRRAP, have similar kinase domains and belong to a family of proteins termed phosphoinositide kinase-related kinases [208]. mTOR also contains an FKBP-rapamycin binding domain adjacent to its kinase domain and N-terminus HEAT motifs that mediate protein-protein interactions in multiprotein complexes [206,208–210]. N-terminus to the FKBP-rapamycin binding domain is an FAT domain, with an FATC domain located at the most C-terminus portion of the protein [207,211]. The function of these two domains is unknown at this time.

mTOR is downstream of kinases such as PI3-K and AKT (protein kinase B) and upstream of proteins such as STAT3, pRb, 4E binding protein (4E-BP1), and p70s6k. When a normal cell is exposed to growth factors and amino acids, mTOR is activated, which leads to activation of p70s6k and inhibition of 4E-BP1 [212,213]. Activation of p70s6k leads to phosphorylation of the 40s ribosomal protein S6, which subsequently leads to translation of 5' terminal oligopyridimine tract (TOP) mRNAs [214]. These mRNAs encode ribosomal proteins and translational apparatus components [215]. In resting cells, inhibitor of eukaryotic initiation factor 4E (eIF4E) and 4E-BP1 are bound together to inhibit translation [208]. mTOR phosphorylates 4E-BP1 and causes the dissociation of these two proteins, which allows eIF4E to help in translation of proteins needed for the cell cycle, including cyclin D and c-myc [216,217]. mTOR also activates RNA polymerase I and RNA polymerase III by possibly inactivating pRb [218–221]. At the same time it upregulates STAT3 [222]. Thus, mTOR upregulates translation and transcription in response to growth factor responses and favorable growth conditions.

Upstream of mTOR are other kinases that are linked to RTKs, such as PI3-K and Akt. In cells treated with rapamycin before stimulation, phosphorylation of mTOR decreased while that of PI3-K and Akt was not affected. When the cells were exposed to the PI3-K inhibitor wortmannin, PI3-K activity decreased, as did Akt phosphorylation [223–226]. Reactive oxygen species also can participate in signal transduction via PI3-K and Akt. Activation of Akt and PI3-K by hydrogen peroxide (H_2O_2) also led to mTOR activation and subsequent cell proliferation [227]. When these cells were exposed to wortmannin and rapamycin before exposure to H_2O_2, similar results were noted, which indicated that Akt is downstream of PI3-K and upstream of mTOR.

Rapamycin also has been shown to cause decreased phosphorylation of 4E-BP1 with rapid association with eIF4E in human tumor cells [228]. Human tumor xenografts in mice also showed association of 4E-BP1 and eIF4E in response to rapamycin exposure. When mTOR is inhibited by rapamycin, cells undergo early G1 phase arrest [229,230]. Cells are no longer able to activate the machinery necessary for translation and transcription, including cyclin D, which is important in getting the cell beyond the restriction point in the G1 phase [231].

mTOR may play an important role in tumorogenesis. No oncogenic form of mTOR has been discovered, but transforming potential has been seen in several of the proteins linked to mTOR signaling, including PI3-K, Akt, and eIF4E. mTOR also regulates c-myc translation, which is dysregulated in several tumor types. Several tumors also have upregulated STAT3, which is controlled by mTOR. Transformation of cells by v-Src occurs via the Ras-MAPK and

PI3-K-mTOR pathways. Inhibiting one pathway allows transformation to occur through the other. Several tumor cell lines have been shown to be sensitive to the effects of rapamycin including pancreatic cancer, glioblastoma, neuroblastoma, and breast cancer [208]. This signaling pathway has yet to be studied in depth in MM cells or cell lines.

MITOGEN-ACTIVATED PROTEIN KINASE PATHWAY

Other pathways include the mitogen-activated protein kinase, extracellular signal-regulated kinases, and p38 kinases. The mitogen-activated protein kinase pathway can be induced by asbestos fibers. Initiation occurs when crocidolite fibers cause aggregation of epidermal growth factor receptors, which leads to autophosphorylation of the receptor [232]. This event leads to a series of phosphorylation events within the cell, which activates the extracellular signal-regulated kinase pathway and eventually activates the mitogen-activated protein kinases [232–235]. This process leads to activation of a family of transcription factors that belong to the activator protein-1 family [236]. These proteins include homo- and heterodimers of the Jun and Fos early response proto-oncogenes [237].

c-fos and c-jun mRNA levels increased in a dose-dependent manner when pleural mesothelial cells from rats were exposed to crocidolite and erionite fibers [238]. Nonfibrous particles failed to increase mRNA levels of c-fos and c-jun, and it is believed that the geometry of the fibers plays an important role in activating cellular pathways [239]. The activation of mRNA transcription has been shown to be mediated through epidermal growth factor receptor. Other proto-oncogenes have been upregulated in mesothelial cells exposed to crocidolite fibers and include c-myc and fra-1 [240]. Confirmed increases in fra-1 occur in activator protein-1 complexes in asbestos-exposed mesothelial cells and MM cells and are extracellular signal-regulated kinase dependent [241].

NUCLEAR FACTOR-κB PATHWAY

Another nuclear transcription factor, nuclear factor-κB, is known to regulate gene expression and cellular proliferation [242]. In hamster tracheal epithelial cells, crocidolite fibers have caused an increase in nuclear factor-κB expression [243]. It also induces redox changes that lead to the activation of nuclear factor-κB and eventual upregulation of proinflammatory cytokines, such as interleukin-6, interleukin-8, and tumor necrosis factor-alpha [244,245].

REACTIVE OXYGEN SPECIES

Reactive oxygen species may play an important role in activation of nuclear transcription factors by asbestos fibers and in cell survival and apoptosis. MM cells are highly resistant to oxidants when compared with non-MM cells [246,247]. Reactive oxygen species can cause cell death, but elimination of these superoxide radicals can have an antiapoptotic effect. Kahlos and colleagues [246] demonstrated that elevated levels of mitochondrial manganese superoxide dismutase occur in MM cells compared with normal mesothelial cells. Mitochondrial manganese superoxide dismutase dismutates superoxide to hydrogen peroxide and oxygen [248]. This molecule has been shown to be upregulated by cytokines, changes in the cellular redox state, and asbestos fibers [249–252]. The upregulation of this molecule may explain the increased resistance of MM cells to radiation and chemotherapeutic agents as reactive oxygen species are generated by these treatment modalities [253,254].

CELLULAR ADHESION MOLECULES

Cellular adhesion molecules play an important role in cell adhesion, cell-cell signaling and recognition, and cell migration. Several studies have shown upregulation of certain cell surface molecules in MM. One in particular, mesothelin, has become of interest in regards to molecular diagnostics and targeted therapies.

Mesothelin is a glycoprotein that is attached to the cell surface. It is produced as a 69-kDa precursor protein that is cleaved into two parts [255]. The first part, a 40-kDa protein, is attached to the cell surface with a phosphatidylinositol linkage and may be important in cell adhesion and cell-cell signaling. The second part, a 31-kDa fragment termed megakaryocyte-potentiating factor is released into serum from the cell. Robinson and colleagues [256] demonstrated a rise in serum concentrations of soluble mesothelin-related proteins in patients with MM. Eighty-four percent of patients who had MM had elevated soluble mesothelin-related protein levels in comparison to 2% of patients with other tumors or inflammatory lung or pleural diseases. Of note, all patients had had prior exposure to asbestos. Twenty-eight controls who had never been exposed to asbestos did not have elevated soluble mesothelin-related protein levels. These levels have been shown to correlate with tumor stage and burden and may prove useful as a diagnostic tool.

MMs also have elevations of other cell surface molecules. Some are unique to mesothelioma. The molecules semaphorin E, integrin β4, and p-cadherin are upregulated in epithelial MM. Sarcomatoid MM shows upregulation of matrix metalloproteinases-9 and tissue plasminogen activator. Neural cell adhesion molecule L1 and chemokine are upregulated in biphasic MM [257].

SV40

SV40 is a DNA tumor virus that is believed to act in conjunction with asbestos to cause MM. The SV40 virus encodes several proteins, including large T antigen (TAg), small t antigen (tAg), and 17kT. TAg is a 90-kDa protein that is located predominately in the nucleus, whereas tAg, a 17-kDa protein, is found primarily in the cytoplasm. TAg has a C-terminus bipartite region that binds p53 and associates with CBP, p300, and p400 [258–263]. The LxCxE motif binds to pRb, p107, and p130 [261,262]. At the N-terminus is the J domain, which binds to hsc70 and is conserved between TAg and tAg [259,263]. The C-terminus of tAg is cysteine rich, which allows it to bind zinc ions and achieve conformational stability [264–266].

TAg causes transformation by binding to and inactivating several different tumor suppressor proteins, including p53, pRb, p107, p130/Rb2, p300, and p400 [258–263]. By inactivating p53, even in the presence of DNA damage, the cell continues to cycle and apoptosis is inhibited. In addition to binding to inactivating p53, TAg is able to induce DNA alterations [267]. TAg also binds to pRb and releases E2F, which leads to transcription of factors needed for cell cycling. Infected cells circumvent checkpoints crucial for controlling the cells entry into the cell cycle. Transformation is helped by tAg inactivating p53, upregulating TAg production, and stimulating AP-1 activity [268–270].

An association between SV40 infection and tumor formation was first observed in the 1960s. Eddy and colleagues [271] observed fibrosarcomas in newborn hamsters at injection sites for SV40-infected rhesus monkey cells. Sixty percent of hamsters injected intracardially with SV40 developed MM [272]. When injected intrapleurally, 100% of the animals developed MM within 3 to 6 months [273].

Possible viral infection of humans might have occurred after polio vaccination with SV40-contaminated vaccines [274,275]. The vaccines were prepared in cell cultures grown on monolayers of infected rhesus monkey kidney cells. The contamination was not discovered until 1960, because this virus is not cytopathic to rhesus monkey kidney cells. It is believed that more than 30 million people in the United States were exposed via vaccination before the virus was discovered [2,274–277]. The virus also may have been transmitted when parenteral adenovirus vaccines contaminated with SV40 were given to military personal in the 1950s and 1960s. It is unknown if human-to-human dissemination can or has ever occurred.

Carbone and colleagues [3] used the polymerase chain reaction (PCR) test to look for SV40 sequences in 48 patient samples, and they observed that 60% of the tissue samples contained SV40-like sequences. These results were soon confirmed independently by 26 other laboratories [278,279]. Scientists at the Finnish Occupational Health Institute were unable to detect any SV40 sequences in their MM samples, which might be because all of the polio vaccines administered in that country were free of SV40 contamination [280].

A recent study has questioned whether SV40 is truly involved in the formation of human MM. Because of inconsistent results obtained while studying the relationship between SV40 and homozygous deletions of CDKN2A, Lopez-Rios and colleagues [281] used several independent techniques to investigate SV40 infection in MM. They extracted high-quality DNA and RNA from 71 frozen MM samples and performed PCR tests using four sets of primers for the SV40 T-antigen gene. Positive results for SV40 were obtained in 56% to 62% of samples when using two primer sets for DNA PCR in a region of the T-antigen gene that contained nucleotides 4100-4713. This region is also known to be present in many common laboratory plasmids. When the two primer sets for DNA PCR were used that did not contain this nucleotide region, only 6% of samples tested positive for SV40 infection. PCR assays confirmed that tumor samples contained SV40 sequences with deletions found only in plasmids and not in native SV40. Using RT-PCR, all 71 MM samples tested negative for SV40 T-antigen, and all samples tested negative for SV40 T-antigen by immunohistochemistry. These data suggest that SV40 may play no role in MM formation and may only be a laboratory anomaly.

SUMMARY

MM is an uncommon tumor with high morbidity and mortality rates. Most cases are caused by asbestos exposure. Transformation occurs either by direct stimulation of pathways through RTKs or by loss of genetic material and tumor suppressors that allow for unchecked proliferation. This article discussed several different genetic and signal pathway alterations that can occur in MM cells and cell lines, but as with other tumor types, these changes are heterogeneous. With increased knowledge of MM cellular pathways, new targeted therapies can be produced and tested with hopes of increasing survival in these patients.

References

[1] Battifora H, McCaughey WTE. Tumors of the serosal membranes. In: Rossi J, Sobin LH, editors. Atlas of tumor pathology. Washington (DC): Armed Forces Institute of Pathology; 1995. p. 17–99.
[2] Testa JR, Pass H, Carbone M. Molecular biology of mesothelioma. In: DeVita V, Hellman S, Rosenberg S, editors. Principles and practice of oncology. Philadelphia: JB Lippincott; 2001. p. 1937–43.
[3] Carbone M, Kratzke RA, Testa JR. The pathogenesis of mesothelioma. Semin Oncol 2002;29(1):2–17.
[4] Wagner JC, Sleggs CA, Marchand P. Diffuse pleural mesothelioma and asbestos exposure in the North Western Cape Province. Br J Ind Med 1960;17:260–71.
[5] McDonald JC. Health implications of environmental exposure to asbestos. Environ Health Perspect 1985;62:319–28.
[6] Peto J, et al. Continuing increase in mesothelioma mortality in Britain. Lancet 1995; 345(8949):535–9.
[7] Britton M. The epidemiology of mesothelioma. Semin Oncol 2002;29(1):18–25.
[8] Selikoff IJ, Hammond EC, Seidman H. Mortality experience of insulation workers in the United States and Canada, 1943–1976. Ann NY Acad Sci 1979;330:91–116.
[9] Jarvholm B, Sanden A. Lung cancer and mesothelioma in the pleura and peritoneum among Swedish insulation workers. Occup Environ Med 1998;55(11):766–70.
[10] Mossman BT, et al. Asbestos: scientific developments and implications for public policy. Science 1990;247(4940):294–301.
[11] Mossman BT, Churg A. Mechanisms in the pathogenesis of asbestosis and silicosis. Am J Respir Crit Care Med 1998;157(5 Pt 1):1666–80.
[12] Nicholson WJ. Comparative dose-response relationships of asbestos fiber types: magnitudes and uncertainties. Ann NY Acad Sci 1991;643:74–84.
[13] Robledo R, Mossman B. Cellular and molecular mechanisms of asbestos-induced fibrosis. J Cell Physiol 1999;180(2):158–66.
[14] Sluis-Kremer G. Asbestos disease at low exposures after long residence times. Ann NY Acad Sci 1991;643:182–93.
[15] Ashcroft T. Epidemiological and quantitative relationships between mesothelioma and asbestos on Tyneside. J Clin Pathol 1973;26(11):832–40.
[16] Hain E, et al. Retrospective study of 150 cases of mesothelioma in Hamburg area. Int Arch Arbeitsmed 1974;33(1):15–37.

[17] McDonald AD, et al. Epidemiology of primary malignant mesothelial tumors in Canada. Cancer 1970;26(4):914–9.

[18] McEwen J, et al. Mesothelioma in Scotland. BMJ 1970;4(735):575–8.

[19] Rubino GF, et al. Epidemiology of pleural mesothelioma in Northwestern Italy (Piedmont). Br J Ind Med 1972;29(4):436–42.

[20] Zielhuis RL, Versteeg JP, Planteijdt HT. Pleura mesothelioma and exposure to asbestos: a retrospective case-control study in the Netherlands. Int Arch Occup Environ Health 1975;36(1):1–18.

[21] McDonald JC. Asbestos. In: McDonald JC, editor. Epidemiology of work related diseases. London: BMJ Books; 2000. p. 85–108.

[22] Coggon D, et al. Differences in occupational mortality from pleural cancer, peritoneal cancer, and asbestosis. Occup Environ Med 1995;52(11):775–7.

[23] Levin JL, et al. Tyler asbestos workers: mortality experience in a cohort exposed to amosite. Occup Environ Med 1998;55(3):155–60.

[24] McDonald JC, et al. Mesothelioma and asbestos fiber type: evidence from lung tissue analyses. Cancer 1989;63(8):1544–7.

[25] Seidman H, Selikoff IJ, Hammond EC. Short term asbestos work exposure and long-term observation. Ann NY Acad Sci 1979;330:61–89.

[26] Baris YI, et al. An outbreak of pleural mesothelioma and chronic fibrosing pleurisy in the village of Karain/Urgup in Anatolia. Thorax 1978;33(2):181–92.

[27] Coplu L, et al. An epidemiological study in an Anatolian village in Turkey environmentally exposed to tremolite asbestos. J Environ Pathol Toxicol Oncol 1996;15(2–4):177–82.

[28] Rohl AN, et al. Endemic pleural disease associated with exposure to mixed fibrous dust in Turkey. Science 1982;216(4545):518–20.

[29] Roushdy-Hammady I, et al. Genetic-susceptibility factor and malignant mesothelioma in the Cappadocian region of Turkey. Lancet 2001;357(9254):444–5.

[30] Murthy SS, Testa JR. Asbestos, chromosomal deletions, and tumor suppressor gene alterations in human malignant mesothelioma. J Cell Physiol 1999;180(2):150–7.

[31] Lu YY, et al. Deletion mapping of the short arm of chromosome 3 in human malignant mesothelioma. Genes Chromosomes Cancer 1994;9(1):76–80.

[32] Seizinger BR, et al. Report of the committee on chromosome and gene loss in human neoplasia. Cytogenetic Cell Genet 1991;58:1080–96.

[33] Shigemitsu K, et al. Genetic alteration of the beta-catenin gene (CTNNB1) in human lung cancer and malignant mesothelioma and identification of a new 3p21.3 homozygous deletion. Oncogene 2001;20(31):4249–57.

[34] Lee WC, et al. Loss of heterozygosity analysis defines a critical region in chromosome 1p22 commonly deleted in human malignant mesothelioma. Cancer Res 1996;56(19):4297–301.

[35] Offit K, et al. 6q deletions define distinct clinico-pathologic subsets of non-Hodgkin's lymphoma. Blood 1993;82(7):2157–62.

[36] Orphanos V, et al. Allelic imbalance of chromosome 6q in ovarian tumours. Br J Cancer 1995;71(4):666–9.

[37] Sheng ZM, et al. Multiple regions of chromosome 6q affected by loss of heterozygosity in primary human breast carcinomas. Br J Cancer 1996;73(2):144–7.

[38] Cher ML, et al. Genetic alterations in untreated metastases and androgen-independent prostate cancer detected by comparative genomic hybridization and allelotyping. Cancer Res 1996;56(13):3091–102.

[39] Osborne RJ, Leech V. Polymerase chain reaction allelotyping of human ovarian cancer. Br J Cancer 1994;69(3):429–38.

[40] Tahara H, et al. Genomic localization of novel candidate tumor suppressor gene loci in human parathyroid adenomas. Cancer Res 1996;56(3):599–605.

[41] Wick W, et al. Evidence for a novel tumor suppressor gene on chromosome 15 associated with progression to a metastatic stage in breast cancer. Oncogene 1996;12(5):973–8.

[42] Heichman KA, Roberts JM. Rules to replicate by. Cell 1994;79(4):557–62.

[43] Wuarin J, Nurse P. Regulating S phase: CDKs, licensing and proteolysis. Cell 1996; 85(6):785–7.

[44] Morgan DO. Principles of CDK regulation. Nature 1995;374(6518):131–4.

[45] Nasmyth K. Control of the yeast cell cycle by the Cdc28 protein kinase. Curr Opin Cell Biol 1993;5(2):166–79.

[46] Nigg EA. Cyclin-dependent protein kinases: key regulators of the eukaryotic cell cycle. Bioessays 1995;17(6):471–80.

[47] Norbury C, Nurse P. Animal cell cycles and their control. Annu Rev Biochem 1992; 61:441–70.

[48] Reed SI. The role of p34 kinases in the G1 to S-phase transition. Annu Rev Cell Biol 1992; 8:529–61.

[49] Sherr CJ. Mammalian G1 cyclins. Cell 1993;73(6):1059–65.

[50] Sherr CJ. G1 phase progression: cycling on cue. Cell 1994;79(4):551–5.

[51] Serrano M, Hannon GJ, Beach D. A new regulatory motif in cell-cycle control causing specific inhibition of cyclin D/CDK4. Nature 1993;366(6456):704–7.

[52] Nobori T, et al. Deletions of the cyclin-dependent kinase-4 inhibitor gene in multiple human cancers. Nature 1994;368(6473):753–6.

[53] Hannon GJ, Beach D. p15INK4B is a potential effector of TGF-beta-induced cell cycle arrest. Nature 1994;371(6494):257–61.

[54] Kamb A, et al. A cell cycle regulator potentially involved in genesis of many tumor types. Science 1994;264(5157):436–40.

[55] Guan KL, et al. Growth suppression by p18, a p16INK4/MTS1- and p14INK4B/MTS2-related CDK6 inhibitor, correlates with wild-type pRb function. Genes Dev 1994;8(24):2939–52.

[56] Hirai H, et al. Novel INK4 proteins, p19 and p18, are specific inhibitors of the cyclin D-dependent kinases CDK4 and CDK6. Mol Cell Biol 1995;15(5):2672–81.

[57] Chan FK, et al. Identification of human and mouse p19, a novel CDK4 and CDK6 inhibitor with homology to p16ink4. Mol Cell Biol 1995;15(5):2682–8.

[58] Ewen ME, et al. Functional interactions of the retinoblastoma protein with mammalian D-type cyclins. Cell 1993;73(3):487–97.

[59] Dowdy SF, et al. Physical interaction of the retinoblastoma protein with human D cyclins. Cell 1993;73(3):499–511.

[60] Kato J, et al. Direct binding of cyclin D to the retinoblastoma gene product (pRb) and pRb phosphorylation by the cyclin D-dependent kinase CDK4. Genes Dev 1993;7(3):331–42.

[61] Weintraub SJ, et al. Mechanism of active transcriptional repression by the retinoblastoma protein. Nature 1995;375(6534):812–5.

[62] Weintraub SJ, Prater CA, Dean DC. Retinoblastoma protein switches the E2F site from positive to negative element. Nature 1992;358(6383):259–61.

[63] Hamel PA, et al. Transcriptional repression of the E2-containing promoters EIIaE, c-myc, and RB1 by the product of the RB1 gene. Mol Cell Biol 1992;12(8):3431–8.

[64] Flemington EK, Speck SH, Kaelin Jr WG. E2F–1-mediated transactivation is inhibited by complex formation with the retinoblastoma susceptibility gene product. Proc Natl Acad Sci U S A 1993;90(15):6914–8.

[65] Lam EW, Watson RJ. An E2F-binding site mediates cell-cycle regulated repression of mouse B-myb transcription. EMBO J 1993;12(7):2705–13.

[66] Koh J, et al. Tumour-derived p16 alleles encoding proteins defective in cell-cycle inhibition. Nature 1995;375(6531):506–10.

[67] Lukas J, et al. Cyclin D1 is dispensable for G1 control in retinoblastoma gene-deficient cells independently of cdk4 activity. Mol Cell Biol 1995;15(5):2600–11.

[68] Lukas J, et al. Retinoblastoma-protein-dependent cell-cycle inhibition by the tumour suppressor p16. Nature 1995;375(6531):503–6.

[69] Medema RH, et al. Growth suppression by p16ink4 requires functional retinoblastoma protein. Proc Natl Acad Sci U S A 1995;92(14):6289–93.

[70] Serrano M, et al. Inhibition of ras-induced proliferation and cellular transformation by p16INK4. Science 1995;267(5195):249–52.

[71] Tam SW, et al. Differential expression and regulation of cyclin D1 protein in normal and tumor human cells: association with CDK4 is required for cyclin D1 function in G1 progression. Oncogene 1994;9(9):2663–74.

[72] Hatakeyama M, et al. Collaboration of G1 cyclins in the functional inactivation of the retinoblastoma protein. Genes Dev 1994;8(15):1759–71.

[73] Hinds PW, et al. Regulation of retinoblastoma protein functions by ectopic expression of human cyclins. Cell 1992;70(6):993–1006.

[74] Mittnacht S, et al. Distinct sub-populations of the retinoblastoma protein show a distinct pattern of phosphorylation. EMBO J 1994;13(1):118–27.

[75] Weinberg RA. The retinoblastoma protein and cell cycle control. Cell 1995;81(3): 323–30.

[76] DeGregori J, Kowalik T, Nevins JR. Cellular targets for activation by the E2F1 transcription factor include DNA synthesis- and G1/S-regulatory genes. Mol Cell Biol 1995;15(8):4215–24.

[77] Duronio RJ, O'Farrell PH. Developmental control of the G1 to S transition in Drosophila: cyclin E is a limiting downstream target of E2F. Genes Dev 1995;9(12):1456–68.

[78] Geng Y, et al. Regulation of cyclin E transcription by E2Fs and retinoblastoma protein. Oncogene 1996;12(6):1173–80.

[79] Johnson DG, Ohtani K, Nevins JR. Autoregulatory control of E2F1 expression in response to positive and negative regulators of cell cycle progression. Genes Dev 1994;8(13): 1514–25.

[80] Neuman E, et al. Transcription of the E2F-1 gene is rendered cell cycle dependent by E2F DNA-binding sites within its promoter. Mol Cell Biol 1994;14(10):6607–15.

[81] Ohtani K, DeGregori J, Nevins JR. Regulation of the cyclin E gene by transcription factor E2F1. Proc Natl Acad Sci U S A 1995;92(26):12146–50.

[82] Schulze A, et al. Cell cycle regulation of the cyclin A gene promoter is mediated by a variant E2F site. Proc Natl Acad Sci U S A 1995;92(24):11264–8.

[83] Clurman BE, et al. Turnover of cyclin E by the ubiquitin-proteasome pathway is regulated by cdk2 binding and cyclin phosphorylation. Genes Dev 1996;10(16):1979–90.

[84] Won KA, Reed SI. Activation of cyclin E/CDK2 is coupled to site-specific autophosphorylation and ubiquitin-dependent degradation of cyclin E. EMBO J 1996;15(16): 4182–93.

[85] Dynlacht BD, et al. Differential regulation of E2F transactivation by cyclin/cdk2 complexes. Genes Dev 1994;8(15):1772–86.

[86] Krek W, et al. Negative regulation of the growth-promoting transcription factor E2F-1 by a stably bound cyclin A-dependent protein kinase. Cell 1994;78(1):161–72.

[87] Krek W, Xu G, Livingston DM. Cyclin A-kinase regulation of E2F-1 DNA binding function underlies suppression of an S phase checkpoint. Cell 1995;83(7):1149–58.

[88] el-Deiry WS, et al. WAF1: a potential mediator of p53 tumor suppression. Cell 1993; 75(4):817–25.

[89] Gu Y, Turck CW, Morgan DO. Inhibition of CDK2 activity in vivo by an associated 20K regulatory subunit. Nature 1993;366(6456):707–10.

[90] Harper JW, et al. The p21 CDK-interacting protein Cip1 is a potent inhibitor of G1 cyclin-dependent kinases. Cell 1993;75(4):805–16.

[91] Lee MH, Reynisdottir I, Massague J. Cloning of p57KIP2, a cyclin-dependent kinase inhibitor with unique domain structure and tissue distribution. Genes Dev 1995;9(6):639–49.

[92] Matsuoka S, et al. p57KIP2, a structurally distinct member of the p21CIP1 CDK inhibitor family, is a candidate tumor suppressor gene. Genes Dev 1995;9(6):650–62.

[93] Noda A, et al. Cloning of senescent cell-derived inhibitors of DNA synthesis using an expression screen. Exp Cell Res 1994;211(1):90–8.

[94] Polyak K, et al. p27Kip1, a cyclin-CDK inhibitor, links transforming growth factor-beta and contact inhibition to cell cycle arrest. Genes Dev 1994;8(1):9–22.

[95] Polyak K, et al. Cloning of p27Kip1, a cyclin-dependent kinase inhibitor and a potential mediator of extracellular antimitogenic signals. Cell 1994;78(1):59–66.

[96] Toyoshima H, Hunter T. p27, a novel inhibitor of G1 cyclin-CDK protein kinase activity, is related to p21. Cell 1994;78(1):67–74.

[97] Xiong Y, et al. p21 is a universal inhibitor of cyclin kinases. Nature 1993;366(6456): 701–4.

[98] Nourse J, et al. Interleukin-2-mediated elimination of the p27Kip1 cyclin-dependent kinase inhibitor prevented by rapamycin. Nature 1994;372(6506):570–3.

[99] Kato JY, et al. Cyclic AMP-induced G1 phase arrest mediated by an inhibitor (p27Kip1) of cyclin-dependent kinase 4 activation. Cell 1994;79(3):487–96.

[100] Agrawal D, et al. Repression of p27kip1 synthesis by platelet-derived growth factor in BALB/c 3T3 cells. Mol Cell Biol 1996;16(8):4327–36.

[101] Hengst L, Reed SI. Translational control of p27Kip1 accumulation during the cell cycle. Science 1996;271(5257):1861–4.

[102] Pagano M, et al. Role of the ubiquitin-proteasome pathway in regulating abundance of the cyclin-dependent kinase inhibitor p27. Science 1995;269(5224):682–5.

[103] Xiong Y, Zhang H, Beach D. Subunit rearrangement of the cyclin-dependent kinases is associated with cellular transformation. Genes Dev 1993;7(8):1572–83.

[104] Jen J, et al. Deletion of p16 and p15 genes in brain tumors. Cancer Res 1994;54(24): 6353–8.

[105] Stone S, et al. Genomic structure, expression and mutational analysis of the P15 (MTS2) gene. Oncogene 1995;11(5):987–91.

[106] Guan KL, et al. Isolation and characterization of p19INK4d, a p16-related inhibitor specific to CDK6 and CDK4. Mol Biol Cell 1996;7(1):57–70.

[107] Okuda T, et al. Molecular cloning, expression pattern, and chromosomal localization of human CDKN2D/INK4d, an inhibitor of cyclin D-dependent kinases. Genomics 1995; 29(3):623–30.

[108] Duro D, et al. A new type of p16INK4/MTS1 gene transcript expressed in B-cell malignancies. Oncogene 1995;11(1):21–9.

[109] Jiang P, et al. Comparative analysis of *Homo sapiens* and *Mus musculus* cyclin-dependent kinase (CDK) inhibitor genes p16 (MTS1) and p15 (MTS2). J Mol Evol 1995; 41(6):795–802.

[110] Mao L, et al. A novel p16INK4A transcript. Cancer Res 1995;55(14):2995–7.

[111] Quelle DE, et al. Cloning and characterization of murine p16INK4a and p15INK4b genes. Oncogene 1995;11(4):635–45.

[112] Stone S, et al. Complex structure and regulation of the P16 (MTS1) locus. Cancer Res 1995;55(14):2988–94.

[113] Quelle DE, et al. Alternative reading frames of the INK4a tumor suppressor gene encode two unrelated proteins capable of inducing cell cycle arrest. Cell 1995;83(6): 993–1000.

[114] Hall M, Bates S, Peters G. Evidence for different modes of action of cyclin-dependent kinase inhibitors: p15 and p16 bind to kinases, p21 and p27 bind to cyclins. Oncogene 1995;11(8):1581–8.

[115] Parry D, et al. Lack of cyclin D-CDK complexes in Rb-negative cells correlates with high levels of p16INK4/MTS1 tumour suppressor gene product. EMBO J 1995;14(3):503–11.

[116] Reymond A, Brent R. p16 proteins from melanoma-prone families are deficient in binding to CDK4. Oncogene 1995;11(6):1173–8.

[117] Matsushime H, et al. Identification and properties of an atypical catalytic subunit (p34PSK-J3/cdk4) for mammalian D type G1 cyclins. Cell 1992;71(2):323–34.

[118] Sewing A, et al. Human cyclin D1 encodes a labile nuclear protein whose synthesis is directly induced by growth factors and suppressed by cyclic AMP. J Cell Sci 1993; 104(Pt 2):545–55.

[119] Shapiro GI, et al. Multiple mechanisms of p16INK4A inactivation in non-small cell lung cancer cell lines. Cancer Res 1995;55(24):6200–9.

[120] Ruas M, Peters G. The p16INK4a/CDKN2A tumor suppressor and its relatives. Biochim Biophys Acta 1998;1378(2):F115–77.

[121] Sherr CJ, Roberts JM. Inhibitors of mammalian G1 cyclin-dependent kinases. Genes Dev 1995;9(10):1149–63.

[122] Kelley MJ, et al. Differential inactivation of CDKN2 and Rb protein in non-small-cell and small-cell lung cancer cell lines. J Natl Cancer Inst 1995;87(10):756–61.

[123] Merlo A, et al. 5' CpG island methylation is associated with transcriptional silencing of the tumour suppressor p16/CDKN2/MTS1 in human cancers. Nat Med 1995;1(7):686–92.

[124] Otterson GA, et al. CDKN2 gene silencing in lung cancer by DNA hypermethylation and kinetics of p16INK4 protein induction by 5-aza 2'deoxycytidine. Oncogene 1995; 11(6):1211–6.

[125] Otterson GA, et al. Absence of p16INK4 protein is restricted to the subset of lung cancer lines that retains wildtype Rb. Oncogene 1994;9(11):3375–8.

[126] Shapiro GI, et al. Reciprocal Rb inactivation and p16INK4 expression in primary lung cancers and cell lines. Cancer Res 1995;55(3):505–9.

[127] Yeager T, et al. Increased p16 levels correlate with pRb alterations in human urothelial cells. Cancer Res 1995;55(3):493–7.

[128] Kamijo T, et al. Tumor suppression at the mouse INK4a locus mediated by the alternative reading frame product p19ARF. Cell 1997;91(5):649–59.

[129] Pomerantz J, et al. The Ink4a tumor suppressor gene product, p19Arf, interacts with MDM2 and neutralizes MDM2's inhibition of p53. Cell 1998;92(6):713–23.

[130] Stott FJ, et al. The alternative product from the human CDKN2A locus, p14(ARF), participates in a regulatory feedback loop with p53 and MDM2. EMBO J 1998;17(17): 5001–14.

[131] Arap W, et al. Functional analysis of wild-type and malignant glioma derived CDKN2Abeta alleles: evidence for an RB-independent growth suppressive pathway. Oncogene 1997;15(17):2013–20.

[132] Liggett Jr WH, et al. p16 and p16 beta are potent growth suppressors of head and neck squamous carcinoma cells in vitro. Cancer Res 1996;56(18):4119–23.

[133] Quelle DE, et al. Cancer-associated mutations at the INK4a locus cancel cell cycle arrest by p16INK4a but not by the alternative reading frame protein p19ARF. Proc Natl Acad Sci U S A 1997;94(2):669–73.

[134] Zhang Y, Xiong Y, Yarbrough WG. ARF promotes MDM2 degradation and stabilizes p53: ARF-INK4a locus deletion impairs both the Rb and p53 tumor suppression pathways. Cell 1998;92(6):725–34.

[135] Cheng JQ, et al. p16 alterations and deletion mapping of 9p21-p22 in malignant mesothelioma. Cancer Res 1994;54(21):5547–51.

[136] Hirao T, et al. Alterations of the p16(INK4) locus in human malignant mesothelial tumors. Carcinogenesis 2002;23(7):1127–30.

[137] Frizelle SP, et al. Re-expression of p16INK4a in mesothelioma cells results in cell cycle arrest, cell death, tumor suppression and tumor regression. Oncogene 1998;16(24): 3087–95.

[138] Yang CT, et al. Adenovirus-mediated p14(ARF) gene transfer in human mesothelioma cells. J Natl Cancer Inst 2000;92(8):636–41.

[139] Comoglio PM. Structure, biosynthesis and biochemical properties of the HGF receptor in normal and malignant cells. EXS 1993;65:131–65.

[140] Comoglio PM, Boccaccio C. The HGF receptor family: unconventional signal transducers for invasive cell growth. Genes Cells 1996;1(4):347–54.

[141] Di Renzo MF, et al. Expression of the Met/HGF receptor in normal and neoplastic human tissues. Oncogene 1991;6(11):1997–2003.

[142] Duh FM, et al. Gene structure of the human MET proto-oncogene. Oncogene 1997; 15(13):1583–6.

[143] Liu Y. The human hepatocyte growth factor receptor gene: complete structural organization and promoter characterization. Gene 1998;215(1):159–69.

[144] Seki T, et al. Organization of the human hepatocyte growth factor-encoding gene. Gene 1991;102(2):213–9.

[145] Ma PC, et al. c-Met: structure, functions and potential for therapeutic inhibition. Cancer Metastasis Rev 2003;22(4):309–25.

[146] Artigiani S, Comoglio PM, Tamagnone L. Plexins, semaphorins, and scatter factor receptors: a common root for cell guidance signals? IUBMB Life 1999;48(5):477–82.

[147] Maestrini E, et al. A family of transmembrane proteins with homology to the MET-hepatocyte growth factor receptor. Proc Natl Acad Sci U S A 1996;93(2):674–8.

[148] Tamagnone L, et al. Plexins are a large family of receptors for transmembrane, secreted, and GPI-anchored semaphorins in vertebrates. Cell 1999;99(1):71–80.

[149] Tamagnone L, Comoglio PM. Signalling by semaphorin receptors: cell guidance and beyond. Trends Cell Biol 2000;10(9):377–83.

[150] Tessier-Lavigne M, Goodman CS. The molecular biology of axon guidance. Science 1996;274(5290):1123–33.

[151] Comoglio PM, Tamagnone L, Boccaccio C. Plasminogen-related growth factor and semaphorin receptors: a gene superfamily controlling invasive growth. Exp Cell Res 1999;253(1):88–99.

[152] Nakashiro K, et al. Hepatocyte growth factor secreted by prostate-derived stromal cells stimulates growth of androgen-independent human prostatic carcinoma cells. Am J Pathol 2000;157(3):795–803.

[153] Stella MC, Comoglio PM. HGF: a multifunctional growth factor controlling cell scattering. Int J Biochem Cell Biol 1999;31(12):1357–62.

[154] Weimar IS, et al. Hepatocyte growth factor/scatter factor (HGF/SF) is produced by human bone marrow stromal cells and promotes proliferation, adhesion and survival of human hematopoietic progenitor cells (CD34 +). Exp Hematol 1998;26(9):885–94.

[155] Yi S, et al. Paracrine effects of hepatocyte growth factor/scatter factor on non-small-cell lung carcinoma cell lines. Br J Cancer 1998;77(12):2162–70.

[156] Hayashi S, et al. Autocrine-paracrine effects of overexpression of hepatocyte growth factor gene on growth of endothelial cells. Biochem Biophys Res Commun 1996;220(3):539–45.

[157] Iwazawa T, et al. Primary human fibroblasts induce diverse tumor invasiveness: involvement of HGF as an important paracrine factor. Jpn J Cancer Res 1996;87(11):1134–42.

[158] Takai K, et al. Hepatocyte growth factor is constitutively produced by human bone marrow stromal cells and indirectly promotes hematopoiesis. Blood 1997;89(5):1560–5.

[159] Furge KA, Zhang YW, Vande Woude GF. Met receptor tyrosine kinase: enhanced signaling through adapter proteins. Oncogene 2000;19(49):5582–9.

[160] Petrelli A, et al. The endophilin-CIN85-Cbl complex mediates ligand-dependent down-regulation of c-Met. Nature 2002;416(6877):187–90.

[161] Lee JH, et al. A novel germ line juxtamembrane Met mutation in human gastric cancer. Oncogene 2000;19(43):4947–53.

[162] Miller M, et al. Structural basis of oncogenic activation caused by point mutations in the kinase domain of the MET proto-oncogene: modeling studies. Proteins 2001;44(1):32–43.

[163] Schmidt L, et al. Germline and somatic mutations in the tyrosine kinase domain of the MET proto-oncogene in papillary renal carcinomas. Nat Genet 1997;16(1):68–73.

[164] Schmidt L, et al. Novel mutations of the MET proto-oncogene in papillary renal carcinomas. Oncogene 1999;18(14):2343–50.

[165] Schmidt L, et al. Two North American families with hereditary papillary renal carcinoma and identical novel mutations in the MET proto-oncogene. Cancer Res 1998;58(8):1719–22.

[166] Peschard P, et al. Mutation of the c-Cbl TKB domain binding site on the Met receptor tyrosine kinase converts it into a transforming protein. Mol Cell 2001;8(5):995–1004.

[167] Tolnay E, et al. Hepatocyte growth factor/scatter factor and its receptor c-Met are

overexpressed and associated with an increased microvessel density in malignant pleural mesothelioma. J Cancer Res Clin Oncol 1998;124(6):291–6.

[168] Harvey P, et al. Hepatocyte growth factor/scatter factor enhances the invasion of mesothelioma cell lines and the expression of matrix metalloproteinases. Br J Cancer 2000;83(9):1147–53.

[169] Klominek J, et al. Hepatocyte growth factor/scatter factor stimulates chemotaxis and growth of malignant mesothelioma cells through c-met receptor. Int J Cancer 1998; 76(2):240–9.

[170] Cacciotti P, et al. SV40 replication in human mesothelial cells induces HGF/Met receptor activation: a model for viral-related carcinogenesis of human malignant mesothelioma. Proc Natl Acad Sci U S A 2001;98(21):12032–7.

[171] Catalano A, et al. Induction of stem cell factor/c-Kit/slug signal transduction in multidrug-resistant malignant mesothelioma cells. J Biol Chem 2004;279(45):46706–14.

[172] Villano JL, et al. A phase II trial of imatinib mesylate in patients (pts) with malignant mesothelioma (MM). J Clin Oncol 2004;22(14S):7200.

[173] Ohta Y, et al. VEGF and VEGF type C play an important role in angiogenesis and lymphangiogenesis in human malignant mesothelioma tumours. Br J Cancer 1999;81(1): 54–61.

[174] Catalano A, et al. Enhanced expression of vascular endothelial growth factor (VEGF) plays a critical role in the tumor progression potential induced by simian virus 40 large T antigen. Oncogene 2002;21(18):2896–900.

[175] Krasnow RE, Wong LL, Adler PN. Dishevelled is a component of the frizzled signaling pathway in Drosophila. Development 1995;121(12):4095–102.

[176] Rothbacher U, et al. Functional conservation of the Wnt signaling pathway revealed by ectopic expression of Drosophila dishevelled in Xenopus. Dev Biol 1995;170(2): 717–21.

[177] Sokol SY. Analysis of dishevelled signalling pathways during Xenopus development. Curr Biol 1996;6(11):1456–67.

[178] Steitz SA, Tsang M, Sussman DJ. Wnt-mediated relocalization of dishevelled proteins. In Vitro Cell Dev Biol Anim 1996;32(7):441–5.

[179] Yanagawa S, et al. The dishevelled protein is modified by wingless signaling in Drosophila. Genes Dev 1995;9(9):1087–97.

[180] Giles RH, van Es JH, Clevers H. Caught up in a Wnt storm: Wnt signaling in cancer. Biochim Biophys Acta 2003;1653(1):1–24.

[181] Lustig B, Behrens J. The Wnt signaling pathway and its role in tumor development. J Cancer Res Clin Oncol 2003;129(4):199–221.

[182] He TC, et al. Identification of c-MYC as a target of the APC pathway. Science 1998;281(5382):1509–12.

[183] Tetsu O, McCormick F. Beta-catenin regulates expression of cyclin D1 in colon carcinoma cells. Nature 1999;398(6726):422–6.

[184] Uthoff SM, et al. Wingless-type frizzled protein receptor signaling and its putative role in human colon cancer. Mol Carcinog 2001;31(1):56–62.

[185] Wodarz A, Nusse R. Mechanisms of Wnt signaling in development. Annu Rev Cell Dev Biol 1998;14:59–88.

[186] Wagner U, et al. Overexpression of the mouse dishevelled-1 protein inhibits GSK-3beta-mediated phosphorylation of tau in transfected mammalian cells. FEBS Lett 1997; 411(2–3):369–72.

[187] Uematsu K, et al. Wnt pathway activation in mesothelioma: evidence of dishevelled overexpression and transcriptional activity of beta-catenin. Cancer Res 2003;63(15): 4547–51.

[188] Boutros M, et al. Dishevelled activates JNK and discriminates between JNK pathways in planar polarity and wingless signaling. Cell 1998;94(1):109–18.

[189] Finch PW, et al. Purification and molecular cloning of a secreted, frizzled-related antagonist of Wnt action. Proc Natl Acad Sci U S A 1997;94(13):6770–5.

[190] Hu E, et al. Tissue restricted expression of two human Frzbs in preadipocytes and pancreas. Biochem Biophys Res Commun 1998;247(2):287–93.

[191] Rattner A, et al. A family of secreted proteins contains homology to the cysteine-rich ligand-binding domain of frizzled receptors. Proc Natl Acad Sci U S A 1997;94(7):2859–63.

[192] Lee AY, et al. Expression of the secreted frizzled-related protein gene family is downregulated in human mesothelioma. Oncogene 2004;23(39):6672–6.

[193] Semenov MV, et al. Head inducer Dickkopf-1 is a ligand for Wnt coreceptor LRP6. Curr Biol 2001;11(12):951–61.

[194] van Es JH, Barker N, Clevers H. You Wnt some, you lose some: oncogenes in the Wnt signaling pathway. Curr Opin Genet Dev 2003;13(1):28–33.

[195] Mao B, et al. Kremen proteins are Dickkopf receptors that regulate Wnt/beta-catenin signalling. Nature 2002;417(6889):664–7.

[196] Lee AY, et al. Dickkopf-1 antagonizes Wnt signaling independent of beta-catenin in human mesothelioma. Biochem Biophys Res Commun 2004;323(4):1246–50.

[197] Mazieres J, et al. Wnt inhibitory factor-1 is silenced by promoter hypermethylation in human lung cancer. Cancer Res 2004;64(14):4717–20.

[198] Suzuki H, et al. Epigenetic inactivation of SFRP genes allows constitutive WNT signaling in colorectal cancer. Nat Genet 2004;36(4):417–22.

[199] Wissmann C, et al. WIF1, a component of the Wnt pathway, is down-regulated in prostate, breast, lung, and bladder cancer. J Pathol 2003;201(2):204–12.

[200] Zhou Z, et al. Up-regulation of human secreted frizzled homolog in apoptosis and its down-regulation in breast tumors. Int J Cancer 1998;78(1):95–9.

[201] Veeman MT, Axelrod JD, Moon RT. A second canon: functions and mechanisms of beta-catenin-independent Wnt signaling. Dev Cell 2003;5(3):367–77.

[202] You L, et al. Inhibition of Wnt-1 signaling induces apoptosis in beta-catenin-deficient mesothelioma cells. Cancer Res 2004;64(10):3474–8.

[203] Brown EJ, et al. A mammalian protein targeted by G1-arresting rapamycin-receptor complex. Nature 1994;369(6483):756–8.

[204] Chiu MI, Katz H, Berlin V. RAPT1, a mammalian homolog of yeast Tor, interacts with the FKBP12/rapamycin complex. Proc Natl Acad Sci U S A 1994;91(26):12574–8.

[205] Sabatini DM, et al. RAFT1: a mammalian protein that binds to FKBP12 in a rapamycin-dependent fashion and is homologous to yeast TORs. Cell 1994;78(1):35–43.

[206] Sabers CJ, et al. Isolation of a protein target of the FKBP12-rapamycin complex in mammalian cells. J Biol Chem 1995;270(2):815–22.

[207] Keith CT, Schreiber SL. PIK-related kinases: DNA repair, recombination, and cell cycle checkpoints. Science 1995;270(5233):50–1.

[208] Schmelzle T, Hall MN. TOR, a central controller of cell growth. Cell 2000;103(2):253–62.

[209] Sekulic A, et al. A direct linkage between the phosphoinositide 3-kinase-AKT signaling pathway and the mammalian target of rapamycin in mitogen-stimulated and transformed cells. Cancer Res 2000;60(13):3504–13.

[210] Andrade MA, Bork P. HEAT repeats in the Huntington's disease protein. Nat Genet 1995;11(2):115–6.

[211] Bosotti R, Isacchi A, Sonnhammer EL. FAT: a novel domain in PIK-related kinases. Trends Biochem Sci 2000;25(5):225–7.

[212] Hara K, et al. Amino acid sufficiency and mTOR regulate p70 S6 kinase and eIF-4E BP1 through a common effector mechanism. J Biol Chem 1998;273(23):14484–94.

[213] Thomas G, Hall MN. TOR signalling and control of cell growth. Curr Opin Cell Biol 1997;9(6):782–7.

[214] Jefferies HB, et al. Rapamycin suppresses 5′TOP mRNA translation through inhibition of p70s6k. EMBO J 1997;16(12):3693–704.

[215] Meyuhas O, Avni D, Shama S. Translational control of ribosomal protein mRNAs in eukaryotes. In: Hershey JWB, Mathews MB, Sonenberg N, editors. Translational control. Cold Spring Harbor (NY): Cold Spring Harbor Laboratory Press; 1996. p. 363–88.

[216] Brunn GJ, et al. The mammalian target of rapamycin phosphorylates sites having a (Ser/Thr)-Pro motif and is activated by antibodies to a region near its COOH terminus. J Biol Chem 1997;272(51):32547–50.

[217] Sonenberg N, Gingras AC. The mRNA 5' cap-binding protein eIF4E and control of cell growth. Curr Opin Cell Biol 1998;10(2):268–75.

[218] White RJ. Regulation of RNA polymerases I and III by the retinoblastoma protein: a mechanism for growth control? Trends Biochem Sci 1997;22(3):77–80.

[219] Mahajan PB. Modulation of transcription of rRNA genes by rapamycin. Int J Immunopharmacol 1994;16(9):711–21.

[220] Leicht M, et al. Okadaic acid induces cellular hypertrophy in AKR-2B fibroblasts: involvement of the p70S6 kinase in the onset of protein and rRNA synthesis. Cell Growth Differ 1996;7(9):1199–209.

[221] Hashemolhosseini S, et al. Rapamycin inhibition of the G1 to S transition is mediated by effects on cyclin D1 mRNA and protein stability. J Biol Chem 1998;273(23): 14424–9.

[222] Yokogami K, et al. Serine phosphorylation and maximal activation of STAT3 during CNTF signaling is mediated by the rapamycin target mTOR. Curr Biol 2000;10(1):47–50.

[223] Cohen P, Alessi DR, Cross DA. PDK1, one of the missing links in insulin signal transduction? FEBS Lett 1997;410(1):3–10.

[224] Dudek H, et al. Regulation of neuronal survival by the serine-threonine protein kinase Akt. Science 1997;275(5300):661–5.

[225] Mendez R, et al. Stimulation of protein synthesis, eukaryotic translation initiation factor 4E phosphorylation, and PHAS-I phosphorylation by insulin requires insulin receptor substrate 1 and phosphatidylinositol 3-kinase. Mol Cell Biol 1996;16(6): 2857–64.

[226] von Manteuffel SR, et al. 4E-BP1 phosphorylation is mediated by the FRAP-p70s6k pathway and is independent of mitogen-activated protein kinase. Proc Natl Acad Sci U S A 1996;93(9):4076–80.

[227] Radisavljevic ZM, Gonzalez-Flecha B. TOR kinase and Ran are downstream from PI3K/Akt in H2O2-induced mitosis. J Cell Biochem 2004;91(6):1293–300.

[228] Dudkin L, et al. Biochemical correlates of mTOR inhibition by the rapamycin ester CCI-779 and tumor growth inhibition. Clin Cancer Res 2001;7(6):1758–64.

[229] Aoki M, Blazek E, Vogt PK. A role of the kinase mTOR in cellular transformation induced by the oncoproteins P3k and Akt. Proc Natl Acad Sci U S A 2001;98(1):136–41.

[230] Podsypanina K, et al. An inhibitor of mTOR reduces neoplasia and normalizes p70/S6 kinase activity in Pten+/− mice. Proc Natl Acad Sci U S A 2001;98(18):10320–5.

[231] Barbet NC, et al. TOR controls translation initiation and early G1 progression in yeast. Mol Biol Cell 1996;7(1):25–42.

[232] Zanella CL, et al. Asbestos causes stimulation of the extracellular signal-regulated kinase 1 mitogen-activated protein kinase cascade after phosphorylation of the epidermal growth factor receptor. Cancer Res 1996;56(23):5334–8.

[233] Goldberg JL, et al. Novel cell imaging techniques show induction of apoptosis and proliferation in mesothelial cells by asbestos. Am J Respir Cell Mol Biol 1997; 17(3):265–71.

[234] Jimenez LA, et al. Role of extracellular signal-regulated protein kinases in apoptosis by asbestos and H2O2. Am J Physiol 1997;273(5 Pt 1):L1029–35.

[235] Seger R, Krebs EG. The MAPK signaling cascade. FASEB J 1995;9(9):726–35.

[236] Karin M. The regulation of AP-1 activity by mitogen-activated protein kinases. J Biol Chem 1995;270(28):16483–6.

[237] Su B, Karin M. Mitogen-activated protein kinase cascades and regulation of gene expression. Curr Opin Immunol 1996;8(3):402–11.

[238] Heintz NH, Janssen YM, Mossman BT. Persistent induction of c-fos and c-jun expression by asbestos. Proc Natl Acad Sci U S A 1993;90(8):3299–303.

[239] Faux SP, et al. Increased expression of epidermal growth factor receptor in rat pleural

mesothelial cells correlates with carcinogenicity of mineral fibres. Carcinogenesis 2000; 21(12):2275–80.

[240] Sandhu H, et al. mRNA expression patterns in different stages of asbestos-induced carcinogenesis in rats. Carcinogenesis 2000;21(5):1023–9.

[241] Ramos-Nino ME, Timblin CR, Mossman BT. Mesothelial cell transformation requires increased AP-1 binding activity and ERK-dependent Fra-1 expression. Cancer Res 2002;62(21):6065–9.

[242] Janssen-Heininger YM, Poynter ME, Baeuerle PA. Recent advances towards understanding redox mechanisms in the activation of nuclear factor kappaB. Free Radic Biol Med 2000;28(9):1317–27.

[243] Janssen YM, et al. Asbestos induces nuclear factor kappa B (NF-kappa B) DNA-binding activity and NF-kappa B-dependent gene expression in tracheal epithelial cells. Proc Natl Acad Sci U S A 1995;92(18):8458–62.

[244] Luster MI, Simeonova PP. Asbestos induces inflammatory cytokines in the lung through redox sensitive transcription factors. Toxicol Lett 1998;102–103:271–5.

[245] Simeonova PP, Luster MI. Asbestos induction of nuclear transcription factors and interleukin 8 gene regulation. Am J Respir Cell Mol Biol 1996;15(6):787–95.

[246] Kahlos K, et al. Generation of reactive oxygen species by human mesothelioma cells. Br J Cancer 1999;80(1–2):25–31.

[247] Kinnula VL, et al. Manganese superoxide dismutase in human pleural mesothelioma cell lines. Free Radic Biol Med 1996;21(4):527–32.

[248] Fridovich I. Superoxide dismutases. Annu Rev Biochem 1975;44:147–59.

[249] Hirose K, et al. Overexpression of mitochondrial manganese superoxide dismutase promotes the survival of tumor cells exposed to interleukin-1, tumor necrosis factor, selected anticancer drugs, and ionizing radiation. FASEB J 1993;7(2):361–8.

[250] Janssen YM, et al. Expression of antioxidant enzymes in rat lungs after inhalation of asbestos or silica. J Biol Chem 1992;267(15):10625–30.

[251] Warner BB, et al. Redox regulation of manganese superoxide dismutase. Am J Physiol 1996;271(1 Pt 1):L150–8.

[252] Wong GH, Goeddel DV. Induction of manganous superoxide dismutase by tumor necrosis factor: possible protective mechanism. Science 1988;242(4880):941–4.

[253] Nakano T, Oka K, Taniguchi N. Manganese superoxide dismutase expression correlates with p53 status and local recurrence of cervical carcinoma treated with radiation therapy. Cancer Res 1996;56(12):2771–5.

[254] Sinha BK, Mimnaugh EG. Free radicals and anticancer drug resistance: oxygen free radicals in the mechanisms of drug cytotoxicity and resistance by certain tumors. Free Radic Biol Med 1990;8(6):567–81.

[255] Chang K, Pastan I. Molecular cloning of mesothelin, a differentiation antigen present on mesothelium, mesotheliomas, and ovarian cancers. Proc Natl Acad Sci U S A 1996; 93(1):136–40.

[256] Robinson BW, et al. Mesothelin-family proteins and diagnosis of mesothelioma. Lancet 2003;362(9396):1612–6.

[257] Kettunen E, et al. L1CAM, INP10, P-cadherin, tPA and ITGB4 over-expression in malignant pleural mesotheliomas revealed by combined use of cDNA and tissue microarray. Carcinogenesis 2005;26(1):17–25.

[258] Eckner R, et al. Association of p300 and CBP with simian virus 40 large T antigen. Mol Cell Biol 1996;16(7):3454–64.

[259] Kierstead TD, Tevethia MJ. Association of p53 binding and immortalization of primary C57BL/6 mouse embryo fibroblasts by using simian virus 40 T-antigen mutants bearing internal overlapping deletion mutations. J Virol 1993;67(4):1817–29.

[260] Lill NL, et al. p300 family members associate with the carboxyl terminus of simian virus 40 large tumor antigen. J Virol 1997;71(1):129–37.

[261] Peden KW, et al. Mutants with changes within or near a hydrophobic region of simian virus 40 large tumor antigen are defective for binding cellular protein p53. Virology 1989;168(1):13–21.

[262] Srinivasan A, Peden KW, Pipas JM. The large tumor antigen of simian virus 40 encodes at least two distinct transforming functions. J Virol 1989;63(12):5459–63.

[263] Zhu J, et al. Transformation of a continuous rat embryo fibroblast cell line requires three separate domains of simian virus 40 large T antigen. J Virol 1992;66(5):2780–91.

[264] Friedmann T, Doolittle RF, Walter G. Amino acid sequence homology between polyoma and SV40 tumour antigens deduced from nucleotide sequences. Nature 1978; 274(5668):291–3.

[265] Goswami R, et al. Effect of zinc ions on the biochemical behavior of simian virus 40 small-t antigen expressed in bacteria. J Virol 1992;66(3):1746–51.

[266] Turk B, et al. Simian virus 40 small-t antigen binds two zinc ions. J Virol 1993;67(6): 3671–3.

[267] Stewart N, Bacchetti S. Expression of SV40 large T antigen, but not small t antigen, is required for the induction of chromosomal aberrations in transformed human cells. Virology 1991;180(1):49–57.

[268] Bikel I, et al. SV40 small t antigen enhances the transformation activity of limiting concentrations of SV40 large T antigen. Cell 1987;48(2):321–30.

[269] Frost JA, et al. Simian virus 40 small t antigen cooperates with mitogen-activated kinases to stimulate AP-1 activity. Mol Cell Biol 1994;14(9):6244–52.

[270] Tiemann F, Deppert W. Immortalization of BALB/c mouse embryo fibroblasts alters SV40 large T-antigen interactions with the tumor suppressor p53 and results in a reduced SV40 transformation-efficiency. Oncogene 1994;9(7):1907–15.

[271] Eddy BE, et al. Identification of the oncogenic substance in rhesus monkey kidney cell culture as simian virus 40. Virology 1962;17:65–75.

[272] Carbone M, et al. The role of small t antigen in SV40 carcinogenesis. In: Nicolini C, editor. Molecular basis of human cancer. New York: Plenum; 1991. p. 191–206.

[273] Cicala C, Pompetti F, Carbone M. SV40 induces mesotheliomas in hamsters. Am J Pathol 1993;142(5):1524–33.

[274] Kops SP. Oral polio vaccine and human cancer: a reassessment of SV40 as a contaminant based upon legal documents. Anticancer Res 2000;20(6C):4745–9.

[275] Rizzo P, et al. Unique strains of SV40 in commercial poliovaccines from 1955 not readily identifiable with current testing for SV40 infection. Cancer Res 1999;59(24):6103–8.

[276] Ali SH, DeCaprio JA. Cellular transformation by SV40 large T antigen: interaction with host proteins. Semin Cancer Biol 2001;11(1):15–23.

[277] Carbone M, et al. New molecular and epidemiological issues in mesothelioma: role of SV40. J Cell Physiol 1999;180(2):167–72.

[278] Jasani B, et al. Association of SV40 with human tumours. Semin Cancer Biol 2001; 11(1):49–61.

[279] Klein G, Powers A, Croce C. Association of SV40 with human tumors. Oncogene 2002; 21(8):1141–9.

[280] Hirvonen A, et al. Simian virus 40 (SV40)-like DNA sequences not detectable in Finnish mesothelioma patients not exposed to SV40-contaminated polio vaccines. Mol Carcinog 1999;26(2):93–9.

[281] Lopez-Rios F, et al. Evidence against a role for SV40 infection in human mesotheliomas and high risk of false-positive PCR results owing to presence of SV40 sequences in common laboratory plasmids. Lancet 2004;364(9440):1157–66.

Hematol Oncol Clin N Am 19 (2005) 1025–1040

HEMATOLOGY/ONCOLOGY CLINICS
OF NORTH AMERICA

Detection of Malignant Mesothelioma in Asbestos-Exposed Individuals: The Potential Role of Soluble Mesothelin-Related Protein

Jenette Creaney, PhD[a],*, Bruce W.S. Robinson, MBBS, MD[a,b]

[a]*School of Medicine and Pharmacology, University of Western Australia, 4th Floor, G-Block, Sir Charles Gairdner Hospital, Nedlands 6009, Western Australia, Australia*
[b]*Western Australian Institute of Medical Research, Nedlands, Western Australia, Australia*

Malignant mesothelioma (MM) is a highly aggressive tumor. Once considered rare, mesothelioma is increasing in incidence. In some countries the peak number of new cases is not predicted to occur until approximately 2015 to 2025 [1]. For practical purposes, MM is universally fatal. Patients who are treated with supportive care have a median survival of 9 months [2], and patients treated with the best available therapy (pemetrexed and cisplatinum) survive 13 to 25 months [3].

The diagnosis of MM generally presents a clinical challenge. It is a tumor of the serosal cavities and tends to present at relatively advanced stages with a broad range of morphologies. Cytology of effusions with immunophenotyping is widely used for diagnosis [4], but histopathologic examination of biopsy tissue is often also required [5]. Major differential diagnostic problems include adenocarcinoma, reactive mesothelium, and fibrinous pleuritis. In some cases there is a long delay between the onset of symptoms and the diagnosis of MM.

MM is strongly associated with asbestos exposure, mostly occupational exposure [6,7], although other assaults, including ionizing radiation and exposure to simian virus 40, have been suggested to cause the disease [8]. Particular occupations at risk for high exposure include those involved in the repair and maintenance of asbestos materials, shipbuilding, asbestos cement production and use, asbestos mining and milling, and insulation manufacture and installation. Navy personnel, railway workers, and boilermakers are also at risk [7]. Passive or low-level exposure also has been implicated because of the deterioration of buildings that contain asbestos. The risk of developing

This work was supported by the National Health and Medical Research Council and the Insurance Commission of Western Australia.
* Corresponding author. *E-mail address:* creaneyj@cyllene.uwa.edu.au (J. Creaney).

0889-8588/05/$ – see front matter
doi:10.1016/j.hoc.2005.09.007

MM varies with the length and intensity of asbestos exposure. The risk of developing mesothelioma in an individual with substantial occupational asbestos-exposure averages 10% over a lifetime [9], although the risk can be much higher in some groups. Since the early 1980s, guidelines and regulations have been put in place in most countries to control the handling of asbestos and set exposure limits.

Historically, the mining of asbestos and manufacture of asbestos products have occurred in somewhat specific geographic regions, and several populations at risk of developing asbestos-related disease have been identified. There are approximately 20 well-studied asbestos-exposed cohorts worldwide, including the Wittenoom crocidolite mining operation and township in Western Australia [10]. The estimated lifetime risk for asbestos-exposed workers in the Wittenoom cohort is at least 17%. Such populations have justifiable anxiety about their risk of developing asbestos-related disease, including MM and lung cancer. Nonmalignant asbestos-related diseases, such as pleural plaques, calcifications, benign effusions, and diffuse pleural thickening, also can cause morbidity in asbestos-exposed populations [11].

SCREENING FOR MESOTHELIOMA

There is little doubt that MM is an important disease, both for the individual and the community. In addition to health benefits, any effective therapy for MM would deliver huge economic advantages because MM is predicted to cost the European and US economies approximately $80 billion [12] and $200 billion [13], respectively, over the next 35 to 40 years. The significance of this disease extends beyond its actual incidence. If effective early intervention or preventive measures could be discovered, they could potentially have a substantial impact on this economic burden, much of which is borne by governments, asbestos companies, and insurers, and could save billions of dollars.

One of the main reasons for developing a screening program for MM would be to begin therapy at an earlier stage than is currently the case. That assumes that therapy would be more effective if given early, as is the case in bowel and breast cancer [14,15]. Difficulties in identifying patients who have early-stage MM have meant that few studies have been performed to demonstrate that early intervention is effective in MM, however. Intracavitary administration of γ-interferon resulted in a 45% response rate in patients with stage I disease and suggested that if MM was detected early, the disease potentially could be treated in a less aggressive manner and more successfully [16]. In a select group of patients who had epithelial, early-stage disease, the 5-year survival rate was 46% after extrapleural pneumonectomy followed by adjunct chemotherapy and radiotherapy [17]. Although there is unavoidable selection bias in these studies and issues of lead-time effects, it does support the notion that early therapy may be more effective than the same therapy given later in the course of the disease. Prospective studies and randomized trials are required to test such a hypothesis, however [18].

AVAILABLE SCREENING TESTS FOR MALIGNANT MESOTHELIOMA HAVE FAILED

Imaging

Several programs have been put in place to screen asbestos-exposed individuals for lung disease. These programs generally involve annual pulmonary function tests and chest radiographs. Neither modality has proved effective at detecting malignancy early, however, although other asbestos-related diseases have been detected [19]. Distinguishing benign from malignant disease is one of the difficulties in detecting early-stage cancers. Obesity, an increasing problem in the developed world, can be associated with subpleural fat and is another confounding factor, often misdiagnosed as pleural thickening or plaques. In 2002, the British Thoracic Society recommended that asbestos-exposed individuals not be screened for MM by annual radiographs [20].

CT is superior to chest radiography in detecting small, potentially curable tumors [21,22]; however, difficulties distinguishing benign from malignant disease are still frequent. It has been suggested that fluorodeoxyglucose positron emission tomography imaging, with its ability to distinguish between malignant and benign conditions, may be a useful alternative [23]. In a small number of studies, positron emission tomography has shown a sensitivity rate of 91% and a specificity rate of 100% for MM [9]. The use of fluorodeoxyglucose positron emission tomography in screening for MM has not been evaluated to date, however, and the cost of such screening is likely to be prohibitive. Concerns have been noted about the ability of positron emission tomography to distinguish epithelial MM with low fluorodeoxyglucose uptake and severe pleural inflammation [9] and possible interpretive problems that occur in early-stage disease because of the nature of MM, which sometimes occurs diffusely as an irregular sheet-like layer rather than a spherical tumor [23].

Biomarker Studies

Several studies have examined biomarkers for patients who have MM. Most of these studies have had few patients at various stages of disease progression. Several biomarkers, including hyaluronic acid, tissue polypeptide antigen (TPA), and ferritin, distinguish the late stages of MM from patients who have asbestosis and age-matched healthy volunteers [24,25]. Serum hyaluronate levels increase during the clinical course of the disease and are primarily elevated only at the advanced stage of the cancer, which makes serum hyaluronate determination of little value for early detection of MM [26].

TPA is a broad-spectrum test that measures cytokeratins-8, -18, and -19 and is routinely used as a marker for tumors of epithelial origin [27]. Measurement of cytokeratin-19 fragments in pleural effusions and serum distinguishes benign from malignant disease, including MM [28]. Serum levels of cytokeratin-19 fragments and TPA in combination were found in a study of 52 patients who had MM to be highly correlated with survival in a univariate analysis [29]. Unfortunately, however, these data have not been validated prospectively, although a recent small-scale study supported a role for TPA in predicting prognosis in patients who have MM [26].

CA125 is a well characterized tumor marker [30]. Serum levels of CA125 are elevated in several benign settings. Such nonspecificity has meant that serum CA125 levels have had little value as a tool for differential diagnosis in patients with suspected malignancy. CA125 seems to be sensitive to changes in tumor bulk, however, and is used routinely to monitor patients who have ovarian cancer. Several studies also have shown that elevations in serum CA125 may occur 18 months or more before clinical presentation of ovarian cancer [31,32], which prompted the establishment of a randomized trial to evaluate the longitudinal change in CA125 levels for early detection of ovarian cancer. Only a few small-scale studies have investigated serum CA125 levels in MM [26,33,34]. In some cases CA125 levels reflect tumor burden.

CANCER SCREENING

Screening programs for the early detection of several non-MM cancers, including cervical, breast, colorectal, and prostate, have been established. Papanicolaou screening (Pap smear) has been widely adopted in many developed countries for screening for cervical cancer. Pap smears are relatively inexpensive, easy to perform, are promoted by the health profession, enable treatment to be provided early in the natural history of the disease, and reduce the likelihood of developing invasive disease. Pap smears represent one of the best available cancer screening technologies currently, and much can be learned about cancer screening from this success. Although there is strong evidence of their role in reducing the morbidity and mortality associated with colorectal cancer, colonoscopies have not been as widely accepted as a screening strategy [15]. In contrast, screening for prostate cancer using a relatively simple, inexpensive, noninvasive blood test for prostate-specific antigen has been used widely, although the efficacy of such screening and the benefits of early intervention strategies have not been demonstrated conclusively [35].

Although each disease, at-risk population, and screening strategy must be evaluated in context, it has been suggested that several key criteria be examined before the recommendation of a particular screening strategy [36]. Simplistically these criteria are as follows:

- The disease is an important health problem
- Treatment of occult disease offers an advantage over current practice
- There is a detectable preclinical phase
- The screening is affordable
- The screening is acceptable to the target population and the health profession
- The screening has an acceptable level of accuracy

Biomarkers

The relatively low invasive nature and inexpensiveness of blood tests make screening of target populations with serum-based biomarkers an attractive strategy. Many current gene and protein expression studies aim to identify clinically useful biomarkers, that is, biomarkers that can be useful in screening, diagnosing, and monitoring treatment and disease progression and can be used as prognostic indicators. To date, many candidate biomarkers have been reported, but their value in a clinical setting is generally still awaiting confirmation.

Guidelines for biomarkers to be used as screening tools for the early detection of cancer have been formalized through the establishment of the Early Detection Research Network by the National Cancer Institute [37]. Five phases have been described to determine if a biomarker is useful in population screening programs. The first three phases are summarized as (1) identification of candidate biomarkers, (2) assessment of biomarker frequency in established disease and controls, and (3) retrospective determination of the biomarker in early disease or before clinical symptoms. The final phases require prospective studies to screen people and will lead to diagnosis and treatment; thus they require different ethical considerations to the first three steps. Phase 4 studies aim to determine the extent and characteristics of the disease when detected and determine the false referral rate. Phase 5 studies quantitate the impact of screening on reducing the burden of disease on the population.

We recently proposed soluble mesothelin-related protein (SMRP)/mesothelin as a candidate biomarker for MM and have begun several studies to determine if the biomarker fulfils the criteria described previously [38].

MESOTHELIN AND SOLUBLE MESOTHELIN-RELATED PROTEIN

Mesothelin is a differentiation molecule of mesothelium. It is a glycophosphatidylinositol-linked cell surface glycoprotein of approximately 40 kDa that was originally described as the antigenic target of a monoclonal antibody (K1) [39]. The biologic role of mesothelin has not been elucidated, although a role in cell adhesion has been suggested [39] and is supported by findings that mesothelin binds CA125/MUC16 [40], another surface glycoprotein expressed on some cancer types, including MM and ovarian cancers.

Molecular Structure

The *MSLN* gene is located on chromosome 16p13.3 and consists of an 1884 bp open reading frame encoded by 17 exons. The locus encodes for a precursor protein with a molecular weight of 69 kDa. This precursor protein includes a furin cleavage site that when processed would yield the 40-kDa (when glycosylated) membrane-bound mesothelin protein that contains the K1 epitope and a 31-kDa soluble protein [39]. The soluble protein was independently identified from the culture medium of a human pancreatic cell line and was designated megakaryocyte potentiating factor (MPF). MPF acts as a novel cytokine and is able to stimulate colony formation of mouse bone marrow cells in the presence of interleukin-3 [41,42]. There has been some speculation in the literature about a role for MPF in the platelet cell elevation seen in patients who have MM, although few supporting data have been found.

Alternative splicing of the *MSLN* gene predicts a third protein product with a molecular weight between 42 kDa and 45 kDa, which has been designated SMRP. The retention of the 82 base pairs of intron 16 of the *MSLN* gene is predicted to lead to a frame-shift mutation that prematurely terminates the protein at amino acid 600. The resulting predicted protein lacks the glycosyl-phosphatidylinositol-linked (GPI) anchor region responsible for cell surface attachment and instead has a unique C-terminal hydrophilic tail that is predicted to make the protein soluble [43]. Analysis of gene sequences in the expressed sequence tag database and reverse transcription-polymerase chain reaction and nucleotide sequencing of ovarian cancer cell lines suggest that the MPF/mesothelin precursor protein is the major product of the *MSLN* gene and that SMR transcripts are less common [44,45].

A fourth reported product of the mesothelin locus, designated mesothelin-variant 2, is 95% identical at the amino acid level to the MPF/mesothelin precursor protein. The major difference between the variants, which does not seem to be caused by sequencing difficulties [44], is the insertion of eight amino acid residues after glutamine 408 in the C-terminal region of the membrane-bound mesothelin protein. This cDNA clone was originally isolated from a HeLa cDNA library level [39] and seems to be an example of the rare use of an alternative splice acceptor site resulting in the retention of the 24 bp of intron 13 [44]. There is the possibility of alternative splicing occurring at other sites in the *MSLN* gene, which may result in protein products with different functions. There is also the possibility that these transcripts are heterogeneous nuclear RNA, which has not been processed completely [44].

Mesothelin in Normal Cells

The K1 monoclonal antibody was generated through immunizing mice with the human ovarian cancer cell line OVCAR-3 [46,47]. In the original studies using cryopreserved specimens and the K1 antibody, mesothelin was shown to be expressed on normal mesothelial cells that lined the pleura, pericardium, and peritoneum. Limited reactivity also was observed on epithelial cells of the trachea, tonsil, and fallopian tube [46]. The expression of mesothelin in normal tissues seems to be in part under transcriptional control, with mesothelium-specific control elements being identified in the mesothelin proximal promoter region in transient transfection analyses [48].

Little is known of the function of mesothelin beyond suggestions of a role in cell adhesion. The generation of mutant mice in which both copies of the mesothelin gene were inactivated revealed no further clues to the protein's function. MSLN −/− mice had no obvious abnormalities and produced viable offspring. The knockout mice had similar growth rates and reproductive functions to their wild-type litter mates. There was no statistical difference in platelet counts between the mesothelin knockout and wild-type mice [49].

Overexpression in Cancer

Serial analysis of gene expression and genetic profiling experiments have demonstrated that products of the *MSLN* locus are overexpressed in various cancers, including MM, ovarian [50,51], pancreatic [52], lung, gastric [53], and colorectal cancers [54], with the highest average expression of *MSLN* mRNA in serous carcinomas of the ovary and adenocarcinomas of the lung [54]. Mesothelin was first isolated from ovarian and pancreatic cell lines.

The original immunohistochemical studies with the K1 monoclonal antibody revealed that mesothelin was expressed on all of 15 pleural epithelial cryopreserved MM tumor samples but not in 4 of 4 sarcomatous MMs examined. In four cases of mixed or biphasic MM, mesothelin staining in each case was observed in regions of epithelial differentiation and not in sarcomatous regions [55]. Aberrant mesothelin expression was seen on ovarian cancers and a significant proportion of pancreatic adenocarcinomas. Mesothelin immunoreactivity also was observed in most endometrioid uterine adenocarcinomas and squamous cell carcinomas of the esophagus, head and neck, vulva, lung, and cervix [39].

Subsequently, a commercial mouse monoclonal antimesothelin antibody, clone 5B2, has been generated by immunizing mice with a recombinant prokaryotic fusion protein that includes 100 amino acids of the membrane-bound mesothelin region. Using this antibody on formalin-fixed paraffin-embedded tissue microarrays that contained 621 carcinomas, mesothelin immunoreactivity was seen in cancers of the ovary (serous papillary, endometrioid, and undifferentiated) and pancreas, with less frequent staining of the endometrium, lung, and stomach/esophagus [54]. A high proportion of lung adenocarcinomas, endometrial carcinoma, biphasic synovial sarcomas, and desmoplastic small, round cell tumors also tested positive for mesothelin [56,57].

Mesothelin Immunotherapy and Cancer

Although mesothelin is not a cancer-specific antigen, the high level of expression in some tumor types and the limited distribution on normal tissues suggests that mesothelin is a suitable candidate for various tumor-specific therapies. Much research has focused on mesothelin antibody-conjugated therapies, work that has been reviewed recently [45]. Currently, a recombinant antimesothelin immunotoxin is undergoing evaluation in patients who have mesothelin-positive tumors.

Mesothelin-specific CD8 + T-cell responses have been demonstrated in patients who have pancreatic cancer who responded to vaccination with an allogenic granulocyte macrophage-colony stimulating factor-transduced pancreatic cell line [58]. No mesothelin-specific T cells were found in patients who did not respond to the vaccine.

Soluble Mesothelin-Related Protein/Mesothelin as a Biomarker

In the late 1990s, the Hellström laboratory in Seattle, Washington developed a panel of monoclonal antibodies to ovarian cancer antigens. The monoclonal antibody OV569 recognized a 42- to 45-kDa protein with an N-terminal amino acid sequence identical to mesothelin. Another monoclonal antibody, 4H3, was raised to the target protein of mAb OV569 and a double-determinant ELISA assay, which measured soluble mesothelin-related proteins, was established [43].

Serum SMRPs were shown to be elevated significantly in 23 of 30 sera from patients who had ovarian carcinoma compared with 0 of 68 sera from healthy controls. SMRP also was elevated in some patients who had breast and lung cancer [43].

Because MM is also a mesothelin-positive tumor and there are some similarities between ovarian cancer and MM, it seemed logical to assess whether patients who had MM had detectable levels of SMRP. In collaboration with the Hellström group we measured SMRP in patients who had MM and several controls, both normal, healthy individuals and clinically relevant patients. Of 44 patients with cytologically or histologically diagnosed MM, 37 (84%) had significantly elevated SMRP in the serum, compared with apparently healthy asbestos-exposed and non–asbestos-exposed controls (Fig. 1).

In these early studies we arbitrarily determined a positive cut-off value for the assay, calculated as the mean plus three standard deviations of the mean of the SMRP values for the non–asbestos-exposed controls. Using this cut-off, 1 of 22 patients with asbestosis and 1 of 22 patients with idiopathic pulmonary fibrosis and 1 of 22 patients with non–small cell lung cancer were SMRP positive; 157 patients with inflammatory or malignant pulmonary or pleural diseases other than MM tested negative. After nearly 4 years of follow-up, the 2 patients who had benign disease have not developed malignancy. In our study, only 1 patient with a non-MM malignant condition was SMRP positive (see Fig. 1)

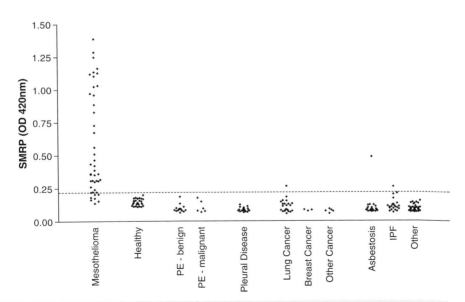

Fig. 1. SMRP concentrations in MM versus other lung and pleural diseases. SMRP for individual patients is plotted as the mean absorbance measurement at 420 nm of duplicate serum samples diluted 1 in 100. Dashed line represents the normal range. IPF, idiopathic pulmonary fibrosis; PE, pleural effusion.

[38]. Scholler and colleagues [43] reported that in addition to ovarian cancer cases, 11 of 35 breast cancers, 6 of 9 lung cancers, 2 of 14 colon cancers, and 6 of 17 leukemias were positive. Further studies are required to evaluate SMRP in patients with other malignant conditions.

Receiver operating characteristic (ROC) curves were generated from these data. ROC curves relate the sensitivity of a marker to the specificity at which it operates. The area under the ROC curve represents the average sensitivity over the entire ROC curve and can be used to quantify marker performance. A value close to 1 is ideal; a value of 0.5 means the test has no discriminatory ability. The area under the ROC curve of SMRP for distinguishing patients who have MM from (1) patients who have asbestosis and pleural plaques is 0.892, (2) patients who have lung cancer is 0.977, and (3) patients who have other pleural disease is 0.994 (Fig. 2).

Soluble Mesothelin-Related Protein in the Detection of Disease Progression

SMRP serum concentration was high in patients with a large tumor burden, as determined from standard thoracic CT scans. Of note, however, approximately half of the patients with a tumor mass less than 1 cm in width had elevated levels, which suggests that the marker may be useful as a marker for early-stage disease. In 20 patients whose SMRP levels were determined in serum samples obtained within a 2-month period of histopathologically confirmed MM diagnosis, 16 had elevated levels. These data support the notion that SMRP is a sensitive marker of disease when MM tumor bulk is small (Fig. 3).

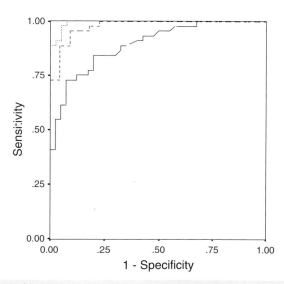

Fig. 2. ROC curves for SMRP for distinguishing patients with MM from patients with asbestosis and pleural plaques (*solid line*), patients with lung cancer (*dashed line*), and patients with other pleural disease (*dotted line*).

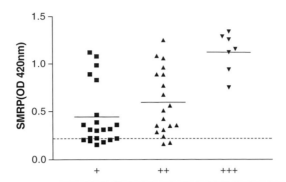

Fig. 3. Serum SMRP levels in relation to tumor size. Horizontal bars are mean absorbance measurement for each group. Tumor mass was estimated from standard thoracic CT scans no mass visible or mass less than 1 cm in width (+); maximum tumor width 1 to 3 cm (++); and maximum tumor width more than 3 cm (+++).

In patients who undergo surgery for MM, SMRP levels initially drop, but subsequently increasing serum SMRP levels can be detected between 5 and 35 weeks before radiologic or clinical recurrence, which again suggests that the SMRP level is sensitive for detecting small tumor volumes [59].

Soluble Mesothelin-Related Protein/Mesothelin in Screening Asbestos-Exposed Individuals

Between 1943 and 1966, approximately 6500 people were employed by the Australian Blue Asbestos Company at the Wittenoom crocidolite mine and mill in Western Australia. A cohort of workers and Wittenoom residents who never worked for the mining company has been assembled and studied. The risk of MM in this group was drastically increased and is one of the highest in the world [10].

We selected 40 random samples from the cohort from individuals who at the time of the blood sample collection were apparently healthy. We found that 7 of these 40 healthy, asbestos-exposed controls had elevated levels of SMRP compared with non–asbestos-exposed controls (Fig. 4). This finding initially suggested that as has been the case with other tumor markers, levels could be elevated in nonmalignant conditions, which reduces the specificity of the assay. When we examined the clinical outcome of these 40 individuals who were followed-up for 8 years after sampling, however, three of the seven who had elevated SMRP levels developed MM at 15, 26, and 69 months after the sample had been taken and died at 3, 6, and 6 years, respectively, after sampling. At the time of sampling, one of these patients was totally free of respiratory symptoms, one had asymptomatic asbestosis, and the third had evidence of pleural thickening. Another patient died of non–small cell lung cancer 4 years after sampling. None of the other three healthy, asbestos-exposed individuals with elevated SMRP levels has evidence of tumor at this 8-year stage of follow-up. None of the remaining 33 asbestos-exposed individuals who had normal

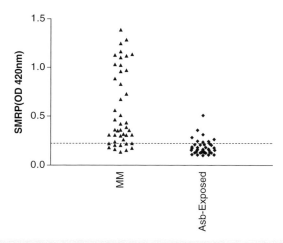

Fig. 4. SMRP concentrations in patients who have MM versus healthy age-matched asbestos-exposed controls. SMRP for individual patients is plotted as the mean absorbance measurement at 420 nm of duplicate serum samples diluted 1 in 100. Dashed line represents the normal range. At the time of serum sampling, controls were apparently healthy with no evidence of disease. Asb-exposed, asbestos-exposed.

SMRP levels developed mesothelioma or other cancer in the 8 years of follow-up. Using the Fisher's exact test, this was a significant difference between the groups ($P = .007$).

To evaluate further whether elevated SMRP levels could predate the clinical presentation of MM, we studied serum SMRP levels in another group of patients who exhibited elevated SMRP levels after diagnosis and for whom sequential prediagnosis samples were available. Approximately 25% to 37% of these patients exhibited increased SMRP levels 12 months before presentation. For the other patients with sequential samples available, however, no early increase in serum SMRP levels was seen. As expected, there was no evidence of transient increases in serum SMRP levels before presentation in individuals who did not show an increase in SMRP levels at the time of progression of their disease.

LESSONS FROM CA125 AND THE EARLY DETECTION OF OVARIAN CANCER

CA125 has many properties that suggest it will be a good marker for the early detection of ovarian cancer, and much can be learned from the extensive work done to evaluate this finding. Approximately 85% of patients with clinically advanced ovarian cancer have elevated serum CA125. Evidence exists that in some patients, deviations in the level of CA125 can be detected 18 months or more before the appearance of symptoms [30]. In individual women, CA125 levels are temporally stable, which enables the development of algorithms designed to detect disease based on small changes in longitudinal CA125 levels [60]. Treatment of early-stage ovarian cancer is more effective than when the cancer is at an advanced stage. Currently, at least two large, randomized clinical trials are underway that aim to estimate the efficacy of screening for ovarian cancer [61].

Only been a few small-scale studies have investigated serum CA125 levels in MM. Elevated levels have been reported in most peritoneal MM cases [33,34]. Three out of a study of ten cases of pleural MM had elevated CA125 serum levels [26]. In our laboratory almost half of the patients who had MM were CA125 positive at diagnosis, which suggested that CA125 may be an early marker of MM and may be useful for screening asbestos-exposed individuals.

A major problem with CA125 in a screening setting is that levels are elevated in several benign conditions, however, including endometriosis, menstruation, early pregnancy, pelvic inflammatory disease, hepatitis, peritonitis, and pleuritis and after surgery [30]. Screening for elevated CA125 detects women with these benign conditions in addition to women who have early-stage ovarian cancer, and all positive findings must undergo further evaluation and possibly surgery. Because specificity is greater in postmenopausal women, screening this population reduces the number of false-positive results. The potential for false-positive results in screening the asbestos-exposed population who are considered to be at risk of developing MM by monitoring serum levels of CA125 would be expected to be low because most are men. Its use in women exposed to asbestos would be limited, however.

Another drawback of screening with CA125 is that approximately 50% of patients who have stage 1 ovarian cancer do not test positive for CA125. It has been suggested that serial measures of the marker also could increase the specificity of CA125 screening. What must be determined is if that level of specificity is acceptable to the individual, the health care profession, and society on a moral and cost level. Jacobs and colleagues [62] suggested that for screening for ovarian cancer, a 10% positive predictive value is acceptable (ie, one cancer identified for ten surgical procedures undergone). It has been calculated that because ovarian cancer has a prevalence of 40 cases per 100,000 in women over age 50 a screening test would require a specificity rate more than 99.6% to have a positive predictive value of 10%, with a sensitivity rate of 75% [30]. Such specificity is greater than that of the biomarker. Several studies have improved specificity by combining CA125 levels with second-line screening, such as transvaginal sonography [61]. Because of the sample size and the length of time that individuals survive, the actual prevalence of MM in the screening target population almost approaches zero. The normal measure for this population is incidence, and in the workers of the Wittenoom cohort the incidence is approximately 7 per 1000 person years. A test developed to screen the asbestos-exposed population for MM would need to be as good as—if not more reliable than—that of CA125 for ovarian cancer.

USES OF MULTIPLE SERUM MARKERS FOR MALIGNANT MESOTHELIOMA

From research into CA125 as a biomarker in ovarian cancer it is clear that CA125 measurements alone will be ineffective as a screening strategy and that the value of screening can be improved by using a combination of independent biomarkers in a longitudinal program with a defined target screening population, followed by a second-line highly sensitive imaging screen. Even then, the screening program must be accepted by the population and the health profession, and a reduction in disease morbidity and mortality must be demonstrated.

It has been suggested that the diagnostic performance of first-line screening for ovarian cancer could be improved by combining CA125 measures with other nonredundant (independent) biomarkers, even if the sensitivity of the additional marker in itself is low [61]. Recently, the Hellström group showed that combining the results for SMRP and CA125 improved the sensitivity for ovarian cancer cases from healthy controls, compared with the sensitivity of each marker individually, yet maintained a level of specificity equal to that of the CA125 marker alone. All three marker measures, the combined measure, and CA125 and SMRP alone were substantially poorer at discriminating between individuals with benign conditions than healthy controls. We have found that combining serum levels of CA125 and SMRP improves the sensitivity of detecting patients who have MM from controls when using ROC curve analysis (unpublished data).

Measurement of SMRP levels in the serum should prove valuable as an adjunct to current tests for the diagnosis of patients who have MM and monitoring of patients after successful treatment strategies for the early detection of disease recurrence. SMRP measures also may be useful in an overall screening program for MM because early results show that some individuals have elevated levels 1 to 4 years before symptom development. Although individuals with occupational and nonoccupational asbestos exposure are justifiably concerned about their risk of developing MM, consideration must be given to the complex issues surrounding screening for this disease, and a more substantial evaluation of the SMRP marker must be undertaken before deciding to promote a mesothelin/SMRP screening program.

References

[1] Musk AW, de Klerk NH. Epidemiology of malignant mesothelioma in Australia. Lung Cancer 2004;45(Suppl 1):S21–3.

[2] Antman K, Pass H, Schiff P. Benign and malignant mesothelioma. In: DeVita VT, Hellman S, Rosenberg S, editors. Cancer: principles and practice of oncology. Philadelphia: Lippincott-Raven; 2001. p. 1943–70.

[3] Vogelzang NJ, et al. Phase III study of pemetrexed in combination with cisplatin versus cisplatin alone in patients with malignant pleural mesothelioma. J Clin Oncol 2003; 21(14):2636–44.

[4] Whitaker D. The cytology of malignant mesothelioma. Cytopathology 2000;11(3): 139–51.

[5] Ordonez NG. The immunohistochemical diagnosis of mesothelioma: a comparative study

of epithelioid mesothelioma and lung adenocarcinoma. Am J Surg Pathol 2003;27(8): 1031–51.

[6] National Occupational Health and Safety Commission. The incidence of mesothelioma in Australia 1997 to 1999: Australian Mesothelioma Register Report. Canberra (Australia): National Occupational Health and Safety Commission; 2002.

[7] Leigh J, Driscoll T. Malignant mesothelioma in Australia, 1945–2002. Int J Occup Environ Health 2003;9(3):206–17.

[8] Lange JH. Mesothelioma trends in the United States: an update based on surveillance, epidemiology, and end results program data for 1973 through 2003. Am J Epidemiol 2004;160(8):823.

[9] Benard F, et al. Metabolic imaging of malignant pleural mesothelioma with fluorodeoxy-glucose positron emission tomography. Chest 1998;114(3):713–22.

[10] Musk AW, et al. Wittenoom, Western Australia: a modern industrial disaster. Am J Ind Med 1992;21(5):735–47.

[11] Chapman SJ, et al. Benign asbestos pleural diseases. Curr Opin Pulm Med 2003;9(4): 266–71.

[12] Shah N, Williams A. Surviving the asbestos epidemic. London: Price Waterhouse Coopers; 2001.

[13] Carroll S, et al. Asbestos litigation costs and compensation: an interim report. Santa Monica (CA): Rank Organisation Publications; 2002.

[14] Elmore JG, et al. Screening for breast cancer. JAMA 2005;293(10):1245–56.

[15] Bromer MQ, Weinberg DS. Screening for colorectal cancer: now and the near future. Semin Oncol 2005;32(1):3–10.

[16] Boutin C, et al. Intrapleural treatment with recombinant gamma-interferon in early stage malignant pleural mesothelioma. Cancer 1994;74(9):2460–7.

[17] Sugarbaker DJ, et al. Resection margins, extrapleural nodal status, and cell type determine postoperative long-term survival in trimodality therapy of malignant pleural mesothelioma: results in 183 patients. J Thorac Cardiovasc Surg 1999;117(1):54–63 [discussion: 63–5].

[18] Treasure T, Sedrakyan A. Pleural mesothelioma: little evidence, still time to do trials. Lancet 2004;364(9440):1183–5.

[19] Hillerdal G. The Swedish experience with asbestos: history of use, diseases, legislation, and compensation. Int J Occup Environ Health 2004;10(2):154–8.

[20] Robinson M, Wiggins J. Statement on malignant mesothelioma in the UK. Thorax 2002; 57(2):187.

[21] Tiitola M, et al. Computed tomography screening for lung cancer in asbestos-exposed workers. Lung Cancer 2002;35(1):17–22.

[22] Peipins LA, et al. Radiographic abnormalities and exposure to asbestos-contaminated vermiculite in the community of Libby, Montana, USA. Environ Health Perspect 2003; 111(14):1753–9.

[23] Haberkorn U. Positron emission tomography in the diagnosis of mesothelioma. Lung Cancer 2004;45(Suppl 1):S73–6.

[24] Ebert W, et al. Monitoring of therapy in inoperable lung cancer patients by measurement of CYFRA 21–1, TPA- TP CEA, and NSE. Anticancer Res 1997;17(4B):2875–8.

[25] Thylen A, Wallin J, Martensson G. Hyaluronan in serum as an indicator of progressive disease in hyaluronan-producing malignant mesothelioma. Cancer 1999;86(10): 2000–5.

[26] Hedman M, et al. Tissue polypeptide antigen (TPA), hyaluronan and CA 125 as serum markers in malignant mesothelioma. Anticancer Res 2003;23(1B):531–6.

[27] Barak V, et al. Clinical utility of cytokeratins as tumor markers. Clin Biochem 2004; 37(7):529–40.

[28] Lee YC, Knox BS, Garrett JE. Use of cytokeratin fragments 19.1 and 19.21 (Cyfra 21–1) in the differentiation of malignant and benign pleural effusions. Aust N Z J Med 1999; 29(6):765–9.

[29] Bonfrer JM, et al. Cyfra 21–1 and TPA as markers in malignant mesothelioma. Anticancer Res 1997;17(4B):2971–3.

[30] Bast Jr RC, et al. CA 125: the past and the future. Int J Biol Markers 1998;13(4):179–87.

[31] Zurawski Jr VR, et al. Serum CA 125 levels in a group of nonhospitalized women: relevance for the early detection of ovarian cancer. Obstet Gynecol 1987;69(4):606–11.

[32] Jacobs IJ, et al. Screening for ovarian cancer: a pilot randomised controlled trial. Lancet 1999;353(9160):1207–10.

[33] Kebapci M, et al. CT findings and serum CA 125 levels in malignant peritoneal mesothelioma: report of 11 new cases and review of the literature. Eur Radiol 2003;13(12): 2620–6.

[34] Simsek H, Kadayifci A, Okan E. Importance of serum CA 125 levels in malignant peritoneal mesothelioma. Tumour Biol 1996;17(1):1–4.

[35] Hernandez J, Thompson IM. Prostate-specific antigen: a review of the validation of the most commonly used cancer biomarker. Cancer 2004;101(5):894–904.

[36] Meissner HI, et al. Promoting cancer screening: learning from experience. Cancer 2004;101(5 Suppl):1107–17.

[37] Sullivan Pepe M, et al. Phases of biomarker development for early detection of cancer. J Natl Cancer Inst 2001;93(14):1054–61.

[38] Robinson BW, et al. Mesothelin-family proteins and diagnosis of mesothelioma. Lancet 2003;362(9396):1612–6.

[39] Chang K, Pastan I. Molecular cloning of mesothelin, a differentiation antigen present on mesothelium, mesotheliomas, and ovarian cancers. Proc Natl Acad Sci U S A 1996; 93(1):136–40.

[40] Rump A, Morikawa Y, Tanaka M, et al. Binding of ovarian cancer antigen CA125/MUC16 to mesothelin mediates cell adhesion. J Biol Chem 2004;279(10):9190–8 [Epub 2003 Dec 15].

[41] Yamaguchi N, et al. A novel cytokine exhibiting megakaryocyte potentiating activity from a human pancreatic tumor cell line HPC-Y5. J Biol Chem 1994;269(2):805–8.

[42] Kojima T, et al. Molecular cloning and expression of megakaryocyte potentiating factor cDNA. J Biol Chem 1995;270(37):21984–90.

[43] Scholler N, et al. Soluble member(s) of the mesothelin/megakaryocyte potentiating factor family are detectable in sera from patients with ovarian carcinoma. Proc Natl Acad Sci U S A 1999;96(20):11531–6.

[44] Muminova ZE, Strong TV, Shaw DR. Characterization of human mesothelin transcripts in ovarian and pancreatic cancer. BMC Cancer 2004;4(1):19.

[45] Hassan R, Bera T, Pastan I. Mesothelin: a new target for immunotherapy. Clin Cancer Res 2004;10(12 Pt 1):3937–42.

[46] Chang K, Pastan I, Willingham MC. Isolation and characterization of a monoclonal antibody, K1, reactive with ovarian cancers and normal mesothelium. Int J Cancer 1992; 50(3):373–81.

[47] Chang K, et al. Characterization of the antigen (CAK1) recognized by monoclonal antibody K1 present on ovarian cancers and normal mesothelium. Cancer Res 1992; 52(1):181–6.

[48] Urwin D, Lake RA. Structure of the mesothelin/MPF gene and characterization of its promoter. Mol Cell Biol Res Commun 2000;3(1):26–32.

[49] Bera TK, Pastan I. Mesothelin is not required for normal mouse development or reproduction. Mol Cell Biol 2000;20(8):2902–6.

[50] Hough CD, et al. Large-scale serial analysis of gene expression reveals genes differentially expressed in ovarian cancer. Cancer Res 2000;60(22):6281–7.

[51] Wang K, et al. Monitoring gene expression profile changes in ovarian carcinomas using cDNA microarray. Gene 1999;229(1–2):101–8.

[52] Argani P, et al. Mesothelin is overexpressed in the vast majority of ductal adenocarcinomas of the pancreas: identification of a new pancreatic cancer marker by serial analysis of gene expression (SAGE). Clin Cancer Res 2001;7(12):3862–8.

[53] Hippo Y, et al. Differential gene expression profiles of scirrhous gastric cancer cells with high metastatic potential to peritoneum or lymph nodes. Cancer Res 2001;61(3):889–95.

[54] Frierson Jr HF, et al. Large-scale molecular and tissue microarray analysis of mesothelin expression in common human carcinomas. Hum Pathol 2003;34(6):605–9.

[55] Chang K, et al. Monoclonal antibody K1 reacts with epithelial mesothelioma but not with lung adenocarcinoma. Am J Surg Pathol 1992;16(3):259–68.

[56] Ordonez NG. Application of mesothelin immunostaining in tumor diagnosis. Am J Surg Pathol 2003;27(11):1418–28.

[57] Miettinen M, Sarlomo-Rikala M. Expression of calretinin, thrombomodulin, keratin 5, and mesothelin in lung carcinomas of different types: an immunohistochemical analysis of 596 tumors in comparison with epithelioid mesotheliomas of the pleura. Am J Surg Pathol 2003;27(2):150–8.

[58] Thomas AM, et al. Mesothelin-specific CD8(+) T cell responses provide evidence of in vivo cross-priming by antigen-presenting cells in vaccinated pancreatic cancer patients. J Exp Med 2004;200(3):297–306.

[59] Pass H. Surgery for mesothelioma at the NCI and KCI: going somewhere very slowly. Presented at the 7th Meeting of the International Mesothelioma Interest Group. Brescia (Italy), June 24–26, 2004.

[60] Skates SJ, et al. Toward an optimal algorithm for ovarian cancer screening with longitudinal tumor markers. Cancer 1995;76(10 Suppl):2004–10.

[61] Urban N, et al. Ovarian cancer screening. Hematol Oncol Clin North Am 2003;17(4):989–1005.

[62] Jacobs I, et al. Prevalence screening for ovarian cancer in postmenopausal women by CA 125 measurement and ultrasonography. BMJ 1993;306(6884):1030–4.

Hematol Oncol Clin N Am 19 (2005) 1041–1052

HEMATOLOGY/ONCOLOGY CLINICS
OF NORTH AMERICA

Prognostic Factors for Mesothelioma

Jeremy P.C. Steele, MD

Bart's Mesothelioma Research Group, St. Bartholomew's Hospital and Medical College, London EC1A 7BE, UK

Malignant mesotheliomas of the pleura and peritoneum are relatively rare tumors with a generally poor prognosis [1]. Chemotherapy is palliative in intent, but recent data from an international phase III randomized trial showed a survival and quality-of-life benefit from the use of a chemotherapy regimen that contained pemetrexed and cisplatin [2]. Poor prognosis is associated with de novo drug resistance that results in short-lived tumor responses [3]. Some patients with low-volume disease and excellent performance status may be considered for radical surgery with extrapleural pneumonectomy (EPP) [4]. This complex and controversial operation carries an acute mortality rate of approximately 5% [5–7]. In Europe, a randomized trial of EPP versus standard palliative therapy (including chemotherapy, radiotherapy, and pleurodesis) is planned to commence in 2005 [8].

Which patients are candidates for radical surgery and which patients fare better than average even without surgery? Clinical prognostic factors can help clinicians and patients when deciding on a treatment plan. Patients in the best prognostic groups may be considered for more intensive or experimental therapy (eg, EPP or intensive drug therapy). Patients with less favorable prognosis should not be considered for high-risk surgery but are candidates for phase II and III clinical trials [9]. Prognostic factors are especially important for clinicians and patients who have malignant mesothelioma because anatomic staging systems are of limited value for most patients. Two of the best known staging systems are the International Mesothelioma Interest Group (IMIG) [10] and Brigham systems [4]. For both of these systems, stage is derived from disease extent at thoracotomy. Radiologic prediction of IMIG or Brigham stage is less accurate and of questionable value. It is likely that the new prognostic and staging protocol being developed by the International Association for the Study of Lung Cancer and IMIG will include clinical and biologic prognostic factors and radiologic and anatomic parameters [11].

CLINICAL PROGNOSTIC FACTOR SCORING SYSTEMS

The best known published prognostic scoring systems are those of the European Organization for the Research and Treatment of Cancer (EORTC) [12]

E-mail address: jeremy.steele@bartsandthelondon.nhs.uk

0889-8588/05/$ – see front matter
doi:10.1016/j.hoc.2005.09.009

and the Cancer and Leukemia Group B (CALGB) in the United States [13]. These systems show that the most important predictors of poor prognosis in pleural mesothelioma are poor performance status, non-epithelioid histology, male gender, low hemoglobin, high platelet count, high white blood cell count, and high lactate dehydrogenase level. These systems are discussed in more detail later.

Cancer and Leukemia Group B System

CALGB examined the individual and joint effect of various pretreatment clinical characteristics on the survival of patients with mesothelioma treated with chemotherapy in a series of sequential phase II trials [13]. Over a 10-year period, 337 untreated patients who had malignant mesothelioma were registered in phase II studies of ten treatment regimens. Median overall survival for the ten regimens ranged from 3.9 to 9.8 months, with 1-year survival rates ranging between 14% and 50%. The investigators then used Cox survival models and exponential regression trees to examine the prognostic importance of pretreatment patient characteristics.

Univariate analyses showed that patients with poor Eastern Cooperative Oncology Group (ECOG) performance status, chest pain at diagnosis, dyspnea, platelet count >400,000/µL, weight loss, serum lactate dehydrogenase level >500 IU/L, pleural involvement, low hemoglobin level, high white blood cell count, and age older than 75 years had the poorest prognosis. Multivariate Cox analyses showed that pleural involvement, lactate dehydrogenase >500 IU/L, poor performance status, chest pain, platelet count >400,000/µL, non-epithelial histology, and age older than 75 years predicted shorter survival. Performance status was the most important prognostic split in the regression tree. Six distinct prognostic subgroups were generated, with median survivals ranging from 1.4 to 13.9 months. The subgroup with the best survival (13.9 months) included patients with a performance status of 0 and age younger than 49 years and patients with performance status of 0, age 49 years or older, and a hemoglobin of 14.6g/dL or more. The worst survival (1.4 months) occurred in patients with a performance status of 1 or 2 and white blood cell count of 15.6/µL or more.

The CALGB prognostic scoring system shows that older patient age, poorer performance status, non-epithelial histology, the presence of chest pain or weight loss, low hemoglobin and high platelet count, high white blood cell count, and high lactate dehydrogenase predict for shorter survival.

European Organization for the Research and Treatment of Cancer Scoring System

The EORTC examined data from 204 adult patients with malignant pleural mesothelioma entered into five consecutive EORTC phase II clinical trials from 1984 to 1993 [12]. The drugs tested were mitoxantrone, epirubicin, etoposide, and paclitaxel. The Cox model was used to assess 13 factors related to biology and disease history with respect to survival. The median survival duration for the complete cohort was 8.4 months from trial entry. In a multivariate analysis, poor prognosis was associated with a poor performance status, a high white blood cell count, a probable/possible histologic diagnosis of mesothelioma, male gender, and having sarcomatoid subtype. Taking these five factors into consideration, the EORTC classified patients into two groups: a good prognosis group (with a 1-year survival rate of 40%) and a poor prognosis group (with a 1-year survival rate of 12%).

VALIDATION OF THE PROGNOSTIC SCORING SYSTEMS OF THE CANCER AND LEUKEMIA GROUP B AND EUROPEAN ORGANIZATION FOR THE RESEARCH AND TREATMENT OF CANCER BY OTHER RESEARCH GROUPS

University of Leicester Hospitals, Leicester, England

In 2000, Edwards and colleagues [14] of Leicester, England, published a retrospective analysis of a series of 142 patients who had mesothelioma. Some of these patients had surgical intervention, whereas others were treated with chemotherapy or supportive care alone. Univariate analysis of prognostic variables was performed using a Cox proportional hazards regression model. Statistically significant variables were analyzed further in a stepwise multivariate model. The authors then derived EORTC prognostic score (EPS) and CALGB prognostic scoring system groups, plotted Kaplan-Meier overall survival, and calculated survival rates from life tables to see if these prognostic groups predicted the established clinical outcomes for the Leicester patients.

Significant poor prognosis factors in univariate analysis included male sex, older age, weight loss, chest pain, poor performance status, low hemoglobin, leukocytosis, thrombocytosis, and non-epithelial cell type. The prognostic significance of cell type, low hemoglobin, high white blood cell count, performance status, and gender were retained in the multivariate model. Overall median

---

Table 1

Patient characteristics in three sequential phase II trials at St. Bartholomew's Hospital

	No. of patients		
	VO	IPM	VIN
Trial size	26	49	70
Male:female ratio	21:5	40:9	64:6
Age (y)			
Median (range)	60 (44–72)	61 (44–75)	59 (29–77)
ECOG PS			
PS 0	6	28	25
PS 1	15	16	30
PS 2	5	5	15
Histology			
Epithelioid	13	36	43
Non-epithelioid	13	13	27

Abbreviations: PS, performance status; VIN, vinorelbine; VO, vinorelbine/oxaliplatin.

Adapted from Fennell DA, Parmar A, Shamash J, et al. Statistical validation of the EORTC prognostic model for malignant pleural mesothelioma based on three consecutive phase II trials. J Clin Oncol 2005; 23(1):185; with permission.

survival was 5.9 months. Median, 1-year, and 2-year survival data within prognostic groups from Leicester were equivalent to the EORTC and CALGB series. The authors concluded that the EORTC and CALGB prognostic scoring systems could be used in the assessment of survival data of series in different countries and the stratification of patients in randomized trials.

St. Bartholomew's Hospital, London, England

Fennell and colleagues [15] from St. Bartholomew's Hospital, London, tested the validity of the EPS as a predictive variable for prognosis in 145 patients treated in three phase II clinical trials between 1999 and 2003. The impact of EPS on objective tumor response and progression-free survival also was determined to gain insight into the differential behavior of malignant mesothelioma between the respective high-risk and low-risk subgroups. One hundred forty-five patients were enrolled in three consecutive, single-center phase II trials between 1999 and 2003. Patients received single-agent vinorelbine [16], vinorelbine and oxaliplatin [17], or irinotecan, cisplatin, and mitomycin C (IPM) [18]. Patient characteristics are summarized in Table 1. EPS was calculated for each patient based on the following formula:

$$EPS = (0.550)a + (0.60)b + (0.52)c + (0.67)d + (0.60)e$$

The descriptors "a" through "e" denote the predictive factors described in the original report from the EORTC: a=if the white blood cell count was more than $8.3 \times 10^9/L$; b=if the ECOG performance status was 1 or 2; c=if the histology was probable; d=if the histology was sarcomatoid; e=if the sex was male. One hundred thirty-four patients were assessable for EPS, which was calculated to allow subgrouping of patients into low-risk (EPS <1.27) and high-risk (EPS >1.27) groups. The cut-off point of 1.27 represents the largest sum that can be calculated from a minimum of two constants in the EPS formula.

Survival Analysis

Kaplan-Meier curves were calculated for overall survival and stratified according to EPS. The log-rank test was used to compare relative survival (level of significance, $P<.05$). EPS was used to divide patients into low-risk and high-risk subgroups; analysis of the overall survival for the low-risk and high-risk subgroups was compared with each of the two phase II trial cohorts and the pooled trials. Kaplan-Meier curves for progression-free survival were stratified according to EPS and compared using the log-rank test. The objective tumor response rate based on Response Evaluation Criteria in Solid Tumors was compared for EPS low-risk and high-risk subgroups using multinomial logistic regression with objective response as the categoric-dependent variable. Goodness of fit was estimated by likelihood ratio test using χ^2 with a significance level of $P<.05$.

EPS was determined for patients treated in the vinorelbine and oxaliplatin, IPM, and vinorelbine trials. Using EPS, patients were assigned into subgroups: low-risk subgroup, with EPS less than 1.27 and high-risk subgroup, with EPS more than 1.27. Kaplan-Meier curves were stratified according to EPS and compared using the log-rank test. Overall survival for patients treated with vinorelbine and oxaliplatin was 10.4 months from diagnosis (95% confidence interval [CI], 8–12.8 months), and 8.8 months from first treatment (95% CI, 6.6–11). A trend to worse survival from diagnosis was observed in the high-risk vinorelbine and oxaliplatin subgroup (overall survival, 10.4 months; 95% CI, 7.7–13.9), compared with the low-risk subgroup (overall survival, 11.3 months; 95% CI, 8.3–14.3; log-rank = 1.0; P = .3). The trend toward worse overall survival from first treatment in the vinorelbine and oxaliplatin trial was 8.4 months (95% CI, 3.3–13.4) versus 7.2 months (95% CI, 6.6–7.8; log-rank = 0.07; P = .8), in the low- versus high-risk subgroups, respectively.

In the IPM trial, overall survival was 16.6 months (95% CI, 10.4–22.8) from diagnosis and 10.1 months (95% CI, 6.6–13.6) from first treatment. The EPS produced a statistically significant separation of the survival curves for patients who received IPM chemotherapy. Overall survival from diagnosis for the low-risk subgroup was 19.2 months (95% CI, 8.3–13.6) and 10.8 months (95% CI, 13.1–25.3) for the high-risk subgroup. From first treatment with IPM, overall survival was 12.7 months (95% CI, 5.4–21.1) for the low-risk subgroup, compared with 8.9 months (95% CI, 5.3–12.5) for the high-risk subgroup; the log-rank score was 4.5, $P < .01$.

In the vinorelbine trial, overall survival was 13.1 months (95% CI, 10.4–13.1) from diagnosis and 9.9 months (95% CI, 7.1–12.7) from first treatment. Kaplan-Meier survival curves were stratified by EPS. Overall survival from first treatment in the vinorelbine trial was 11.7 months (95% CI, 4.2–19.4) for the low-risk subgroup compared with 7.3 months (95% CI, 5–9.5) for the high-risk subgroup (log-rank = 10.3; $P < .01$). Overall survival for the three pooled phase II trials was 12.7 months from diagnosis (95% CI, 10.7–16.7) (Table 2) and 9.9 months from first treatment (95% CI, 8.5–11.3). Overall survival from diagnosis, stratified by EPS, was 18.2 months (95% CI, 14.4–22.8) for the low-risk group versus 10.4 months for the high-risk group (95% CI, 8.8–12; log-rank = 25; $P < .0001$). Overall survival from treatment, stratified by EPS, was 11.8 months for the low-risk group (95% CI, 7.6–16.1) versus 8.4 months for the high-risk group (95% CI, 6.8–10; log-rank = 15.5; $P < .0001$).

Table 2
Survival from diagnosis: high-risk EPS group or low-risk EPS group

| | EPS >1.27 | | EPS <1.27 | | | |
| | Survival | | Survival | | | |
	Months	(95% CI)	Months	(95% CI)	Log-rank	P value
VO	10.4	(7.7–13.9)	11.3	(8.3–14.3)	1.0	.3
IPM	10.8	(8.3–13.6)	19.2	(13.1–25.3)	7.0	<.01
VIN	9.9	(8.5–11.3)	19.1	(14.6–23.8)	13.4	<.01

Abbreviations: VIN, vinorelbine; VO, vinorelbine/oxaliplatin.

Adapted from Fennell DA, Parmar A, Shamash J, et al. Statistical validation of the EORTC prognostic model for malignant pleural mesothelioma based on three consecutive phase II trials. J Clin Oncol 2005; 23(1):186; with permission.

To confirm a correlation between EPS cutoff and overall survival, the distribution of EPS scores was divided into thirds using the thirty-third percentile (EPS = 1.15) and sixty-sixth percentile (EPS = 1.75). The frequency distribution was parametric. Kaplan-Meier curves were plotted for each subgroup (EPS < 1.15, 1.15 < EPS < 1.75, and EPS > 1.75) and showed a trend toward worse survival with increasing EPS (log-rank = 16.4; P = .0003). The individual effects of each EPS variable on overall survival was then determined: EPS did not predict response to chemotherapy when tested by multinomial logistic regression, using partial remission, stable disease, and progressive disease as the categoric-dependent variables and EPS as covariate (χ^2 for model 2.56; P = .28).

The St. Bartholomew's Hospital data provide strong evidence to support the use of the EPS as a statistically valid method to predict survival in patients with pleural mesothelioma. The EPS is robust and seems to be able to stratify small trials. It is simple to derive and interpret, which may be an advantage over the CALGB prognostic scoring system, which yields six strata for risk and requires a large sample size to ensure statistically significant subgroup separation. The survival rate from diagnosis for low-risk patients treated with vinorelbine or IPM was more than 19 months; however, it is uncertain what the survival of untreated patients in this subgroup would be.

The British Thoracic Society MS-01 trial [19], which will be complete in Fall 2005, is a randomized phase III study that compares chemotherapy (vinorelbine alone or the combination of mitomycin C, vinblastine, and cisplatin [20]) with active supportive care. It is of great interest to determine the survival of patients who receive active supportive care with respect to the EPS to understand better the impact of chemotherapy in this subgroup. The EPS is a valuable tool for predicting outcome in patients who have pleural mesothelioma. It is useful for interpreting the benefit of chemotherapy in clinical trials and should be used prospectively in future trials.

The EORTC and CALGB data show the importance of biologic measures of disease activity in prognosis. Low hemoglobin, high white blood cell count, high platelet count, and elevated lactate dehydrogenase were shown to be important by the CALGB, and high white blood cell count was important in the EORTC system. These parameters are apparently markers of mesothelioma biologic activity and may prove more useful than some of the prognostic factors described previously, such as age and radiologic clinical stage.

Many other possible biologic prognostic factors are under investigation, but none, as yet, has a proven role [21]. An example is glucose tranporter-1, which is a molecule that recently was shown to correlate with outcome [22] and is explained by the importance of core-apoptosis resistance in mesothelioma [3]. Apoptosis and glycolysis are closely linked, and glucose tranporter-1 is inherent to the glycolytic pathway. Glucose tranporter-1 overexpression reflects core-apoptosis resistance and correlated for poor clinical outcome in a group of 51 mesothelioma samples as efficiently as the EPS. Cyclo-oxygenase-2 overexpression also has been shown to correlate with poor survival and independently with CALGB and EPS [23].

Soluble mesothelioma-related protein (commonly known as mesothelin) is an exciting discovery that is under investigation worldwide [24]. The hope is that this protein will allow early detection of malignant mesothelioma in asbestos-exposed individuals and monitoring of therapy in patients who already have developed mesothelioma. Mesothelin also may be relevant in prognostication, although more research is needed.

MOLECULAR PROGNOSTIC MARKERS IN MALIGNANT MESOTHELIOMA

In the last 3 years, pivotal research has been published on the molecular genetic profile of malignant mesothelioma. Data acquired by genomics technology should produce fundamental insights into all aspects of the tumor's biology. Prognostication and treatment will improve when the key genetic events in mesothelioma initiation and propagation are understood. Mesothelioma has an unusual molecular biology, with loss of tumor suppressor genes being especially significant. The P16INK4A, P14ARF, and NF2 genes are lost more frequently than the more usual p53 and Rb. Several groups have performed the gene expression analyses on human mesothelioma samples [1].

Pass and colleagues [25] performed gene expression analyses with the U95 Affymetrix (Santa Clara, California) gene chip on tumor samples from 21 patients who had malignant mesothelioma that was treated with cytoreductive surgery and adjuvant therapy. Using dChip and Sam, neural networks constructed a common 27 gene classifier, which was associated with a high-risk and low-risk group of patients. Results were confirmed by real-time polymerase chain reaction and immunohistochemistry. The 27 gene classifier was then validated on a separate set of 17 patients who had mesothelioma. The groups predicted by the gene classifier mirrored the actual time to progression and survival of the test set with an accuracy of 95%. Clinical outcomes were independent of histology. The gene classifier had a 76% accuracy in the validation set of tumor samples.

Gordon and colleagues [26] analyzed gene expression in a conceptually similar fashion to the previously described report. This group acquired gene expression data from a new cohort of human mesothcliomas from 39 patients undergoing similar treatments. The relative expression levels for specific genes also were determined using reverse transcription polymerase chain reaction. A training set of 23 human mesothelioma samples was used to identify candidate prognostic molecular markers and gene ratio-based prognostic tests. The prognostic power of these newly discovered markers and gene ratio-based prognostic tests was tested on an independent group of tumors ($n=52$). The results showed that the mesothelioma prognostic genes and gene ratio-based prognostic tests were able to predict the clinical outcome in the 39 independent malignant pleural mesothelioma tumor specimens in a statistically significant manner. The authors showed the value of gene expression data for the prediction of outcome in mesothelioma.

Lopez-Rios and colleagues [27] used the dataset generated by Pass to classify prognosis in a sample of 99 mesotheliomas. They also examined differential gene expression using microarray technology and were able to identify some previously unrecognized genes, including uroplakins and kallikrein 11. The authors also examined gene expression profiles with regard to the diagnosis of mesothelioma.

Gene expression technology is evolving rapidly and will allow us to define prognostic groups for mesothelioma with a new level of precision. In addition to important prognostic insights, the technology will lead to fundamental biologic insights and effective therapies.

PREDICTORS OF SURVIVAL IN PATIENTS TREATED SURGICALLY

A brief review of the surgical prognostic predictors is included from the two largest series available. From 1980 to 1997, 183 patients underwent EPP followed by adjuvant chemotherapy and radiotherapy (various protocols were used) at Brigham and Women's Hospital in Boston [4,6]. There were seven (3.8%) acute deaths, and a morbidity rate of 50% was quoted. The 2-year survival rate was 38% in the 176 remaining patients. The 5-year survival rate was 15% and the median overall survival was 19 months. The authors conducted univariate and multivariate analyses on the survival data and concluded that patients with epithelial mesotheliomas, negative resection margins, and extrapleural nodes free from tumor resection had longer survival. Based on these data, few units would recommend EPP for patients with non-epithelioid histology. The issue of nodal involvement remains open, although positron emission tomographic (PET) imaging may, in the future, help clarify this.

Researchers at Memorial Sloan-Kettering Cancer Center recently presented data on 945 patients who had malignant pleural mesothelioma [28]. Variables, including patient demographics, symptoms, histology, smoking history, asbestos exposure, CT scan findings, stage, surgical procedure, and adjuvant therapy, were obtained retrospectively from the patient records. The primary outcome of interest was overall survival. A Kaplan-Meier analysis was performed on all variables, and significant variables were included in a multivariable Cox proportional hazard analysis. Survival data are presented in Fig. 1.

Five hundred fifty-eight patients were treated surgically with EPP, pleurectomy/decortication, or exploratory thoracotomy only. Of 939 patients for whom survival data were available, the median overall survival was 12.5 months. Of 313 patients with epithelioid subtype, the overall survival was 16.3 months, compared with 6.1 months for sarcomatoid subtype (44 patients) and 9.5 months ($P < .001$) for mixed subtype (99 patients). Four hundred eighty-three patients were unclassified for pathologic subtype. Overall survival was 20.2 months in patients with lower pathologic stage (AJCC [American Joint Committee on Cancer] stage 1-2) compared with 12.3 months ($P < .001$) for patients with more extensive stage (AJCC 3 or 4). These staging data probably should be considered with some caution in view of the difficulty of staging mesothelioma. Female patients ($n = 190$) survived for a median 17.3 months compared with 11.8 months for male patients ($P < .001$). Longer survival also was associated

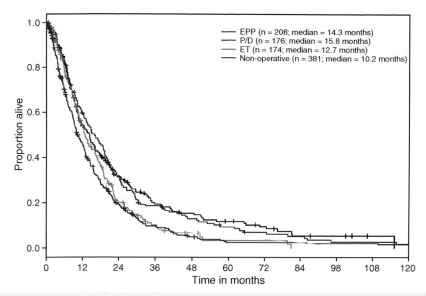

Fig. 1. Overall survival for all patients in the Memorial Sloan-Kettering surgical series according to type of surgical procedure performed. EPP, extrapleural pneumonectomy; ET, exploratory thoracotomy; P/D, pleurectomy/decortication.

with being asymptomatic at presentation, never having smoked, not knowingly being exposed to asbestos, and having a left-sided tumor.

Analysis of survival according to type of surgical procedure performed showed that longest survival was associated with pleurectomy/decortication (15.8 months). Patients who underwent EPP lived for a median 14.3 months, and patients who underwent exploratory thoracotomy only lived for a median 12.7 months. The superior survival of patients who underwent pleurectomy/decortication was possibly explained by the fact that these patients generally have less extensive disease than patients treated by EPP. Patients not treated

Table 3

Malignant pleural mesothelioma: survival predictors and surgery (Cox proportional hazards model)

Variable	Hazard ratio	95% CI	P value
Surgical resection versus exploration only	0.75	0.62–0.91	.003
Nonsmokers	0.77	0.61–0.97	.023
No asbestos exposure	0.95	0.77–1.19	.600
Female gender	0.63	0.51–0.77	.001
No pain at diagnosis	0.77	0.69–0.91	.008
Epithelioid histology	0.59	0.46–0.71	.001
Left-sided tumor	0.84	0.72–0.98	.020
Stage (I + II)	0.84	0.68–1.05	.100

Total number of patients was 939.
  Data courtesy of R. Flores, MD, New York, NY.

with any surgical procedure lived for a median 10.2 months. Table 3 summarizes these data. These results also should be viewed with caution because the data are nonrandomized and cover many decades of clinical practice. The patients would have been exposed to numerous additional variables that cannot be assessed easily or corrected for, including different operating surgeons and advances in critical care practice. The data provide an invaluable overview of a remarkably large series of patients who had mesothelioma.

The authors concluded that in addition to histologic subtype and stage (clinical or pathologic), important predictors of survival included gender (women live longer), laterality (left-sided tumors are better), asbestos exposure (non-exposed individuals live longer), and smoking (nonsmokers live longer). Patients who presented without symptoms at diagnosis lived longer than patients with symptoms. Multimodality treatment produced superior overall survival than a surgical approach performed without additional radiotherapy or chemotherapy ($P < .001$). The authors also suggested that surgical resection was associated with improved survival. Pleurectomy/decortication and EPP demonstrated similar survival when correction was made for stage. The authors suggested that if surgery is to be performed, it should occur within a clinical trial setting and that a multimodality treatment approach should be preferred.

OTHER PROGNOSTIC PREDICTORS FOR MESOTHELIOMA
PET is established as an important staging modality in many cancers, and PET standard update value (SUV) is reported as a prognostic indicator in several malignancies. The role of PET in prognostication of mesothelioma is unclear, however. From 1998 to 2003, 65 patients who had pleural mesothelioma at Memorial Sloan-Kettering Cancer Center underwent PET scans [29]. Median PET SUV in the primary tumor was 6.6 (range, 2–23), and the median follow-up for all surviving patients was 16 months. Median survivals were 14 and 24 months for the high-SUV and low-SUV groups, respectively. In a multivariate analysis, high-SUV tumors were associated with a 3.3-fold greater risk of death than low SUV tumors ($P = .03$). The authors concluded that an SUV more than 4 was a poor risk factor in malignant pleural mesothelioma.

Asbestos and erionite-related malignant pleural mesotheliomas are serious health issues in Turkey. In the Cappadocia region, erionite-associated mesothelioma is the center of much research interest because familial clustering of malignant mesothelioma in erionite-exposed individuals has suggested a genetic predisposition to mesothelioma [30]. One study from Turkey also showed a survival advantage for patients with asbestos-induced mesothelioma compared with erionite-induced mesothelioma [31]. This finding could be used as an independent prognostic factor for patients from this region who have malignant pleural mesothelioma.

SUMMARY
Knowledge of the clinical behavior, treatment, and molecular biology of malignant mesothelioma is accumulating rapidly. The disease is no longer considered

an untreatable rarity but rather is an interesting disease of known origin (in most cases) that will provide crucial insights into cancer biology. Treatment is improving, with palliative two-drug chemotherapy being an established approach for fitter patients. A small proportion of patients are candidates for radical surgery, although defining operability is difficult. Prognostic factors are essential, because they allow us to select patients for the most appropriate treatment. The EORTC and CALGB systems are the most useful clinical prognostic systems and are unlikely to be improved upon. Recent data clearly validated the EORTC system in the prediction of outcome in chemotherapy-treated patients. Future prospects are exciting, with gene expression profiling likely to provide a new level of accuracy in diagnosis and prognostication. Beyond this, understanding of the molecular biology of mesothelioma will generate new targets for effective therapy.

Acknowledgments

The author thanks the following persons for their assistance in providing data for this article: Raja Flores, MD (New York, NY) and Dean Fennell, MD, PhD (Belfast, Northern Ireland).

References

[1] Robinson BW, Musk AW, Lake RA. Malignant mesothelioma. Lancet 2005;366(9483): 397–408.

[2] Vogelzang NJ, Rusthoven JJ, Symanowski J, et al. Phase III study of pemetrexed in combination with cisplatin versus cisplatin alone in patients with malignant pleural mesothelioma. J Clin Oncol 2003;21(14):2636–44.

[3] Fennell DA, Rudd RM. Defective core-apoptosis signalling in diffuse malignant pleural mesothelioma: opportunities for effective drug development. Lancet Oncol 2004;5(6): 354–62.

[4] Sugarbaker DJ, Flores RM, Jaklitsch MT, et al. Resection margins, extrapleural nodal status, and cell type determine postoperative long-term survival in trimodality therapy of malignant pleural mesothelioma: results in 183 patients. J Thorac Cardiovasc Surg 1999; 117(1):54–63.

[5] Rusch VW, Rosenzweig K, Venkatraman E, et al. A phase II trial of surgical resection and adjuvant high-dose hemithoracic radiation for malignant pleural mesothelioma. Thorac Cardiovasc Surg 2001;122(4):788–95.

[6] Sugarbaker DJ, Jaklitsch MT, Bueno R, et al. Prevention, early detection, and management of complications after 328 consecutive extrapleural pneumonectomies. J Thorac Cardiovasc Surg 2004;128(1):138–46.

[7] Stewart DJ, Martin-Ucar AE, Edwards JG, et al. Extra-pleural pneumonectomy for malignant pleural mesothelioma: the risks of induction chemotherapy, right-sided procedures and prolonged operations. Eur J Cardiothorac Surg 2005;27(3):373–8.

[8] National Cancer Research Network (UK): Trials database. Available at: http://www.ncrn. org.uk/portfolio/. Accessed August 31, 2005.

[9] Steele JP, Rudd RM. Malignant mesothelioma: predictors of prognosis and clinical trials. Thorax 2000;55(9):725–6.

[10] Rusch VW. A proposed new international TNM staging system for malignant pleural mesothelioma from the International Mesothelioma Interest Group. Lung Cancer 1996; 14(1):1–12.

[11] van Meerbeeck JP, Boyer M. Consensus report: pretreatment minimal staging and treatment of potentially resectable malignant pleural mesothelioma. Lung Cancer 2005; 49(Suppl 1):S123–7.

[12] Curran D, Sahmoud T, Therasse P, et al. Prognostic factors in patients with pleural mesothelioma: the European Organization for Research and Treatment of Cancer experience. J Clin Oncol 1998;16(1):145–52.

[13] Herndon JE, Green MR, Chahinian AP, et al. Factors predictive of survival among 337 patients with mesothelioma treated between 1984 and 1994 by the Cancer and Leukemia Group B. Chest 1998;113(3):723–31.

[14] Edwards JG, Abrams KR, Leverment JN, et al. Prognostic factors for malignant mesothelioma in 142 patients: validation of CALGB and EORTC prognostic scoring systems. Thorax 2000;55(9):731–5.

[15] Fennell DA, Parmar A, Shamash J, et al. Statistical validation of the EORTC prognostic model for malignant pleural mesothelioma based on three consecutive phase II trials. J Clin Oncol 2005;23(1):184–9.

[16] Steele JP, Shamash J, Evans MT, et al. Phase II study of vinorelbine in patients with malignant pleural mesothelioma. J Clin Oncol 2000;18(23):3912–7.

[17] Fennell DA, Steele JP, Shamash J, et al. Phase II trial of vinorelbine and oxaliplatin as first-line therapy in malignant pleural mesothelioma. Lung Cancer 2005;47(2):277–81.

[18] Fennell D, Steele J, Shamash J, et al. A phase II study of irinotecan, cisplatin, and mitomycin C (IPM) in malignant pleural mesothelioma [abstract P517]. Lung Cancer 2003; 41(Suppl 2):S221.

[19] Muers MF, Rudd RM, O'Brien ME, et al. BTS randomised feasibility study of active symptom control with or without chemotherapy in malignant pleural mesothelioma. Thorax 2004;59(2):144–8.

[20] Middleton GW, Smith IE, O'Brien ME, et al. Good symptom relief with palliative MVP (mitomycin-C, vinblastine and cisplatin) chemotherapy in malignant mesothelioma. Ann Oncol 1998;9(3):269–73.

[21] Kumar P, Kratzke RA. Molecular prognostic markers in malignant mesothelioma. Lung Cancer 2005;49(Suppl 1):S53–60.

[22] Fennell DA, Klabatsa A, Sheaff MT, et al. Identification of glucose transporter type 1 overexpression as a predictor of survival in patients with malignant pleural mesothelioma [abstract 7199]. J Clin Oncol 2004;22:14S.

[23] Edwards JG, Faux SP, Plummer SM, et al. Cyclooxygenase-2 expression is a novel prognostic factor in malignant mesothelioma. Clin Cancer Res 2002;8(6):1857–62.

[24] Robinson BW, Creaney J, Lake R, et al. Mesothelin-family proteins and diagnosis of mesothelioma. Lancet 2003;362(9396):1612–6.

[25] Pass HI, Liu Z, Wali A, et al. Gene expression profiles predict survival and progression of pleural mesothelioma. Clin Cancer Res 2004;10(3):849–59.

[26] Gordon GJ, Rockwell GN, Godfrey PA, et al. Validation of genomics-based prognostic tests in malignant pleural mesothelioma. Clin Cancer Res 2005;11(12):4406–14.

[27] Lopez-Rios F, Chuai S, Hussain S, et al. Gene expression profiling of malignant mesothelioma for prognostic prediction and identification of potential therapeutic targets and differential diagnostic markers [abstract O78]. Lung Cancer 2005;49(Suppl 2):S29.

[28] Flores R, Zakowski M, Venkatramen E, et al. Malignant pleural mesothelioma (MPM): new predictors of survival and analysis of the impact of current treatment [abstract O75]. Lung Cancer 2005;49(Suppl 2):S28.

[29] Flores RM. The role of PET in the surgical management of malignant pleural mesothelioma. Lung Cancer 2005;49(Suppl 1):S27–32.

[30] Roushdy-Hammady I, Siegel J, Emri S, et al. Genetic-susceptibility factor and malignant mesothelioma in the Cappadocian region of Turkey. Lancet 2001;357(9254):444–5.

[31] Emri S, Demir AU. Malignant pleural mesothelioma in Turkey, 2000–2002. Lung Cancer 2004;45(Suppl 1):S17–20.

Hematol Oncol Clin N Am 19 (2005) 1053–1066

ELSEVIER
SAUNDERS

The Radiologic Measurement of Mesothelioma

Samuel G. Armato III, PhD[a],*, Geoffrey R. Oxnard, MD[b]

[a]Department of Radiology, University of Chicago, 5841 South Maryland Avenue, MC 2026, Chicago, IL 60637, USA
[b]Department of Medicine, Massachusetts General Hospital, Boston, MA, USA

T he need to visualize the internal structure and function of the human body has increased dramatically since Wilhelm Roentgen produced the first x-ray image of human anatomy shortly after his 1895 discovery, and the technology to bring about such visualization has advanced at an equally dramatic pace. Whether the need to visualize has driven technology or technologic improvements have stimulated the desire to visualize, the radiologic evaluation of disease is ubiquitous in modern clinical medicine. Radiologic evaluation generally consists of two standard tasks: (1) the presence of an abnormality must be established or ruled out and (2) lesion classification (eg, malignant potential) must be assessed. The role of radiologic imaging of mesothelioma for these two tasks was reviewed recently [1,2]. In addition to the detection and classification of abnormalities, the notion of radiologic evaluation has expanded to include the quantification of disease.

The subjective, qualitative interpretation of imaging studies has been augmented by demands for objective, quantitative analysis of those same studies, but even a quantitative interpretation is necessarily subjective when performed by a human observer. A greater degree of reliability is inherently associated with numeric, rather than qualitative, descriptions. Those numbers, however, must be considered in the proper context. How were those numbers obtained? What subjective decisions were made by the radiologist or clinician during the acquisition of those numbers? How reproducible is the process? Intra- and inter-observer variability is ubiquitous.

The unique circumferential and often scalloped morphology of mesothelioma distinguishes it from other thoracic neoplasms. Unlike bronchogenic lung cancer, for example, mesothelioma is not a focal, intraparenchymal lesion amenable to visual separation from normal anatomic structures. The general radiographic

Dr. Armato holds warrants to stock in R2 Technology, Inc. (Sunnyvale, California).
* Corresponding author. E-mail address: s-armato@uchicago.edu (S.G. Armato III).

progression of mesothelioma, as described by Yilmaz and colleagues [3], conveys the morphologic complexities of this disease:

> The radiographic appearance of malignant mesothelioma is variable. In the early stages of the disease, a large pleural effusion is often the only finding. Subtle pleural thickening or small discrete pleural-based masses may be seen on CT [computed tomography]. A dominant pleural-based mass may be the initial presentation, but ultimately the involvement of the pleura is always diffuse. Subsequently, larger pleura-based masses become evident, and are often associated with multiloculated effusions. Eventually, a thick irregular, pleural rind encases the lung and obliterates the pleural space. Mediastinal adenopathy, direct extension of the tumor into the mediastinum, involvement of the pericardium with pericardial effusion, [or] extension into the chest wall or through the diaphragm are seen in very locally advanced tumors.

In light of this varied presentation, the challenges of measuring mesothelioma are many. In this article we explore the demands, the current standard of clinical practice, and the opportunities associated with the radiologic measurement of mesothelioma.

MEASURING LESIONS

The notion of tumor response is fundamental in oncology. Assessment of disease progression or response to therapy is necessary for patient management and the evaluation of drug efficacy during clinical trials. The radiologic assessment of patients enrolled in clinical trials provides endpoints that have gained acceptance as a substitute for patient survival during the regulatory approval process [4,5]. This radiologic assessment, however, necessitates quantitative tumor measurements and the standardization of tumor response criteria based on such measurements. The quantification of tumor response has been promoted as a broad clinical biomarker [6].

The standardization of lesion measurements has evolved over time, beginning with the World Health Organization (WHO) guidelines of 1981. These guidelines recommended the radiologic quantification of solid tumors through bidimensional measurements comprising the product of (1) the length of the longest in-plane diameter of the lesion and (2) the length of the longest diameter perpendicular to the longest in-plane diameter [7]. Tumor response is determined from a comparison of bidimensional measurements across temporally sequential imaging studies. Under WHO guidelines, a tumor is classified as demonstrating (1) partial response (PR) if the sum of the bidimensional measurements of all lesions in a follow-up study decreases by more than 50% of the sum from the baseline study, (2) progressive disease (PD) if the sum of bidimensional measurements in the follow-up study increases by more than 25% of the sum from the baseline study, (3) stable disease if the extent of measurement reduction is not great enough to qualify as PR or the extent of measurement increase is not great enough to qualify as PD, or (4) complete response if the follow-up study demonstrates resolution of all lesions. The interval development of new lesions also represents PD.

The Response Evaluation Criteria in Solid Tumors (RECIST) guidelines were later developed to replace the bidimensional tumor measurements of WHO with more straightforward unidimensional measurements; each measurable lesion is represented by the length of its single longest diameter [8,9]. According to RECIST, tumor response is classified as (1) PR if the sum of the unidimensional measurements of all lesions in a follow-up CT scan demonstrates a decrease of more than 30% from the baseline scan sum, (2) PD if the unidimensional measurement sum in the follow-up CT scan demonstrates an increase of more than 20% from the baseline scan sum (or if new lesions develop), (3) stable disease if the extent of measurement reduction is not great enough to qualify as PR or the extent of measurement increase is not great enough to qualify as PD, or (4) complete response if all lesions have resolved [9].

The WHO and RECIST guidelines both present (1) a tumor measurement technique and (2) a set of tumor response criteria. These guidelines attempt to standardize how measurements are acquired and how the acquired measurements are to be interpreted. The interpretation of measurements fundamentally depends on the manner in which the measurements were acquired, such that a change in measurement technique necessitates mathematical computation of corresponding response criteria. The RECIST response criteria were developed for spherical-tumor-based mathematical consistency with the WHO criteria (although practical considerations resulted in modifications) but with a streamlined measurement technique that requires only a single measurement. Consistency between both facets of the guidelines is important, and consistency in their execution must be maintained.

CLINICAL TRIAL MEASUREMENTS OF MESOTHELIOMA

Like the measurement of other solid tumors, the measurement of mesothelioma has changed much over the last few decades. Chemotherapy studies in the 1980s and early 1990s frequently applied the WHO guidelines for tumor measurement and response classification [7]. Generally, these studies required the bidimensional measurement of all measurable disease, and response classification was determined from the change in the sum of bidimensional measurements across serial imaging studies, including chest radiographs, CT, and ultrasound [10–16].

Some chemotherapy trials undertook unidimensional measurement of mesothelioma before the emergence of the RECIST literature. In a study that assessed treatment of malignant mesothelioma with chemotherapy in combination with high-dose radiation of the affected hemithorax, Mattson and colleagues [17] measured mesothelioma on CT and designated PD as a "doubling in thickness of contrast medium-enhanced mesothelioma plaque" and PR as a "decrease in thickness of the plaque-like lesion by one half." These response criteria were used later in a study of oral etoposide [18].

Unidimensional measurement of mesothelioma was further advanced when Byrne and colleagues [19] published their phase II study of cisplatin and gemcitabine in 1999, which yielded one of the highest response rates (47.6%) reported in the mesothelioma literature. In addition to evaluating all bidimensionally measurable lesions, their protocol explicitly required unidimensional measurement of the pleural tumor on three separate sections of the CT scan. This approach circumvented the proscribed measurement of all measurable lesions, which, for mesothelioma, can be a vague task because of its circumferential growth and appearance on numerous CT sections. The unidimensional measurements were acquired to capture the thickness of the pleural tumor, and the sum of these measurements was evaluated for change. This study maintained the WHO definition of PD (an increase of more than 25%) but changed the criteria for PR to require a decrease of more than 30% (rather than 50%). This measurement protocol was subsequently used in a study of pemetrexed by Vogelzang and colleagues [20]. Another chemotherapy study obtained unidimensional tumor thickness measurements on three separate CT sections, as did Byrne and colleagues, but applied the WHO tumor response criteria for PD and PR [21].

The RECIST criteria [9] provide rules for the standardization of unidimensional measurement of solid tumors, and beginning in 2000, chemotherapy trials for mesothelioma incorporated the RECIST recommendations. In studying vinorelbine, Steele and colleagues [22] acquired all tumor measurements on CT and distinctly addressed mass lesions and pleural lesions. Up to five mass lesions were followed with unidimensional measurement of the lesion's longest diameter. In the absence of obvious mass lesions, pleural tumor was evaluated at three separate levels (as described by Byrne and colleagues [19]) by unidimensional measurement of tumor thickness. The total sum of unidimensional measurements was compared over time using the RECIST criteria for response: a decrease of 30% was considered PR, whereas an increase of 20% was considered PD.

RESPONSE EVALUATION CRITERIA IN SOLID TUMORS (RECIST) AND MESOTHELIOMA

Growing evidence suggests that the measurement aspect of RECIST is not appropriate for the unique circumferential growth pattern and often scalloped morphology of mesothelioma [23,24]. The RECIST guidelines present (1) a tumor measurement technique and (2) a set of tumor response criteria. In a case study of four mesothelioma patients, Monetti and colleagues [23] noted potential problems with "longest diameter" (the RECIST measurement technique) in the assessment of mesothelioma on CT because of the circumferential extension of mesothelioma along the chest wall. These authors noted that tumor regression tends to occur along the short-axis dimension (ie, the dimension perpendicular to the chest wall: thickness) rather than along the long-axis dimension. In all four cases reported by Monetti and colleagues, the WHO guidelines (bidimensional measurements) yielded PR classifications, whereas the RECIST guidelines (unidimensional measurements along the long axis) resulted in stable disease classifications. When the RECIST response criteria were applied to thickness (rather than long-axis) measurements, all four cases were reclassified as PR (the same as the WHO classifications).

Van Klaveren and colleagues [24] applied the RECIST long-axis measurement technique to a larger sample of mesothelioma patients and also found tumor response classifications that differed from those of WHO. Serial tumor measurements were acquired from the CT scans of 34 patients. Comparison of WHO and RECIST response classifications demonstrated discordance in 27% of cases, largely because of underscoring by RECIST (eg, PD or PR classified as stable disease). The percentage of patients in whom one or more discordant classifications were obtained was 47%. The authors noted that misclassification could cause undue chemotherapy exposure to a subset of patients. Like Monetti and colleagues [23], these authors found that measurement of tumor thickness instead of largest tumor diameter (long axis) generated response classifications more consistent with those of WHO.

To confront the confusion and inconsistencies of mesothelioma measurement, Byrne and Nowak [25] recently published "modified RECIST criteria" specifically for the assessment of mesothelioma. More accurately, the authors modified the tumor measurement technique of RECIST rather than the tumor response criteria, which remain a decrease of at least 30% for PR and an increase of at least 20% for PD as specified by RECIST. Similar to the approach used in the gemcitabine/cisplatin clinical trial [19], the new measurement technique entails the acquisition of multiple measurements on three separate CT sections with a minimum axial separation of 1 cm, in which these measurements extend perpendicular to the chest wall or mediastinum to capture tumor thickness (Fig. 1). Follow-up measurements are then acquired from corresponding sites on a follow-up CT scan. To validate this approach, measurements were acquired from the CT scans of 73 patients who had mesothelioma using the WHO criteria and the Byrne (modified RECIST) measurement technique. Discordant tumor response classifications were demonstrated in 9% of patients, although the overall response rate was the same for WHO and modified RECIST. An analysis of survival showed a statistically significant difference between patients classified as responders and nonresponders using modified RECIST.

Although the tumor thickness measurement technique of Byrne and Nowak [25] (modified RECIST) seems to capture properly the extent of mesothelioma in the selected CT sections, the most appropriate tumor response criteria remain uncertain despite the reported concordance rate. The use of the RECIST response criteria (30% decrease for PR, 20% increase for PD) is complicated by the degree of variability present in the acquisition of mesothelioma tumor thickness measurements. Armato and colleagues [26] obtained 95% limits of agreement for relative interobserver difference of mesothelioma tumor thickness measurements that spanned a range of 30% (see later discussion). With this degree of variability in the measurement of mesothelioma, reproducible response classification may necessitate tumor response criteria that require larger thickness changes.

Tumor geometry represents another factor that complicates the use of RECIST response criteria for mesothelioma. In spherical tumors for which

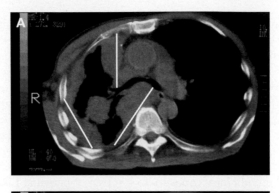

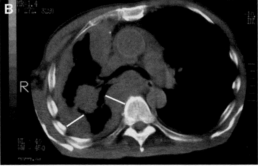

Fig. 1. Line segments represent mesothelioma tumor measurements on the same CT section based on (A) the longest diameter as specified by RECIST and (B) the dimension perpendicular to the chest wall or mediastinum ("thickness") as suggested by the modified RECIST technique. (*From* Byrne MJ, Nowak AK. Modified RECIST criteria for assessment of response in malignant pleural mesothelioma. Ann Oncol 2004;15(2):258; with permission.)

the RECIST criteria were developed, the 30% decrease in unidimensional measurement that was classified as PR corresponds to a 65.7% decrease in tumor volume, whereas the 20% increase that was classified as PD corresponds to a 72.8% increase in tumor volume. The relationship between change in unidimensional measurements and change in volume, however, may be substantially different for nonspherical tumor geometries, particularly mesothelioma with its plate-like growth. A new set of response criteria for use with mesothelioma tumor thickness measurements is likely warranted to achieve volumetric consistency with RECIST or WHO. The validity of response classification based on these volumetric changes for a tumor with the natural history of mesothelioma, however, remains an unexplored question of a more fundamental nature.

MEASUREMENT VARIABILITY
The actual manner in which tumor measurement protocols are implemented raises issues of consistency and reproducibility across clinicians and between methods [27–31]. Because longitudinal measurements obtained from serial im-

aging studies provide essential information regarding tumor progression or response to therapy, consistency of measurements acquired across temporally sequential CT scans is central to the accurate assessment of tumor response. Consistency, however, may be compromised by several factors, including inter- and intraobserver variability in the measurement process, variability in the location of anatomically equivalent measurement sites between scans, and misinterpretation of baseline scan measurements. In studies of intraparenchymal solid tumors (mostly metastases) unrelated to mesothelioma, inter- and intraobserver variability in the selection and measurement of lesions in CT scans has been reported [27,28,30]. The complex morphology of mesothelioma would render its measurement susceptible to potentially unacceptable levels of variability.

The manual measurement of mesothelioma in CT scans has been described as a three-step process that involves (1) selection of a limited number of CT sections in which the disease is most prominent, (2) identification of specific locations within the selected sections that demonstrate the greatest extent of pleural thickening, and (3) the actual measurement of tumor thickness at those locations [26]. The third step may be divided further in that the acquisition of a tumor thickness measurement requires (1) selection of a specific point along the outer tumor margin at which to initiate the measurement, (2) determination of the direction that captures the most appropriate dimension of the tumor, and (3) location of a point along the inner tumor margin encountered in that direction [26].

Armato and colleagues [26] conducted a study in which three attending radiologists and two attending oncologists served as observers to assess variability in the last two of the substeps described previously. The first observer to participate reviewed all 22 CT scans on a computer interface. In accordance with a clinical protocol for the measurement of mesothelioma on CT scans, the first observer selected the three sections from which measurements would be acquired on each scan, selected up to three measurement sites on each section, and acquired thickness measurements by constructing tumor-spanning line segments specified by an initial endpoint along the chest wall or mediastinal aspect of the tumor and a terminal endpoint along the visceral aspect of the tumor. The other observers each independently viewed the same 22 CT scans through the interface, which also displayed on the appropriate sections the initial measurement endpoints chosen by the first observer, although the actual line segments and terminal endpoints of the first observer were not shown. The task of the other observers was as follows: Given a specific location on a specific CT section, construct a line segment that most appropriately measures mesothelioma tumor thickness. Interobserver variability in the selection of CT section and measurement location was eliminated, and only variability of the actual tumor thickness measurements at the fixed sites was captured. Tumor thickness measurements were compared among all five observers. Differences in the measurements acquired by four of these observers are demonstrated in Fig. 2. The 95% limits of agreement for relative interobserver difference spanned a range of 30%, and the 95% limits of agreement for relative intraobserver

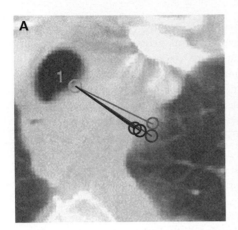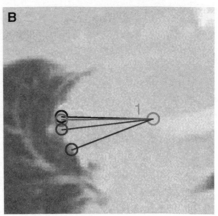

Fig. 2. The process of obtaining a tumor thickness measurement at a measurement site involves an interpretation of the location of the inner tumor margin and an interpretation of the direction that captures the most appropriate dimension of the tumor (ie, the direction at which the line segment should extend from the initial endpoint). (*A*) Observers constructed line segments oriented in nearly the same direction, but differences in perceived inner tumor margin are evident. (*B*) Observers interpreted the inner tumor margin consistently, but line segments were constructed over a wide range of angles. (*From* Armato III SG, Oxnard GR, MacMahon H, et al. Measurement of mesothelioma on thoracic CT scans: a comparison of manual and computer-assisted techniques. Med Phys 2004;31(5):1108; with permission.)

difference spanned a range of 27%. The reported variability in measurements made on the same scans likely would have been exaggerated had observers been allowed to implement all three steps of the measurement process and had temporally sequential scans of the patients been evaluated as they are in actual clinical practice.

A study by Armato and colleagues [32] examined the effect of baseline scan measurement presentation on the variability of subsequent measurements. The previously measured baseline CT scans along with the corresponding follow-up scans of 22 patients who had mesothelioma were presented to four radiologists and clinicians. Each observer independently manually measured tumor thickness in the follow-up scans through a computer interface that allowed for side-by-side viewing of baseline and follow-up scans. Observers acquired follow-up scan measurements during two separate sessions that differed in the manner in which baseline scan measurements were presented. During one session, baseline measurements were visually displayed as line segments superimposed across the measurement sites on the baseline scan, whereas during the other session, a written report of baseline measurements was used without a visual aid. For the baseline scan measurements shown in Figs. 3A and B depict the tumor thickness measurements acquired by an observer in the corresponding follow-up scan section based on a written report of the baseline scan measurements and with the benefit of the visual aid. The potential for substantially different tumor thickness measurements with and without the visual aid

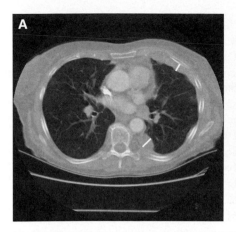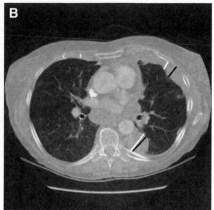

Fig. 3. (A) Baseline scan measurements are shown superimposed on one section of a baseline CT scan. (B) Tumor thickness measurements acquired by an observer in the corresponding follow-up scan section based on a written report of the baseline scan measurements (*black line segments*) and with the benefit of the visual aid (*white line segments*). The potential for substantially different tumor thickness measurements is evident.

is evident. Tumor response classification was determined from the percent change in summed linear measurements between the two scans of each patient in accordance with the RECIST criteria. With the visual aid, concordant tumor response classifications were obtained in 84.8% of the pair-wise comparisons among the four observers, whereas an 82.6% concordance rate was obtained when the written report was used. The written report and visual aid methods demonstrated statistically significant differences in percent measurement change between baseline and follow-up scans across observers $(P < .01)$.

In the evaluation of mesothelioma tumor response through measurements on CT scans, the selection of anatomically equivalent sections between baseline and follow-up scans is required, whereas for the evaluation of focal, intra-parenchymal lesions, the lesion itself represents the anatomic landmark for comparison, which obviates the need for section selection. To appreciate this difference, consider the evaluation of response in a focal lesion. The lesion that was measured in the baseline scan is identified (relocalized) in the follow-up scan, and the follow-up measurement is acquired. The decision in this scenario is which CT section demonstrates the greatest extent of the lesion in accordance with the RECIST measurement guidelines. This decision, however, is based on the local region occupied by the lesion and may be made regardless of surrounding patient anatomy. Assessment of focal lesion response is effectively immune from differences in patient positioning or differences in respiratory effort between the two scans. The unique morphology and growth patterns of mesothelioma, however, have forced modifications of the standard one lesion/one measurement paradigm, so that a single, contiguous bulk of tumor mass may be represented by multiple linear thickness measurements across three separate

CT sections. Global anatomic features between the two CT scans—and not the tumor itself—must be used to relocalize measurement sites, which necessitates the selection of anatomically equivalent sections as the first step of the measurement process for tumor response assessment.

Sensakovic and colleagues [33] evaluated variability in the manual selection of anatomically equivalent CT sections. Five radiologists and oncologists were presented independently with the three sections on which measurements had been acquired in each of 22 baseline CT scans that demonstrated mesothelioma. The observers selected the best anatomically matched section in the corresponding follow-up scan for each of these 66 baseline scan sections so that appropriate follow-up scan measurements could be acquired. All observers selected for measurement the exact same section of the follow-up scan for only 14 of the 66 (21.2%) baseline scan sections. For 31 of the 66 (47%) baseline scan sections, the selected follow-up scan sections comprised a range of two contiguous sections, and for 12.1% (8 of 66) of the baseline scan sections, the selected follow-up scan sections comprised a range of four or more contiguous sections. The investigators then developed an automated method to select anatomically matched sections based on the mathematical concept of mutual information. The automated method was applied to the same 66 baseline scan sections that were presented to the observers and selected equivalent sections that were within the observers' range for 60 of the 66 sections (90.9%).

COMPUTER-ASSISTED MEASUREMENTS

The computerized analysis of medical images has been the subject of intense research and clinical interest. Techniques for the computerized detection and classification of abnormalities on CT scans (and images from other multidimensional imaging modalities) have been supplemented with techniques for the computerized quantification of lesions, with the potential to facilitate implementation of tumor measurement protocols. Although such computerized tumor measurement methods have been reported for intraparenchymal and lymph node–based tumor masses [29,34,35], the evaluation of mesothelioma only recently has begun to benefit from this progress.

Armato and colleagues [26] have developed computerized techniques for the semiautomated measurement of mesothelioma tumor thickness in CT scans. During the initial phase of this research, a user interface was constructed to facilitate the softcopy visualization of CT scans. Similar to interfaces that are currently available with commercial CT scanners, this interface was designed to allow manual measurement of structures in the images. A measurement is obtained from the length of a line segment constructed by the user within a selected CT section image. The initial endpoint of the line segment is placed when the user clicks the mouse at the desired image location, and the terminal endpoint is established when, after dragging the mouse to create a visible line segment extending from the initial endpoint, the user releases the mouse button. Any number of line segments may be created within any number of sections. The corresponding lengths of the line segments are displayed through the interface, and data associated with each line segment (ie, length, section number, and coordinates of the initial and terminal endpoints) are stored for comparison of measurements among observers or across temporally sequential scans.

The interface serves as the front end of a semiautomated mesothelioma measurement system in which user-identified points along the parietal or mediastinal aspect of the tumor (the outer tumor boundary) are automatically connected to computer-identified points along the visceral aspect of the tumor (the inner tumor boundary) to provide tumor thickness measurements. Automated segmentation of the lungs in the CT scan isolates the lungs from surrounding structures based on gray-level thresholding techniques and provides the basis for tumor measurement, because the outer boundary of the lung serves as a surrogate for the inner tumor boundary. The lung segmentation regions and spatial positions of pixels along the lung boundary are used to identify automatically a terminal endpoint for a given initial endpoint [26]. Six algorithms were used to identify terminal endpoints based on logical approaches to the measurement of mesothelioma with its highly variable local morphology. An example of one such algorithm is shown in Fig. 4.

The semiautomated algorithms were applied to 134 measurement sites manually identified in the CT scans of 22 patients who had mesothelioma. The resulting tumor thickness measurements closely approximated the average measurements of five radiologists and oncologists. Of all semiautomated tumor thickness measurements, 83% were within 15% of the length of the corresponding average

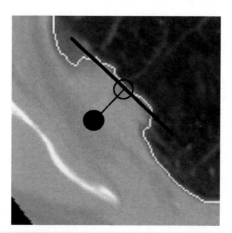

Fig. 4. Illustration of one of the algorithms used to identify the terminal endpoint (*open circle*) associated with a given initial endpoint (*closed circle*) for the generation of computer-assisted tumor thickness measurements. A magnified view of a CT section is shown, with a portion of the lung contour (*white pixels*) visible. The "normal-to-lung-boundary" algorithm selects the lung contour pixel with a local tangent line (*thick black line*) that yields a perpendicular that extends through the initial endpoint. (*From* Armato III SG, Oxnard GR, MacMahon H, et al. Measurement of mesothelioma on thoracic CT scans: A comparison of manual and computer-assisted techniques. Med Phys 2004;31(5):1109; with permission.)

manual measurements [26]. In a follow-up study, the frequency with which observers accepted semiautomated measurements without modification was as high as 86% [36]. Such computer-assisted approaches are expected to enhance greatly the use of CT scans in the management of patients who have mesothelioma, reduce data-acquisition time during clinical trials, and make the radiologic assessment of mesothelioma more efficient.

VOLUMETRIC MEASUREMENTS

Despite the volumetric capabilities of CT, tumor volume is not considered in the clinical assessment of mesothelioma, although some investigators have begun to explore the prognostic potential of tumor volume. Pass and colleagues [37] conducted a phase III trial of surgery and postoperative immunochemotherapy with or without intraoperative photodynamic therapy in which progression or recurrence of disease was established based on tumor volume measurements manually extracted from follow-up CT scans. An ancillary study explored the association of tumor volume with survival, time to first recurrence, nodal status, and postoperative International Mesothelioma Interest Group staging [38]. A statistically significant difference between the survival of patients with a preoperative tumor volume more than 100 cc and patients with a volume less than 100 cc was observed (11 months and 22 months, respectively); a significant difference in progression-free survival was obtained between patients with a preoperative volume more than and less than 51 cc. Tumor volumes were significantly smaller for patients without nodal metastases, and the median preoperative tumor volumes correlated well with postoperative International Mesothelioma Interest Group staging. A correlation of 0.91 was obtained between preoperative volume measurements and the sum of bidimensional measurements acquired from mesothelioma tumor present in each of four quadrants defined within the individual CT sections.

Studies of metastatic tumors have demonstrated that volume measurement yields response classifications that differ from those of RECIST [35,39]. The extent to which unidimensional measurements sufficiently capture the often asymmetric and nonuniform three-dimensional growth of a morphologically complex tumor such as mesothelioma is questionable and may cast doubt on the ability of linear measurements to serve as accurate surrogates for tumor volume. For example, a consistent relationship between change in mesothelioma tumor thickness and change in axial extent of the tumor may not exist so that axial growth may require direct measurement to accurately assess change in tumor volume. Volume measurements, however, are impractical to obtain through manual approaches, so the eventual incorporation of volume measurements into the clinical evaluation of mesothelioma patients will require some degree of automation.

References

[1] Truong MT, Erasmus JJ, Marom EM, et al. Imaging evaluation in the diagnosis and staging of malignant pleural mesothelioma. Semin Roentgenol 2004;39(3):386–96.

[2] Armato III SG, MacMahon H, Oxnard GR, et al. Radiologic assessment of mesothelioma. In: Pass HI, Vogelzang NJ, Carbone M, editors. Malignant mesothelioma. New York: Springer; 2005. p. 433–53.

[3] Yilmaz UM, Utkaner G, Yalniz E, et al. Computed tomographic findings of environmental asbestos-related malignant pleural mesothelioma. Respirology 1998;3(1):33–8.

[4] Saini S. Radiologic measurement of tumor size in clinical trials: past, present, and future. AJR Am J Roentgenol 2001;176(2):333–4.

[5] Johnson JR, Williams G, Pazdur R. End points and United States Food and Drug Administration approval of oncology drugs. J Clin Orthod 2003;21(7):1404–11.

[6] Frank R, Hargreaves R. Clinical biomarkers in drug discovery and development. Nature Reviews 2003;2(7):566–80.

[7] Miller AB, Hogestraeten B, Staquet M, et al. Reporting results of cancer treatment. Cancer 1981;47(1):207–14.

[8] James K, Eisenhauer E, Christian M, et al. Measuring response in solid tumors: unidimensional versus bidimensional measurement. J Natl Cancer Inst 1999;91(6):523–8.

[9] Therasse P, Arbuck SG, Eisenhauer EA, et al. New guidelines to evaluate the response to treatment in solid tumors. J Natl Cancer Inst 2000;92(3):205–16.

[10] Dimitrov NV, Egner J, Balcueva E, et al. High-dose methotrexate with citrovorum factor and vincristine in the treatment of malignant mesothelioma. Cancer 1982;50(7):1245–7.

[11] Lerner HJ, Schoenfeld DA, Martin A, et al. Malignant mesothelioma: the Eastern Cooperative Oncology Group (ECOG) experience. Cancer 1983;52(11):1981–5.

[12] Colbert N, Vannetzel JM, Izrael V, et al. A prospective study of detorubicin in malignant mesothelioma. Cancer 1985;56(9):2170–4.

[13] Zidar BL, Metch B, Balcerzak SP, et al. A phase II evaluation of ifosfamide and mesna in unresectable diffuse malignant mesothelioma: a Southwest Oncology Group study. Cancer 1992;70(10):2547–51.

[14] Chahinian AP, Antman K, Goutsou M, et al. Randomized phase II trial of cisplatin with mitomycin or doxorubicin for malignant mesothelioma by the Cancer and Leukemia Group B. J Clin Orthod 1993;11(8):1559–65.

[15] Vogelzang NJ, Weissman LB, Herndon Jr JE, et al. Trimetrexate in malignant mesothelioma: a Cancer and Leukemia Group B Phase II study. J Clin Orthod 1994;12(7):1436–42.

[16] Kindler HL, Millard F, Herndon Jr JE, et al. Gemcitabine for malignant mesothelioma: a phase II trial by the Cancer and Leukemia Group B. Lung Cancer 2001;31(2–3):311–7.

[17] Mattson K, Holsti LR, Tammilehto L, et al. Multimodality treatment programs for malignant pleural mesothelioma using high-dose hemithorax irradiation. Int J Radiat Oncol Biol Phys 1992;24(4):643–50.

[18] Tammilehto L, Maasilta P, Mantyla M, et al. Oral etoposide in the treatment of malignant mesothelioma: a phase II study. Ann Oncol 1994;5(10):949–50.

[19] Byrne MJ, Davidson JA, Musk AW, et al. Cisplatin and gemcitabine treatment for malignant mesothelioma: a phase II study. J Clin Orthod 1999;17(1):25–30.

[20] Vogelzang NJ, Rusthoven J, Symanowski J, et al. A phase III study of pemetrexed in combination with cisplatin vs. cisplatin alone in patients with malignant pleural mesothelioma. J Clin Orthod 2003;21(14):2636–44.

[21] Bakhshandeh A, Bruns I, Traynor A, et al. Ifosfamide, carboplatin and etoposide combined with 41.8 degrees C whole body hyperthermia for malignant pleural mesothelioma. Lung Cancer 2003;39(3):339–45.

[22] Steele JP, Shamash J, Evans MT, et al. Phase II study of vinorelbine in patients with malignant pleural mesothelioma. J Clin Orthod 2000;18(23):3912–7.

[23] Monetti F, Casanova S, Grasso A, et al. Inadequacy of the new Response Evaluation Criteria in Solid Tumors (RECIST) in patients with malignant pleural mesothelioma: report of four cases. Lung Cancer 2004;43(1):71–4.

[24] van Klaveren RJ, Aerts JGJV, de Bruin H, et al. Inadequacy of the RECIST criteria for response evaluation in patients with malignant pleural mesothelioma. Lung Cancer 2004; 43(1):63–9.

[25] Byrne MJ, Nowak AK. Modified RECIST criteria for assessment of response in malignant pleural mesothelioma. Ann Oncol 2004;15(2):257–60.
[26] Armato III SG, Oxnard GR, MacMahon H, et al. Measurement of mesothelioma on thoracic CT scans: a comparison of manual and computer-assisted techniques. Med Phys 2004;31(5):1105–15.
[27] Hopper KD, Kasales CJ, van Slyke MA, et al. Analysis of interobserver and intraobserver variability in CT tumor measurements. AJR Am J Roentgenol 1996;167(4):851–4.
[28] Thiesse P, Ollivier L, Di Stefano-Louineau D, et al. Response rate accuracy in oncology trials: reasons for interobserver variability. J Clin Orthod 1997;15(12):3507–14.
[29] Schwartz LH, Ginsberg MS, DeCorato D, et al. Evaluation of tumor measurements in oncology: use of film-based and electronic techniques. J Clin Orthod 2000;18(10): 2179–84.
[30] Erasmus JJ, Gladish GW, Broemeling L, et al. Interobserver and intraobserver variability in measurement of non-small-cell carcinoma lung lesions: implications for assessment of tumor response. J Clin Orthod 2003;21(13):2574–82.
[31] Schwartz LH, Mazumdar M, Brown W, et al. Variability in response assessment in solid tumors: effect of number of lesions chosen for measurement. Clin Cancer Res 2003;9(12): 4318–23.
[32] Armato III SG, Ogarek JL, Starkey A, et al. Variability in mesothelioma tumor response classification. AJR Am J Roentgenol, in press.
[33] Sensakovic WF, Armato III SG, Starkey A, et al. Automated matching of temporally sequential CT sections. Med Phys 2004;31(12):3417–24.
[34] Kostis WJ, Reeves AP, Yankelevitz DF, et al. Three-dimensional segmentation and growth-rate estimation of small pulmonary nodules in helical CT images. IEEE Trans Med Imaging 2003;22(10):1259–74.
[35] Tran LN, Brown MS, Goldin JG, et al. Comparison of treatment response classifications between unidimensional, bidimensional, and volumetric measurements of metastatic lung lesions on chest computed tomography. Acad Radiol 2004;11(12):1355–60.
[36] Armato III SG, Oxnard GR, Kocherginsky M, et al. Evaluation of semi-automated measurements of mesothelioma tumor thickness on CT scans. Acad Radiol 2005;12(10):1301–9.
[37] Pass HI, Temeck BK, Kranda K, et al. Phase III randomized trial of surgery with or without intraoperative photodynamic therapy and postoperative immunochemotherapy for malignant pleural mesothelioma. Ann Surg Oncol 1997;4(8):628–33.
[38] Pass HI, Temeck BK, Kranda K, et al. Preoperative tumor volume is associated with outcome in malignant pleural mesothelioma. J Thorac Cardiovasc Surg 1998;115(2):310–7.
[39] Prasad SR, Jhaveri KS, Saini S, et al. CT tumor measurement for therapeutic response assessment: comparison of unidimensional, bidimensional, and volumetric techniques. Initial observations. Radiology 2002;225(2):416–9.

Hematol Oncol Clin N Am 19 (2005) 1067–1087

HEMATOLOGY/ONCOLOGY CLINICS
OF NORTH AMERICA

Nonpleural Mesotheliomas: Mesothelioma of the Peritoneum, Tunica Vaginalis, and Pericardium

Raffit Hassan, MD[a],*, Richard Alexander, MD[b]

[a]Laboratory of Molecular Biology, Center for Cancer Research, National Cancer Institute,
National Institutes of Health, 37 Convent Drive, Room 5116, Bethesda, MD 20892-4264, USA
[b]Surgery Branch, Center for Cancer Research, National Cancer Institute, National Institutes of Health,
Bethesda, MD, USA

Mesotheliomas are tumors that arise from the mesothelial cells of the pleura, peritoneum, pericardium, or tunica vaginalis. Although the number of new mesothelioma cases diagnosed each year in the United States seems to be leveling off or decreasing, several other countries are projected to have continued increased incidence of mesothelioma over the next several years [1,2]. Of the approximately 2500 new cases of mesothelioma in the United States each year, most are pleural mesotheliomas. The peritoneum is the second most common site of mesothelioma development and accounts for approximately 10% to 20% of all mesotheliomas [3]. Mesotheliomas that involve the pericardium or originate from the tunica vaginalis are rare tumors. Given the rarity of these tumors, it is difficult to obtain precise information regarding their incidence, natural history, and optimal management.

PERITONEAL MESOTHELIOMA
Epidemiology
Information regarding incidence of peritoneal mesothelioma in the United States is obtained from the Surveillance, Epidemiology, and End Results (SEER) Program. This database contains information from nine cancer registries from 1973 to 1991 and 11 cancer registries from 1992 to 2000 [4]. A recent analysis of the SEER database estimated approximately 250 new cases of peritoneal mesothelioma each year in the United States [3]. Although the overall incidence of peritoneal mesothelioma was higher in men than women, a higher proportion of women develop mesothelioma that involves the peritoneum compared with men. Peritoneal mesothelioma accounted for 17% of all mesotheliomas in women and 7% of all mesotheliomas in men.

* Corresponding author. E-mail address: hassanr@mail.nih.gov (R. Hassan).

0889-8588/05/$ – see front matter
doi:10.1016/j.hoc.2005.09.005

Published by Elsevier Inc.
hemonc.theclinics.com

Like pleural mesothelioma, exposure to asbestos is also believed to play a role in the development of peritoneal mesothelioma. The evidence that asbestos exposure is related to the development of peritoneal mesothelioma is greater in men than women. In a case control study by Spirtas and colleagues [5], 88% of pleural mesotheliomas and 58% of peritoneal mesotheliomas among men were directly attributable to past asbestos exposure. For women, only 20% of cases (both pleural and peritoneal mesothelioma) were related to past asbestos exposure. In a study using data from the Swedish Cancer Environment Registry, 35 pathologically confirmed cases of peritoneal mesothelioma were noted in gainfully employed Swedish men from 1961 to 1979. Almost 40% of these cases were in men who worked in the construction industry, with insulation workers at especially high risk [6]. An increased risk of peritoneal mesothelioma among insulation workers also has been reported in other studies. In a study that examined the occupational risks for peritoneal cancer using a job-exposure matrix, researchers observed an increased incidence among male insulators and found that the risk increased significantly by probability and intensity of exposure to asbestos [7]. Another study that prospectively followed 17, 800 asbestos insulation workers noted 175 deaths caused by mesothelioma. A higher proportion of these deaths were caused by peritoneal (64%) rather than pleural (36%) mesothelioma [8]. Increased incidence of peritoneal mesothelioma also has been noted in workers at the Wittenoom crocidolite mines of Western Australia, although pleural mesothelioma was seven times more common in these workers than peritoneal mesothelioma [9]. Cases of peritoneal mesothelioma caused by environmental exposure from asbestos contaminated soil in Anatolia, Turkey also have been reported [10].

Many patients who have peritoneal mesothelioma do not report direct or indirect exposure from family members to asbestos, however, and other factors are involved in its causation. A few cases of peritoneal mesothelioma after external beam radiation were described. They usually involved men with a history of testicular carcinoma, although cases of peritoneal mesothelioma after radiation for ovarian teratocarcinoma and cervical cancer have been reported [11–14]. A case of peritoneal mesothelioma after administration of thorotrast also was reported [15]. Although simian virus 40 has been implicated in the causation of some mesotheliomas, its role in the causation of peritoneal mesothelioma is unclear [16].

Pathology

The common tumors to be considered in the pathologic differential diagnosis of peritoneal mesothelioma include ovarian cancer, colon cancer, and other tumors metastatic to the peritoneum. The diagnosis in most cases can be established by immunohistochemistry using a panel of mesothelioma and adenocarcinoma markers [17,18]. In small biopsy specimens, however, it may be difficult to differentiate benign from malignant mesothelial proliferations [19]. It is important that the pathology report accurately describe the subtype of peritoneal mesothelioma, because it has a direct bearing on patient treatment and prognosis. Pathologic features of some of the subtypes of peritoneal mesothelioma are shown in Fig. 1 and briefly described later.

Diffuse Malignant Peritoneal Mesothelioma

Unless otherwise specified, the term "peritoneal mesothelioma" generally refers to diffuse malignant peritoneal mesothelioma that has histologic similarities to pleural mesothelioma [20,21]. Histologically, most of these tumors are epithelial and typically have a characteristic tubulopapillary pattern. These tumors show true signs of malignancy, such as stromal invasion. Immunohistochemical

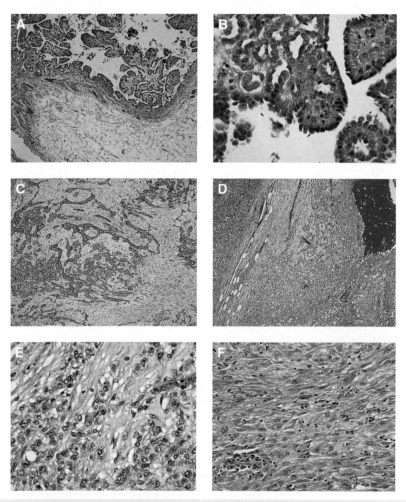

Fig. 1. Histopathology of peritoneal mesothelioma. (*A, B*) Low-grade, tubulopapillary type, without deep tissue invasion or desmoplasia. (*C*) Low-grade, tubulopapillary type, with deep invasion and desmoplasia. (*D, E*) High-grade, epithelioid type, with deep invasion and desmoplasia. (*F*) High-grade, sarcomatoid type. (*A, C,* and *D*, original magnification, ×100; *B* and *E*, original magnification, ×600; *F*, original magnification ×400).

markers similar to those used in pleural mesotheliomas help establish the diagnosis. Peritoneal sarcomatous mesotheliomas are much less common than pleural sarcomatous mesotheliomas.

Deciduoid Peritoneal Mesothelioma

A variant of epithelial diffuse malignant peritoneal mesothelioma, composed of cells with abundant glassy eosinophilic cytoplasm, resembles a decidual reaction [22]. In some cases this variant has been described in patients during or after pregnancy, and researchers believe that pregnancy-induced peritoneal deciduosis and diffuse mesothelial proliferation caused by hormonal changes may be responsible [23]. Cases of deciduous mesothelioma also have been reported in men and elderly women, however [24,25]. The treatment of these patients is similar to that of patients who have diffuse malignant peritoneal mesothelioma, but it is characterized by an aggressive clinical course and poor prognosis.

Well-differentiated Papillary Mesothelioma of the Peritoneum

On pathologic examination, these tumors are characterized by uniform appearance of tumor cells without multilayering and absence of nuclear features of malignancy [21]. It is more common in young women, and patients may present with multiple peritoneal nodules [26,27]. Association with asbestos exposure is not well established [26,28]. In the largest reported series, patients had a prolonged survival, and in view of the favorable prognosis, treatment is generally not recommended unless a patient is symptomatic or there is evidence of tumor progression [26]. There are reports that these lesions can recur or progress to malignant mesothelioma with distant metastases, however [29].

Multicystic (Cystic) Mesothelioma

Typically these patients present with an abdominal or pelvic mass and at the time of surgery are noted to have multiple translucent, grape-like clusters of fluid-filled cysts. On microscopic examination the cysts are lined by a single layer of flattened or cuboidal mesothelial cells [21,30,31]. It is much more common in women than men [32]. In general, these tumors have a benign clinical course but are characterized by a high recurrence rate after surgical resection, and a recent report showed malignant transformation in a patient who had multicystic mesothelioma [33,34]. These tumors are believed to be hormone sensitive, and some case reports have reported reduction in cyst volume and clinical improvement in patients treated with leuprolide and tamoxifen [35,36]. Multicystic mesothelioma of other serosal sites, such as pleura or tunica vaginalis, have been reported [37,38].

Adenomatoid Tumor (Benign Mesothelioma)

The adenomatoid tumor is a benign tumor that arises from the mesothelium and forms gland-like structures. Although these tumors could be confused with carcinomas, the cells do not exhibit nuclear atypia and mitotic figures are absent [21]. The tumors are usually confined to the genital tract, with the epididmyis being the most common site in men and the uterus, fallopian tubes, and ovaries being the most common sites in women. These lesions are generally solitary and less than 2 cm in size. Clinically, patients are asymptomatic, and rarely do the tumors recur after adequate excision [20].

Clinical Presentation

The clinical presentation of patients can be varied, and they may have symptoms and signs for several months before a diagnosis is made. Patients typically present with abdominal distension, pain, bloating, alteration in bowel habits, and weight loss, with ascites present in most patients at diagnosis [39,40]. Occasionally, patients may present with fever [41]. Laboratory studies often show leukocytosis and thrombocytosis [42,43]. There is no reliable tumor marker for the diagnosis and follow-up of patients who have peritoneal mesothelioma. A few case reports have described elevated serum CA-125 in patients with peritoneal mesothelioma, however, which in some instances was associated with a close correlation with tumor response [44–46].

Abdominal and pelvic CT scans are important imaging modalities for the diagnosis and follow-up of patients who have peritoneal mesothelioma [47]. Findings on CT scan can be varied and show ascites, localized disease, or diffuse peritoneal involvement [48,49]. A recent study suggested that the CT scan can be a valuable aid in determining if a patient is a surgical candidate [50]. The role of other imaging modalities, such as positron emission tomography or positron emission tomographic CT in peritoneal mesothelioma, is unclear.

Surgical Treatment Protocols of Cytoreduction and Hyperthermic Chemotherapy

Patients who have peritoneal mesothelioma experience morbidity and mortality almost exclusively secondary to disease progression in the abdominal cavity, and various regional therapeutic strategies have been developed to specifically control this component of disease. In general, regional therapies have the advantage of allowing intensive and directed measures to control tumor while minimizing unnecessary systemic toxicity. Until the later stages of tumor growth, peritoneal mesothelioma usually progresses as a diffuse and superficially spreading condition in the abdominal cavity that, in many circumstances, can be nearly or completely grossly resected by using systematic peritonectomy procedures or local ablative measures. Many investigators have combined intraperitoneal (IP) administration of chemotherapeutics or biologic agents intraoperatively with hyperthermia or as a dwell in the early postoperative period. There are several advantages of continuous hyperthermic peritoneal perfusion (CHPP), also commonly referred to as hyperthermic intraoperative peritoneal chemotherapy. After all or most or the peritoneal tumor has been removed and no adhesions are present is perhaps the optimal time to achieve uniform distribution of topical chemotherapy to a complex surface such as the peritoneal cavity. This timing takes advantage of the well-established pharmacokinetic advantage of IP therapy because the clearance of many drugs from the peritoneum is far less than plasma clearance [51,52]. Conversely, topically applied IP chemotherapy may have unpredictable or incomplete tumor penetration and may have regional toxicity, such as fibrosis [53]. Early postoperative IP chemotherapy, usually administered as a dwell, shares these advantages of intraoperative chemotherapy because it is administered before the development of any intra-abdominal adhesions. Hyperthermia has established direct tumoricidal activity and can augment significantly the cytotoxicity of various chemotherapeutics in experimental models [54,55]. By rapidly recirculating the chemotherapy solution, or perfusate, by using a circuit that consists of a heat exchanger, reservoir, and roller pump, one can achieve moderate levels of hyperthermia in the superficial peritoneal tissues consistently.

The techniques of peritonectomy and CHPP have been described in detail [56]. For patients who have peritoneal mesothelioma, a complete omentectomy is required and en bloc splenectomy or other organ resection is required in almost one third of patients [57]. Small volume gross disease is usually left in situ in most individuals, but by using careful patient selection criteria, the frequency of leaving large (>2 cm) tumor deposits in most series is less than 15%. Formal peritonectomy of the pelvis, lesser sac, and upper quadrants are performed, and implants on the bowel mesentery or serosa are usually treated with electrofulgaration. The technique of CHPP, type and dose of chemotherapy, duration of treatment, and degree of hyperthermia used are not consistent from one series to another. Generally, large-bore catheters are placed at either end of the peritoneal cavity (ie, above the liver and in the pelvis) and are connected to the perfusion circuit. IP temperature probes are used to document the level of hyperthermia. Some investigators advocate the use of an open or "coliseum" technique, in which a plastic sheet is sewn to the fascial edges of the incision and the surgeon's gloved hand is placed through a hole in the sheet to agitate the abdominal contents manually [58]. We and others use a closed system, in which the abdominal fascia is closed temporarily before CHPP. By virtue of the rapid perfusate flow rates and gentle external agitation of the abdominal cavity, distribution of the IP chemotherapy is achieved [57].

Several centers have reported results using operative cytoreduction and CHPP for individuals with peritoneal mesothelioma (Table 1). Despite the fact that there are no standard criteria for patient selection and treatment parameters, the results of these different institutional experiences have been remarkably consistent in some aspects. For example, all the series report a fairly impressive overall survival that seems to be better than the anticipated natural history of the condition, and the ability of this type of therapy to palliate the secondary malignant ascites in most individuals who present with this condition (Fig. 2). Investigators from Columbia-Presbyterian Hospital have reported preliminary results of an intensive regional therapy program that consists of initial surgical debulking, 4 months of IP chemotherapy using cisplatin and doxorubicin, and a second-look procedure to resect residual tumor and apply a CHPP using cisplatin and mitomycin C administered for 1 hour [59]. Because the number of patients is small ($n=3$), meaningful interpretation of complications and outcome is difficult. A series of 19 patients who had benign and malignant peritoneal mesothelioma treated with cytoreduction and CHPP using cisplatin with either mitomycin C or doxorubicin has been reported by investigators from

Table 1
Studies of operative cytoreduction and continuous hyperthermic peritoneal perfusion for treatment of peritoneal mesothelioma

Study [reference]	No. of patients	CHPP agents	Residual disease status	Median survival	Comments
Washington Cancer Institute, 2003 [58]	68	Cisplatin + doxorubicin	60% <2.5 cm	67 mo	OS greater for women than men
National Cancer Institute, 2003 [62]	49	Cisplatin	88% <1 cm	92 mo	OS better for patients ≤60 y; Minimal residual disease; History of previous debulking
Wake Forest University Baptist Medical Center, 2001 [61]	12	MMC	66% <2 cm	34.2 mo	86% ascites palliated
National Cancer Institute of Milan, 2003 [60]	19	Cisplatin + MMC or cisplatin + doxorubicin	75% <2.5 mm	NR	94% ascites palliated

Abbreviations: MMC, mitomycin C; NR, not reported; OS, overall survival.

Pre-CHPP

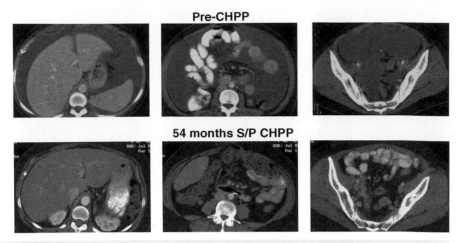

54 months S/P CHPP

Fig. 2. Axial abdominal CT scans show complete resolution of ascites in a patient with malignant mesothelioma after treatment on the National Cancer Institute protocol of tumor resection and CHPP. (*Top panels*) Pre-CHPP. (*Bottom panels*) Fifty-four months after CHPP.

the National Cancer Institute of Milan [60]. They quantitated area under the curve ratios for the various drugs that were indicated for use between 60 and 90 minutes under hyperthermic conditions and observed favorable concentrations ratios (IP versus systemic) of 23.5 for mitomycin C, 500 for doxorubicin, and 14 for cisplatin. The 3-year actuarial survival rate was 69% at a mean follow-up of 27 months. Of note, 94% of patients had complete resolution of their malignant ascites for the duration of their follow-up. A comparably sized series also was reported by investigators from Wake Forest University [61]. In their cohort of 12 patients, all of whom had malignant mesothelioma, treatment consisted of cytoreduction and a 2-hour CHPP using 30 mg of mitomycin C and another 10 mg added after 1 hour of perfusion. Median survival was 34.2 months with a median follow-up of 45 months, and 86% of patients had permanent control of malignant ascites.

The two largest series were reported from the Washington Hospital Center and the National Cancer Institute in Bethesda, Maryland. The Washington Hospital Center series consisted of 68 patients, some of whom had systemic metastases, who were treated over a 15-year interval (1989–2003). Fifty-five of these patients were treated with cytoreduction and various regimens of CHPP using cisplatin and doxorubicin with or without early postoperative IP chemotherapy consisting of IP paclitaxel [58]. The median overall survival of all 68 patients was 67 months, and in this series only 47% of patients had resolution of ascites. Of note, women had a significantly longer survival than men but also presented to the Washington Hospital Center with a longer time interval between diagnosis and treatment and a smaller burden of disease. The National Cancer Institute reported results in 49 patients with malignant peritoneal mesothelioma treated with cytoreduction and CHPP using cisplatin administered for 90 minutes [62]. Thirty-five patients also received early postoperative IP dwell with paclitaxel and 5-fluorouracil. At a median follow-up time of 28 months, the median overall survival was 92 months. Fifteen of 26 patients who presented with ascites had palliation for a median duration of 25 months. Using a backward selection process, an analysis was performed of the data to identify prognostic factors that were independently and significantly associated with progression-free or overall survival. For progression-free survival, the presence of deep invasion, defined as invasion of tumor more than 0.5 mm from a defined mesothelial surface, and no history of a previous debulking procedure were adverse prognostic factors associated with short progression-free survival (Table 2). With respect to overall survival, those two factors plus age older than 60 years and residual disease masses at the end of cytoreduction larger than 1 cm in diameter were significantly associated with poor outcome (Fig. 3).

Although morbidities after cytoreduction and CHPP are related to the operative procedure and chemotherapy, most treatment mortalities seem to be related primarily to the extent of the operative procedure rather than IP chemotherapy and range from 0% to 7% [60,62]. For example, in the series from the Washington Hospital Center, mortalities were secondary to postoperative sepsis or pulmonary embolism. Morbidities are related to the operation and chemotherapy; most series report a complication rate of approximately 25%. Careful patient selection and the use IP chemotherapy regimens established in carefully designed clinical trials serve to minimize morbidity and mortality. The extent of surgical procedure (ie, concomitant organ resection or routine total peritonectomy) necessary for prolonged survival is not known. Most series indicate that complete gross cytoreduction is achieved in only 15% to 20% of operations; however, minimal gross residual disease (ie, all tumor nodules <1 cm) has been identified as an independent predictor of good outcome [62]. Despite the

Table 2
Adverse prognostic significance of clinicopathologic variables based on Cox Proportional Hazards Model Analysis

End point	Variable (in terms of poor prognosis)	Parameter estimate	SE	P	Hazard ratio	95% CI
Progression-free survival	No previous debulking versus debulking	1.55	0.43	.0003	4.70	2.02–10.9
	Deep invasion versus no deep invasion	1.28	0.44	.003	3.60	1.53–8.48
Overall survival	Age >60 y versus ≤60 y	1.29	0.61	.034	3.65	1.10–12.1
	No previous debulking versus debulking	1.67	0.80	.036	5.33	1.12–25.4
	Deep invasion versus no deep invasion	1.44	0.71	.041	4.24	1.06–16.9
	Residual disease >1 cm versus none <1 cm	1.75	0.82	.032	5.76	1.16–28.5

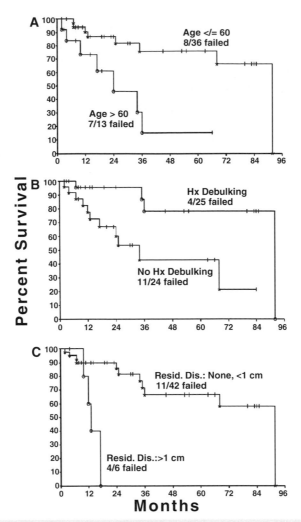

Fig. 3. Effects of (A) age, (B) history (Hx) of previous debulking, and (C) status of residual disease after debulking on overall survival after treatment, for patients treated on the National Cancer Institute protocol of cytoreduction and CHPP.

intensity of this form of therapy, quality-of-life measures after cytoreduction and CHPP have been reported. Investigators from Wake Forest University reported that 10 of 17 patients who had survived more than 3 years after surgery and CHPP reported their health as good or better, and 90% of the entire group reported no limitations on moderate activity [63]. In 10 patients for whom pretreatment quality-of-life data were available, there was a significant improvement in physical and functional senses of well-being. The National Cancer Institute reported results of an analysis of health-related quality of life in patients who underwent laparotomy and CHPP [64]. Seventy-three patients were prospectively studied with standard tools to assess mental and physical well-being at baseline (pretreatment) and at regular intervals during a follow-up interval of almost 1 year. The physical scores were lower at 6 weeks after treatment, which reflected the impact of the surgical procedure on quality of life; however, physical and mental quality of life and FACT-C scores showed a significant and sustained improvement over baseline after 3 months throughout the study.

Taken together, these studies demonstrate that in selected patients, the use of surgical resection and CHPP can palliate ascites and is associated with long-term survival and improved quality of life in many individuals. Additional studies are being conducted to refine and improve this type of approach further for patients who have peritoneal mesothelioma.

Intraperitoneal and Systemic Chemotherapy for Peritoneal Mesothelioma

Because all newly diagnosed patients who have peritoneal mesothelioma are not candidates for surgery and many of the patients treated with surgery ultimately relapse, these patients are candidates for systemic chemotherapy or phase I studies. The optimal chemotherapeutic regimen or route of drug administration (IP versus intravenous) for treatment of peritoneal mesothelioma is unclear because there have been no prospectively designed clinical trials specific for this disease. Treatment regimens that have been used incorporate drugs that have shown some activity in pleural mesothelioma.

Because the disease is mostly confined to the peritoneal cavity, several studies have evaluated IP chemotherapy in peritoneal mesotheliomas because it has the potential advantage of increased drug concentration in the peritoneal cavity with less systemic toxicity [51,65]. The drawbacks of this approach include poor penetration in tumors >1 cm and the need for an indwelling catheter, however, with risk of complications including infection and blockage [66]. IP chemotherapeutic agents that have been used include cisplatin, mitomycin, 5-fluouracil, adriamycin, and taxol [65]. In one of the largest studies of IP chemotherapy in peritoneal mesothelioma, 19 patients were treated with IP administration of cisplatin (100 mg/m^2 every 28 days) and mitomycin (5–10 mg/treatment given 7 days after each IP administration of cisplatin) [67]. Of the 15 patients with malignant ascites, 7 (47%) experienced control of fluid reaccumulation that ranged from 2 to more than 73 months. Four patients survived more than 3 years from the initiation of therapy. No objective tumor responses were noted. This study showed that a subset of patients who had peritoneal mesothelioma with small volume disease after surgical resection might benefit from IP chemotherapy, especially in terms of decreasing fluid collection. Another study of IP cisplatin and etoposide in patients who had peritoneal mesothelioma showed a median survival of 22 months in patients whose tumor was debulked to less than 2 cm before administration of chemotherapy compared with a median survival of 5 months for patients with measurable surgically inaccessible disease [68]. This study, like the Markman study [67], showed that cisplatin-based IP chemotherapy may be of value in patients with decreased tumor bulk after cytoreductive surgery.

Initial studies of systemic chemotherapy in peritoneal mesothelioma evaluated doxorubicin-containing regimens that showed some activity but also significant toxicity [41]. A recent study tested the combination of cisplatin and irinotecan in peritoneal mesothelioma. In a retrospective review of 17 patients treated at a single institution, patients received the combination of intravenous (IV) or IP cisplatin, 50 or 60 mg/m^2, on day 1 and irinotecan, 50 or 60 mg/m^2 IV, on days 1, 8, and 15 given every 4 weeks for 6 cycles [69]. Fifteen patients received two or more cycles of treatment, and 8 patients each received IV or IP cisplatin, whereas 1 patient received both IV and IP cisplatin. The treatment was well tolerated, with toxicity consisting predominately of nausea, emesis, granulocytopenia, and anemia. The overall response rate was 24%, with 4 patients achieving a partial response and 9 patients having stable disease.

Based on the results of the phase III clinical trial of cisplatin plus pemetrexed versus cisplatin alone in pleural mesothelioma that showed an increased response rate and an increase in overall survival in favor of the combination, many oncologists also would consider this regimen for the treatment of patients who have peritoneal mesothelioma who are not surgical candidates or who experience relapse after surgery [70]. There is no published information on the effectiveness of this combination in peritoneal mesothelioma except for the preliminary results of the Eli Lilly and Company–sponsored expanded access program for pemetrexed [71]. This nonrandomized study started in June 2002 and was designed to obtain additional efficacy and safety data on pemetrexed alone or in combination with cisplatin in mesotheliomas. Of the 1056 patients who had mesothelioma who were treated on this study, 98 (9.2%) had peritoneal mesothelioma. Newly diagnosed patients were treated with a combination of cisplatin, 75 mg/m^2, and pemetrexed, 500 mg/m^2, given every 21 days for a maximum of six cycles. Patients who received prior treatment were treated with pemetrexed alone. Of the 73 patients who had peritoneal mesothelioma who were evaluable for response, there were 4 complete and 15 partial responses for an overall objective response rate of 26%. The proportion of these responses in patients who received the combination treatment versus patients treated with pemetrexed alone was not described. From these limited data it is difficult to make any definitive conclusions except that pemetrexed and cisplatin seem to have activity in peritoneal mesothelioma that merits further investigation.

Radiation and Biologic Agents for Treatment of Peritoneal Mesothelioma

The role of radiation alone for the treatment of peritoneal mesothelioma is unclear. It has been evaluated as a component of aggressive treatment strategies consisting of surgery, chemotherapy, and whole abdominal radiotherapy, however. This approach is based on the initial results seen in a small number of patients treated at Dana-Farber Cancer Institute in the early 1980s [72]. Of the 14 patients with malignant peritoneal mesothelioma treated at that institute between 1982 and 1984, 6 patients had nonbulky disease limited to the peritoneal cavity. These patients underwent surgery with omentectomy with maximal tumor resection, followed by IP and IV chemotherapy and 30 Gy whole abdominal radiotherapy in 5 of the 6 patients. All 6 of these patients were alive at 9 to 36 months with no evidence of disease by CT scan. In a retrospective report from the same institute on patients who had peritoneal mesothelioma who were seen between 1984 and 1999, treatment details were available for 17 patients with early-stage mesothelioma. These patients underwent cytoreductive surgery followed by IP chemotherapy with doxorubicin and cisplatin. Of the 11 patients who had a response, further treatment with 30 Gy total abdominal radiation ($n=3$), IV chemotherapy ($n=3$), or both ($n=4$) was administered. The median survival of this group of patients was 27.6 months [73]. Taub and colleagues [74] at Columbia University College of Physicians and Surgeons recently presented results of their prospectively designed clinical trial of surgery, chemotherapy, immunotherapy, and whole abdominal radiotherapy in patients who have peritoneal mesothelioma. The treatment regimen consisted of surgical debulking followed by IP administration of doxorubicin, cisplatin, and gamma interferon, second laparotomy with attempted resection of any residual disease and intraoperative hyperthermic perfusion with cisplatin and mitomycin followed subsequently by whole abdominal radiotherapy. The median overall survival of the 27 patients treated on this study was 68 months. The contribution of radiotherapy to the improved overall survival of these patients is unclear because these results are not significantly different from other surgical series using cytoreduction and CHPP without radiation [58,62].

Some patients who have peritoneal mesothelioma have been treated with biologic agents usually as part of phase I studies. In a phase I study of IP administration of recombinant human interleukin-12 in patients with peritoneal carcinomatosis a complete response was noted in a patient with epithelial papillary mesothelioma [75]. In a phase I study of Flt3 ligand administered IP or subcutaneous no responses were noted in the four patients with peritoneal mesothelioma treated on the study [76]. Other biologic therapies, including immunotoxins that target the tumor antigen mesothelin, are also undergoing clinical evaluation in patients who have peritoneal mesothelioma [77].

Prognosis

The prognosis of peritoneal mesothelioma depends on tumor histology. It is important to separate diffuse malignant mesothelioma from the well-differentiated papillary mesotheliomas that usually have indolent behavior and therefore a prolonged survival [26]. Patients who have solitary tumors have a better prognosis than patients who have diffuse disease [78]. In patients who have resectable disease who undergo extensive tumor debulking followed by intraoperative hyperthermic chemotherapy the median overall survival is longer than 5 years [58,62]. These data are similar to an earlier report showing that patients with nonbulky disease who underwent surgical debulking and IP and IV chemotherapy followed by whole abdominal radiotherapy had prolonged survival [72].

Many patients are not candidates for surgical resection, however, and prognosis of such patients is not clear. Some studies have suggested that in contrast to pleural mesothelioma, which has a uniformly poor prognosis, the prognosis of patients with diffuse epithelial peritoneal mesothelioma is varied. In a retrospective study of 25 patients who had peritoneal mesothelioma, the patients were divided into two groups based on survival less than or longer than 4 years [79]. The median survival of the short-term survivors (ie, <4 years) was 12 months, whereas for the 10 long-term survivors the median survival was 7 years. Although complete information regarding the surgical and postoperative treatment was not available in all cases, it seemed that the differences in survival in the two groups were independent of the treatments received. This finding suggests that a proportion of patients with peritoneal mesothelioma have prolonged survival, which is in contrast to pleural mesothelioma, in which few long-term survivors are seen.

MESOTHELIOMA OF THE TUNICA VAGINALIS

During normal embryonic development, an outpouching of the peritoneum traverses through the inguinal canal as processus vaginalis and surrounds the testis. The processus vaginalis then atrophies, except the portion that surrounds the testis, and is called the tunica vaginalis [80]. Histologically the cells that line the tunica vaginalis are similar to those that line the pleura, peritoneum, and pericardium and are at risk of developing mesothelioma. Tunica vaginalis mesotheliomas are rare tumors and are mostly reported in the literature as case reports, with Barbera and Rubino [81] first describing a case in 1957. A detailed review of this tumor was published by Plas and colleagues [82], who reviewed the world literature from 1966 to 1997 and found 73 case reports during that time period. Of the 11,629 malignant mesothelioma deaths recorded in the UK Health and Safety Executive Mesothelioma Register from 1968 to 1991, only 0.09% of the deaths were caused by mesothelioma of the tunica vaginalis [83].

Epidemiology and Clinical Presentation

Some case reports and reviews on this subject have noted an association between asbestos exposure and development of the tumor. Antman and colleagues [84] described six cases of tunica vaginalis mesothelioma, in which four cases had previous exposure to asbestos. There was a latent period of 8 to 40 years from the first exposure to asbestos and development of mesothelioma. In a report by Jones and colleagues [85] of 27 cases of tunica vaginalis mesothelioma, a positive occupational history for asbestos exposure was noted in 41% of the cases. In the review by Plas and colleagues [82] of 73 cases of tunica vaginalis testis reported in the literature, a positive history of exposure to asbestos was present in 34% of the cases.

Although the peak incidence of tunica vaginalis mesotheliomas is in men older than 50 years, approximately 10% of the cases occur in men younger than 25 years [82]. It usually presents as a unilateral testicular mass, with the most common preoperative diagnosis being a hydrocele or testicular tumor. At the time of surgery the tumor typically presents as papillary exophytic excrescences of the tunica vaginalis, although it also can invade the adjacent structures. The right and left tunica vaginalis are involved in equal proportion, with bilateral tunica vaginalis mesothelioma being rare [82]. Although the typical presentation is that of a local testicular mass, in rare cases the mesothelioma can spread to draining lymph nodes, peritoneum, and the liver [84,86,87].

Treatment and Prognosis

Given the rarity of the disease, it is difficult to develop treatment guidelines based on clinical protocols developed specifically for this tumor. Treatments are based on those used for mesothelioma at other and as anecdotal case reports [88]. Surgery is the treatment of choice, especially in patients with a localized tumor. The type of surgery performed bears a relationship to local tumor recurrence. In patients who undergo only resection of the hydrocele wall, the recurrence rate is as high as 35.7% compared with recurrence rates of 10.5% and 11.5% after scrotal and inguinal orchiectomy, respectively [82]. Because preoperative diagnosis is often difficult, most surgeons approach this as a testicular tumor and perform an inguinal orchiectomy, which avoids disruption of the scrotal lymphatics and allows complete removal of the spermatic cord [88]. In cases in which biopsy or hydrocele surgery was performed initially, hemiscrotectomy and inguinal orchiectomy are recommended. The role of adjuvant therapy after surgery is not clear. In patients who are not surgical candidates or have tumor recurrence and metastatic disease, chemotherapy has been used with little benefit [84,89]. Given the activity of cisplatin and pemetrexed combination in pleural mesothelioma, evaluation of this regimen in tunica vaginalis mesothelioma is appropriate.

Individual case reports vary in the prognosis of patients, with some researchers noting prolonged survival after surgery and others reporting aggressive behavior of the tumor. In the review of 73 patients with malignant mesothelioma of the tunica vaginalis, Plas and colleagues [82] noted a median survival of 23 months and an overall recurrence rate (local and distant) of 52.5%, with most of these recurrences occurring in the first 2 years of follow-up. Tumor recurrences as late as 5 to 10 years from diagnosis have been reported, however [84]. In the review by Plas and colleagues [82], the most important prognostic factor for survival was patient age at diagnosis, with significantly better survival in patients younger than 60 years compared with patients older than 60 years ($P<.01$). An aggressive clinical course with recurrent local disease and systemic metastasis has been noted in some young patients, however [86].

PERICARDIAL MESOTHELIOMA

Although pericardial mesothelioma is a rare tumor with only a few hundred cases reported in the literature, it is one of the commonest pericardial tumors [90]. In an autopsy series of 500,000 cases, the incidence of pericardial mesothelioma was $<0.0022\%$ [91]. Most of these tumors are diagnosed postmortem. In a review of 140 cases of pericardial mesothelioma, Kaul and colleagues [92] noted that antemortem diagnosis was made in only 40 (28.5%) cases. Some published series reported prior occupational exposure to asbestos in many of these patients, which suggested that like mesotheliomas at other sites, asbestos also may play a role in the development of pericardial mesotheliomas [93–95]. There have been case reports of pericardial mesothelioma occurring after mantle field radiotherapy for Hodgkin's disease [96].

The median age of patients who have pericardial mesothelioma at presentation is 48 years (range, 12–77 years), with a male-to-female ratio of 2:1 [97]. The clinical presentation can be varied to include symptoms of dyspnea, fever, and night sweats [92,97]. Patients also can develop signs of congestive heart failure or constrictive pericarditis because the tumor encases the heart [98,99]. Occasionally patients present with pericardial effusion with or without tampo-nade or acute myocardial infarction [100,101]. Given the diffuse nature of the disease, imaging studies, such as echocardiography and CT, may fail to reveal the tumor [102]. Some case reports suggest that MRI might be a better modality for diagnosing this tumor [103].

Pericardial mesothelioma is an aggressive disease with poor prognosis, and most patients die within a few months of diagnosis [92,97]. Surgical excision can result in temporary relief of symptoms, and except in cases with a discrete tumor mass, it is difficult to excise the tumor completely [104,105]. In cases in which chemotherapy or radiotherapy was used, little clinical benefit was observed [92,97].

References

[1] Weill H, Hughes JM, Churg AM. Changing trends in US mesothelioma incidence. Occup Environ Med 2004;61(5):438–41.
[2] Peto J, Decarli A, La Vecchia C, et al. The European mesothelioma epidemic. Br J Cancer 1999;79(3–4):666–72.
[3] Price B, Ware A. Mesothelioma trends in the United States: an update based on surveillance, epidemiology, and end results program data from 1973 through 2003. Am J Epidemiol 2004;159(2):107–12.
[4] National Cancer Institute. The Surveillance Epidemiology and End Results (SEER) program. Available at: http://seer.cancer.gov. Accessed May 4, 2005.
[5] Spirtas R, Heineman EF, Bernstein L, et al. Malignant mesothelioma: attributable risk of asbestos exposure. Occup Environ Med 1994;51(12):804–11.
[6] Malker HS, McLaughlin JK, Weiner JA, et al. Peritoneal mesothelioma in the construction industry in Sweden. J Occup Med 1987;29(12):979–80.
[7] Cocco P, Dosemeci M. Peritoneal cancer and occupational exposure to asbestos: results from the application of a job-exposure matrix. Am J Ind Med 1999;35(1):9–14.
[8] Selikoff IJ, Hammond EC, Seidman H. Mortality experience of insulation workers in the United States and Canada, 1943–1976. Ann NY Acad Sci 1979;330:91–116.
[9] Berry G, de Klerk NH, Reid A, et al. Malignant pleural and peritoneal mesotheliomas in former miners and millers of crocidolite at Wittenoom, Western Australia. Occup Environ Med 2004;61(4):e14.
[10] Manavoglu O, Orhan B, Evrensel T, et al. Malignant peritoneal mesothelioma following asbestos exposure. J Environ Pathol Toxicol Oncol 1996;15(2–4):191–4.
[11] Antman K, Corson JM, Li FP, et al. Malignant mesothelioma following radiation exposure. J Clin Oncol 1983;1(11):695–700.

[12] Amin A, Mason C, Rowe P. Diffuse malignant mesothelioma of the peritoneum following abdominal radiotherapy. Eur J Surg Oncol 2001;27(2):214–5.

[13] Gilks B, Hegedus C, Freeman H, et al. Malignant peritoneal mesothelioma after remote abdominal radiation. Cancer 1988;61(10):2019–21.

[14] Babcock TL, Powell DH, Bothwell RS. Radiation-induced peritoneal mesothelioma. J Surg Oncol 1976;8(5):369–72.

[15] Maurer R, Egloff B. Malignant peritoneal mesothelioma after cholangiography with thorotrast. Cancer 1975;36(4):1381–5.

[16] Shah KV. Causality of mesothelioma: SV40 question. Thorac Surg Clin 2004;14(4): 497–504.

[17] Ordonez NG. Role of immunohistochemistry in distinguishing epithelial peritoneal mesotheliomas from peritoneal and ovarian serous carcinomas. Am J Surg Pathol 1998;22(10):1203–14.

[18] Bollinger DJ, Wick MR, Dehner LP, et al. Peritoneal malignant mesotheliomas versus serous papillary adenocarcinoma: a histochemical and immunohistochemical comparison. Am J Surg Pathol 1989;13(8):659–70.

[19] Churg A, Colby TV, Cagle P, et al. The separation of benign and malignant mesothelial proliferations. Am J Surg Pathol 2000;24(9):1183–200.

[20] Clement PB. Diseases of the peritoneum (including endometriosis). In: Kurman RJ, editor. Blaustein's pathology of the female genital tract. New York: Springer-Verlag; 1994. p. 647–703.

[21] Mok SC, Schorge JO, Welch WR, et al. Peritoneal tumours. In: Tavassoli FA, Devilee P, editors. World Health Organization classification of tumours: pathology and genetics of tumours of the breast and female genital organs. Lyons (France): IARC Press; 2003. p. 197–202.

[22] Nascimento AG, Keeney GL, Fletcher CD. Deciduoid peritoneal mesothelioma: an unusual phenotype affecting young females. Am J Surg Pathol 1994;18(5):439–45.

[23] Urbanczyk K, Hajduk A, Stachura J. Pregnancy-associated diffuse malignant fibrous mesothelioma of peritoneum: immunohistochemical studies of ectopic decidual reaction and concomitant myofibroblastic and mesothelial proliferations. Pol J Pathol 1996;47(4): 233–7.

[24] Sugarbaker PH, Acherman YIZ, Brun E. Deciduoid peritoneal mesothelioma. Contemp Surg 2002;58(7):341–6.

[25] Shanks JH, Harris M, Barerjee SS, et al. Mesotheliomas with deciduoid morphology: a morphologic spectrum and a variant not confined to young females. Am J Surg Pathol 2000;24(2):285–94.

[26] Daya D, McCaughey WT. Well-differentiated papillary mesothelioma of the peritoneum: a clinicopathologic study of 22 cases. Cancer 1990;65(2):292–6.

[27] Wunsch L, Flemming P, Reiter A. Long-term follow-up of a well-differentiated mesothelioma of the peritoneum in a 2-year-old girl. Med Pediatr Oncol 1998;31(2):123–4.

[28] Hoekman K, Tognon G, Risse EK, et al. Well-differentiated papillary mesothelioma of the peritoneum: a separate entity. Eur J Cancer 1996;32A(2):255–8.

[29] Burrig KF, Pfitzer P, Hort W. Well-differentiated papillary mesothelioma of the peritoneum: a borderline mesothelioma: report of two cases and review of literature. Virchows Arch A Pathol Anat Histopathol 1990;417(5):443–7.

[30] Sawh RN, Malpica A, Deavers MT, et al. Benign cystic mesothelioma of the peritoneum: a clinicopathologic study of 17 cases and immunohistochemical analysis of estrogen and progesterone receptor status. Hum Pathol 2003;34(4):369–74.

[31] van Ruth S, Bronkhorst MW, van Coevorden F, et al. Peritoneal benign cystic mesothelioma: a case report and review of the literature. Eur J Surg Oncol 2002;28(2):192–5.

[32] Weiss SW, Tavassoli FA. Multicystic mesothelioma: an analysis of pathologic findings and biologic behavior in 37 cases. Am J Surg Pathol 1988;12(10):737–46.

[33] Horn LC, Schutz A, Heinemann K, et al. Multicystic peritoneal mesothelioma of the omentum. Eur J Obstet Gynecol Reprod Biol 2004;116(2):246–7.

[34] Gonzalez-Moreno S, Yan H, Alcorn KW, et al. Malignant transformation of "benign" cystic mesothelioma of the peritoneum. J Surg Oncol 2002;79(4):243–51.

[35] Letterie GS, Yon JL. Use of a long-acting GnRH agonist for benign cystic mesothelioma. Obstet Gynecol 1995;85(5, Pt 2):901–3.

[36] Letterie GS, Yon JL. The antiestrogen tamoxifen in the treatment of recurrent benign cystic mesothelioma. Gynecol Oncol 1998;70(1):131–3.

[37] Ball NJ, Urbanski SJ, Green FH, et al. Pleural multicystic mesothelial proliferation: the so-called multicystic mesothelioma. Am J Surg Pathol 1990;14(4):375–8.

[38] Lane TM, Wilde M, Schofield J, et al. Benign cystic mesothelioma of the tunica vaginalis. BJU Int 1999;84(4):533–4.

[39] Acherman YI, Welch LS, Bromley CM, et al. Clinical presentation of peritoneal meso-thelioma. Tumori 2003;89(3):269–73.

[40] van Gelder T, Hoogsteden HC, Versnel MA, et al. Malignant peritoneal mesothelioma: a series of 19 cases. Digestion 1989;43(4):222–7.

[41] Antman KH, Pomfret EA, Aisner J, et al. Peritoneal mesothelioma: natural history and response to chemotherapy. J Clin Oncol 1983;1(6):386–91.

[42] Melero M, Lloveras J, Waisman H, et al. Malignant peritoneal mesothelioma: an infrequent cause of prolonged fever syndrome and leukocytosis in a young adult. Medicina (B Aires) 1995;55(1):48–50.

[43] Jori GP, Turrisi E, Perrone Donnorso R. Thrombocytosis with peritoneal mesothelioma. Lancet 1968;2(7565):463.

[44] Simsek H, Kadayifci A, Okan E. High serum level of CA125 in malignant peritoneal mesothelioma. Eur J Cancer 1995;31A(1):129.

[45] Almudevar Bercero E, Garcia-Rostan Perez GM, Garcia Bragado F, et al. Prognostic value of high serum levels of CA125 in malignant secretory peritoneal mesotheliomas affecting young women: a case report with differential diagnosis and review of the literature. Histopathology 1997;31(3):267–73.

[46] Simsek H, Kadayifci A, Okan E. Importance of serum CA125 levels in malignant peritoneal mesothelioma. Tumour Biol 1996;17(1):1–4.

[47] Whitley NO, Brenner DE, Antman KH, et al. CT of peritoneal mesothelioma: analysis of eight cases. AJR Am J Roentgenol 1982;138(3):531–5.

[48] Kebapci M, Vardareli E, Adapinar B, et al. CT findings and serum ca 125 levels in malignant peritoneal mesothelioma: report of 11 new cases and review of the literature. Eur Radiol 2003;13(12):2620–6.

[49] Smith TR. Malignant peritoneal mesothelioma: marked variability of CT findings. Abdom Imaging 1994;19(1):27–9.

[50] Yan TD, Haveric N, Carmignani CP, et al. Abdominal computed tomography scans in the selection of patients with malignant peritoneal mesothelioma for comprehensive treatment with cytoreductive surgery and perioperative intraperitoneal chemotherapy. Cancer 2005;103(4):839–49.

[51] Markman M. Intraperitoneal belly bath´chemotherapy. In: Lokich J, editor. Cancer chemotherapy by infusion. 2nd edition. Chicago: Precept Press; 1990. p. 552–74.

[52] Dedrick RL. Theoretical and experimental bases of intraperitoneal chemotherapy. Semin Oncol 1985;12(3 Suppl 4):1–6.

[53] Dedrick RL, Flessner MF. Pharmacokinetic problems in peritoneal drug administration: tissue penetration and surface exposure. J Natl Cancer Inst 1997;89(7):480–7.

[54] Barlogie B, Corry PM, Drewinko B. In vitro thermochemotherapy of human colon cancer cells with cis-dichlorodiammineplatinum (II) and mitomycin C. Cancer Res 1980;40(4):1165–8.

[55] Miller RC, Richards M, Baird C, et al. Interaction of hyperthermia and chemotherapy agents: cell lethality and oncogenic potential. Int J Hyperthermia 1994;10(1):89–99.

[56] Sugarbaker PH. Peritonectomy procedures. Surg Oncol Clin N Am 2003;12(3):703–27.

[57] Alexander HR, Buell JF, Fraker DL. Rationale and clinical status of continuous hy-perthermic peritoneal perfusion (CHPP) for the treatment of peritoneal carcinomatosis.

In: DeVita V, Hellman S, Rosenberg S, editors. Principles and practices of oncology up-
dates. 9th edition. Philadelphia: JB Lippincott; 1995. p. 1–9.

[58] Sugarbaker PH, Welch LS, Mohamed F, et al. A review of peritoneal mesothelioma
at the Washington Cancer Institute. Surg Oncol Clin N Am 2003;12(3):605–21, xi.

[59] Mongero LB, Beck JR, Kroslowitz RM, et al. Treatment of primary peritoneal mesothelioma by hyperthermic intraperitoneal chemotherapy. Perfusion 1999;14(2):141–5.

[60] Deraco M, Casali P, Inglese MG, et al. Peritoneal mesothelioma treated by induction
chemotherapy, cytoreductive surgery, and intraperitoneal hyperthermic perfusion. J Surg
Oncol 2003;83(3):147–53.

[61] Loggie BW, Fleming RA, McQuellon RP, et al. Prospective trial for the treatment of
malignant peritoneal mesothelioma. Am Surg 2001;67(10):999–1003.

[62] Feldman AL, Libutti SK, Pingpank JF, et al. Analysis of factors associated with outcome
in patients with malignant peritoneal mesothelioma undergoing surgical debulking and
intraperitoneal chemotherapy. J Clin Oncol 2003;21(24):4560–7.

[63] McQuellon RP, Loggie BW, Lehman AB, et al. Long-term survivorship and quality of life
after cytoreductive surgery plus intraperitoneal hyperthermic chemotherapy for peritoneal
carcinomatosis. Ann Surg Oncol 2003;10(2):155–62.

[64] Dan A, Saha S, Wiese D, et al. Upstaging of early colon cancer (T1 & T2) by sentinel
lymph node (SLN) mapping. Ann Surg Oncol 2004;11(Suppl 2):S109–10.

[65] Vlasveld LT, Gallee MP, Rodenhuis S, et al. Intraperitoneal chemotherapy for malignant
peritoneal mesothelioma. Eur J Cancer 1991;27(6):732–4.

[66] Los G, Mutsaers PH, van der Vijgh WJ, et al. Direct diffusion of cis-diamminedichloro-
platinum (II) in intraperitoneal rat tumors after intraperitoneal chemotherapy: compari
son with systemic chemotherapy. Cancer Res 1989;49(12):3380–4.

[67] Markman M, Kelsen D. Efficacy of cisplatin-based intraperitoneal chemotherapy as
treatment of malignant peritoneal mesothelioma. J Cancer Res Clin Oncol 1992;118(7):
547–50.

[68] Langer CJ, Rosenblum N, Hogan M, et al. Intraperitoneal cisplatin and etoposide in
peritoneal mesothelioma: favorable outcome with a multimodality approach. Cancer
Chemother Pharmacol 1993;32(3):204–8.

[69] Le DT, Deavers M, Hunt K, et al. Cisplatin and irinotecan (CPT-11) for peritoneal
mesothelioma. Cancer Invest 2003;21(5):682–9.

[70] Vogelzang NJ, Rusthoven JJ, Symanowski J, et al. Phase III study of pemetrexed in
combination with cisplatin versus cisplatin alone in patients with malignant pleural
mesothelioma. J Clin Oncol 2003;21(14):2636–44.

[71] Bloss J, Wozniak TF, Janne PA, et al. Survival update on a subset of peritoneal mesothelioma (PM) patients in an expanded access program (EAP) of pemetrexed (P) alone
or combined with cisplatin in the treatment of malignant mesothelioma (MM). In:
2005 ASCO Annual Meeting Proceedings, Orlando, 2005. J Clin Oncol 2005;
23(16S Part I):663s.

[72] Antman KH, Osteen RT, Klegar KL, et al. Early peritoneal mesothelioma: a treatable
malignancy. Lancet 1985;2(8462):977–81.

[73] Waxman AK, Gos GA, Merriam P, et al. Survival for patients with peritoneal mesothelioma: aggressive multimodality therapy for early stage disease [abstract 2223].
Proc Am Soc Clin Oncol 2000;19:564a.

[74] Taub RN, Hesdorffer ME, Keohan ML, et al. Combined resection, intraperitoneal
chemotherapy, and whole abdominal radiation for malignant peritoneal mesothelioma
(MPM). In: 2005 ASCO Annual Meeting Proceedings, Orlando, 2005. J Clin Oncol
2005;23(16S Part I):664s.

[75] Lenzi R, Rosenblum M, Verschraegen C, et al. Phase I study of intraperitoneal recombinant human interleukin 12 in patients with müllerian carcinoma, gastrointestinal
primary malignancies and mesothelioma. Clin Cancer Res 2002;8(12):3686–95.

[76] Freedman RS, Vadhan-Rai S, Butts C, et al. Pilot study of Flt3 ligand comparing intraperitoneal with subcutaneous routes on hematologic and immunologic responses in pa-

tients with peritoneal carcinomatosis and mesotheliomas. Clin Cancer Res 2003;9(14): 5228–37.

[77] Hassan R, Bera T, Pastan I. Mesothelin: a new target for immunotherapy. Clin Cancer Res 2004;10(12 Pt 1):3937–42.

[78] Goldblum J, Hart WR. Localized and diffuse mesotheliomas of the genital tract and peritoneum in women: a clinicopathological study of nineteen true mesothelial neoplasms other than adenomatoid tumors, multicystic mesotheliomas and localized fibrous tumors. Am J Surg Pathol 1995;19(10):1124–37.

[79] Kerrigan SA, Turnnir RT, Clement PB, et al. Diffuse malignant epithelial mesotheliomas of the peritoneum in women: a clinicopathologic study of 25 patients. Cancer 2002; 94(2):378–85.

[80] Heyns CF. The gubernaculum during testicular descent in the human fetus. J Anat 1987;153:93–112.

[81] Barbera V, Rubino M. Papillary mesothelioma of the tunica vaginalis. Cancer 1957; 10(1):183–9.

[82] Plas E, Riedl CR, Pfluger H. Malignant mesothelioma of the tunica vaginalis testis: review of the literature and assessment of prognostic parameters. Cancer 1998;83(12): 2437–46.

[83] Attanoos RL, Gibbs AR. Primary malignant gonadal mesotheliomas and asbestos. Histopathology 2000;37(2):150–9.

[84] Antman K, Cohen S, Dimitrov NV, et al. Malignant mesothelioma of the tunica vaginalis testis. J Clin Oncol 1984;2(5):447–51.

[85] Jones MA, Young RH, Scully RE. Malignant mesothelioma of the tunica vaginalis: a clinicopathologic analysis of 11 cases with review of the literature. Am J Surg Pathol 1995;19(7):815–25.

[86] Sebbag G, Yan H, Shmookler BM, et al. Malignant mesothelioma of the male genital tract: report of two cases. Urol Oncol 2001;6(6):261–4.

[87] Iczkowski KA, Katz G, Zander DS, et al. Malignant mesothelioma of tunica vaginalis testis: a fatal case with liver metastasis. J Urol 2002;167(2 Pt 1):645–6.

[88] Gupta NP, Kumar R. Malignant gonadal mesothelioma. Curr Treat Options Oncol 2002;3(5):363–7.

[89] Gupta NP, Agrawal AK, Sood S, et al. Malignant mesothelioma of the tunica vaginalis testis: a report of two cases and review of literature. J Surg Oncol 1999;70(4):251–4.

[90] Burke A, Virmani R. Malignant mesothelioma of the pericardium. In: Rosai J, Sobin LH, editors. Tumors of the heart and great vessels: atlas of tumor pathology, third series, fascicle 16. Washington (DC): Armed Forces Institute of Pathology; 1996. p. 181–94.

[91] Cohen JL. Neoplastic pericarditis. Cardiovasc Clin 1976;7(3):257–69.

[92] Kaul TK, Fields BL, Kahn DR. Primary malignant pericardial mesothelioma: a case report and review. J Cardiovasc Surg (Torino) 1994;35(3):261–7.

[93] Kahn EO, Rohl A, Barrett EW, et al. Primary pericardial mesothelioma following exposure to asbestos. Environ Res 1980;23(2):270–81.

[94] Churg A, Warnock ML, Bensch KG. Malignant mesothelioma arising after direct application of asbestos and fiberglass to the pericardium. Am Rev Respir Dis 1978;118(2): 419–24.

[95] Beck B, Konetzke G, Ludwig V, et al. Malignant pericardial mesotheliomas and asbestos exposure: a case report. Am J Ind Med 1982;3(2):149–59.

[96] Velissaris TJ, Tang AT, Millward-Sadler GH, et al. Pericardial mesothelioma following mantle field radiotherapy. J Cardiovasc Surg (Torino) 2001;42(3):425–7.

[97] Thomason R, Schlegel W, Lucca M, et al. Primary malignant mesothelioma of the pericardium. Tex Heart Inst J 1994;21(2):170–4.

[98] Suman S, Schofield P, Large S. Primary pericardial mesothelioma presenting as pericardial constriction: a case report. Heart 2004;90(1):e4.

[99] Eryilmaz S, Sirlak M, Inan MB, et al. Primary pericardial mesothelioma. Cardiovasc Pathol 2001;10(3):147–9.

[100] Gopez EV, Carey M, Klatt E. Cardiac tamponade as the initial manifestation of primary pericardial malignant mesothelioma. Acta Cytol 2002;46(6):1171–3.
[101] Chun PK, Leeburg WT, Coggin JT, et al. Primary pericardial malignant epithelioid mesothelioma causing acute myocardial infarction. Chest 1980;77(4):559–61.
[102] Quinn DW, Qureshi F, Mitchell IM. Pericardial mesothelioma: the diagnostic dilemma of misleading imaging. Ann Thorac Surg 2000;69(6):1926–7.
[103] Gossinger HD, Siostrzonek P, Zangeneh M, et al. Magnetic resonance imaging findings in a patient with pericardial mesothelioma. Am Heart J 1988;115(6):1321–2.
[104] Nambiar CA, Tareif HE, Kishore KU, et al. Primary pericardial mesothelioma: one-year event-free survival. Am Heart J 1992;124(3):802–3.
[105] Sane AC, Roggli VL. Curative resection of a well-differentiated papillary mesothelioma of the pericardium. Arch Pathol Lab Med 1995;119(3):266–7.

Hematol Oncol Clin N Am 19 (2005) 1089–1097

HEMATOLOGY/ONCOLOGY CLINICS
OF NORTH AMERICA

Multimodality Treatments in the Management of Malignant Pleural Mesothelioma: An Update

Raphael Bueno, MD[a,b,*]

[a]*Division of Thoracic Surgery, Brigham and Women's Hospital, 75 Francis Street, Boston, MA 02115, USA*
[b]*Department of Surgery, Harvard Medical School, Boston, MA, USA*

M alignant pleural mesothelioma (MPM) is a highly malignant pleural cancer for which there are few effective treatments and an overall 99% five-year mortality rate. Approximately 3000 patients are diagnosed with MPM in the United States annually, and the incidence worldwide is projected to rise substantially in the next two decades [1,2]. The most common cause for MPM (70%–80%) is previous industrial asbestos exposure [3]. Despite the elimination of asbestos from industrial use, it is still present in countless buildings where it has been used for insulation and as a fire retardant. It continues to be a potential health hazard in circumstances such as asbestos exposure and the destruction of the World Trade Center on September 11, 2001, when 10 million New York residents were potentially exposed to this carcinogen [4]. Other proposed causes for MPM include radiation therapy and infection with SV40 through contaminated polio vaccines [5,6].

MPM is relatively unique among cancers, since the local and regional disease rather than the systemic disease usually contributes to death, which occurs for two major reasons. First, because of its multifocal distribution in the chest, MPM progresses locally by compressing the lung, heart, and major vessels, and causes death by cardiac tamponade and lung collapse physiology. Second, the therapy for this aggressive local malignancy is currently inadequate. In most cases there is insufficient time for systemic disease to develop or contribute to mortality. The first order of therapy in MPM is currently, as it has been for decades, to control effectively the tumor's locoregional spread and then deal with controlling the distant disease [7].

Without any treatment, the expected median survival of patients who present with MPM is between 4 and 12 months [8,9]. MPM is exceedingly resistant to most chemotherapy regimens. Pemetrexed and cisplatin combination chemotherapy recently was shown in a prospective randomized trial to be a superior

* Division of Thoracic Surgery, Brigham and Women's Hospital, 75 Francis Street, Boston, MA 02115. *E-mail address:* rbueno@partners.org

0889-8588/05/$ – see front matter
doi:10.1016/j.hoc.2005.09.011

chemotherapy regimen compared with single-agent cisplatin for MPM. This combination only increased median survival from 9 to 12 months, however [10]. Radiation therapy alone is generally ineffective as a primary treatment because the multifocal nature of the tumor makes the proposed treatment field too large to allow for sufficient dosages [7]. The dosages required for definitive treatment clearly cause intolerable lung and potentially cardiac toxicities. Radiation therapy and chemotherapy alone and in combinations have been used for adjuvant and palliative therapy with some degrees of success.

As a result of the inadequate chemotherapy and radiation therapy options for local control of MPM, surgical therapy has been explored as a therapeutic modality. One initial approach has been removal of the pleura or ablation of the pleural space to prevent recurrent pleural effusions. Pleurectomy (or pleurectomy with decortication) and pleurodesis are palliative operations that generally improve symptoms without substantially impacting survival [11–14]. Pleurectomy is an operation in which the pleural tumor is removed. The degree of resection varies among centers. The pleurectomy resection cannot be completed sufficiently in most patients because of tumor invasion of the lung parenchyma and interlobar fissures. A small subset of patients with minimal tumor burden (often confined to the parietal pleura) may derive excellent results from a pleurectomy [7,15,16].

A pleurectomy is usually performed through an extended thoracotomy incision with the lung inflated. The major portion of the sixth rib is removed and an extrapleural plane is developed manually and extended down to the diaphragm, cephalad to the apex of the hemithorax, posteriorly to the level of the azygos vein, and anteriorly to the pericardium. The lung is then deflated and the dissection continues from the apex to the pericardium and hilum, baring the superior vena cava and the internal thoracic vessels. The azygos vein and esophagus are left behind and the posterior dissection continues to the hilum of the lung. The diaphragm is taken completely, partially, or not at all based on involvement. The pericardium is treated in the same manner. The pleura is opened and the lung inspected. In rare cases in which the visceral pleura is completely uninvolved, it is left behind. Usually, the visceral pleura is resected carefully with the lung inflated or not. Usually a plane can be identified and manually developed to free the tumor down to the hilum, where it is resected. Extra care must be exercised in the fissures to avoid injury to the pulmonary arteries or veins. The lung must be mobilized and decorticated completely. After accomplishing a complete macroscopic tumor resection, bleeding is controlled, the pericardium is reconstructed if necessary, and the tumor bed is treated with an argon beam coagulator. Chest drains are strategically placed, the lung is inflated, and the chest cavity is closed [16].

Pleurodesis is a surgical procedure in which the pleural space is mechanically or pharmacologically obliterated to prevent recurrent lung collapse from pleural effusion. Chemotherapy regimens often are added to these surgical procedures. Pleurectomy and pleurodesis patients are still not candidates for whole chest radiation therapy at high doses, because the lung remains in place. In some instances of early disease, in which the parietal pleura is the only portion of the thoracic cavity involved, a near complete extirpation of the tumor can be affected by pleurectomy. This approach has been advocated by some surgeons because it is a less morbid operation; however, the approach itself is not sufficient because most patients suffer from recurrent local disease.

The more aggressive surgical approach is extrapleural pneumonectomy (EPP), which is a major en bloc resection of the lung, all involved pleura, the diaphragm, and pericardium of the ipsilateral thoracic cavity. This procedure has been used in thoracic surgery for the management of advanced tuberculosis and resection of some tumors, such as thymomas. It was proposed for the extirpation of mesothelioma several decades ago, and it is the only procedure that comes close to removing all potential tumor cells [7,15,17–22].

EPP is performed like a pleurectomy through an extended thoracotomy incision and the bed of the resected sixth rib. The initial approach is identical to that of a pleurectomy with the development of an extrapleural plane. The entire ipsilateral diaphragm and a portion of the pericardium are routinely removed, however. The specimen remains en bloc and the lung is not visualized. The pulmonary veins are divided intrapericardially. The pulmonary artery and bronchus are then divided and the specimen—including the lung—is removed. The tumor bed is then ablated with the argon beam coagulator to ensure complete macroscopic resection [23]. There are several limitations to EPP in the management of MPM that specifically require preoperative consideration of physiologic requirements, complication rates, and the degree of cancer resection.

From a physiologic standpoint, patients must be able to tolerate the removal of their lung and ipsilateral diaphragm, which is a particular risk for older patients who may have had substantial tobacco exposure. Regardless of cardiopulmonary function, older age (older than 70) is an independent risk factor for mortality after EPP. The physiologic requirements to withstand EPP are straightforward. Patients should have sufficient pulmonary reserve to function without a lung and the ipsilateral diaphragm. The predicted postoperative FEV_1 should be at least 1 L/min and the DLCO (diffusing capacity of the lung for carbon monoxide) should be near normal. Surgical candidates should have normal cardiac function without significant coronary artery disease or pulmonary hypertension. Pulmonary hypertension or insufficient cardiac reserve can preclude survival after this surgery because of inability of the remaining lung to cope with the entire pulmonary blood flow. Every candidate for EPP should be evaluated with pulmonary function studies and an echocardiogram, including Doppler evaluation of the pulmonary artery pressures. In circumstances in which the pulmonary functions are believed to be marginal, surgical candidates can be evaluated further with pulmonary stress tests and right heart catheterization and balloon occlusion of the ipsilateral pulmonary artery [15,18–20].

Careful patient staging is undertaken before surgery. All patients are evaluated with mediastinoscopy to exclude nodal disease. The tissue diagnosis is confirmed with pleuroscopy. Chest CT, positron emission tomography, and MRI are obtained to assess for diaphragmatic involvement, chest wall involvement, and the extent of the disease. Patients with suspected extension to the abdomen should undergo laparoscopic evaluation.

The morbidity of the EPP operation even in younger patients is substantial. When initially described, this operation was reported to have a high mortality rate. Since then, specialized centers developed in which attention to details, growing experience, and better selection decreased the mortality rate substantially. The morbidity rates remain relatively high, however, and require vigilance and experience for identification and successful treatment. This is one operation that should be performed only by experienced surgeons in high volume centers. The mortality rate has been reported as low as 3.2% in experienced centers and more than 10% in less experienced centers. Some complications, such as atrial fibrillation, cardiac tamponade, deep venous thrombosis, and pulmonary embolus, are caused by the cancer and altered physiology created by the operation. Other complications are technical and include empyema, bronchopleural fistula, and gastric herniation, which are well described in a recent publication from the Brigham and Women's Hospital group in Boston [15,18–20]. To reduce the rate of complication, this group has made some modifications in their treatment regimens. All patients receive beta blockers pre- and postoperatively. Preoperative lower extremity venous ultrasounds are obtained routinely and repeated upon discharge. Pericardial patches are fenestrated routinely, and diaphragmatic patches are sewn in loosely and securely.

A limitation of EPP surgery from the cancer point of view has been that the margin of resection for EPP is usually a single tissue plane that consists frequently of a single cell layer (if that much). It is often likely that some cells from an effusion or the cancer remain embedded in the tissues left behind. The margins of EPP resection (ie, esophagus, aorta, heart, spine, chest wall, trachea, vena cava, liver) are major structures that, with the exception of the chest wall, cannot be removed even if the tumor is too close, which is the usual case. Even the removal of a major portion of the chest wall or tracheal carina is ill advised concomitantly with an EPP because of the risk of infection and nonhealing. Seemingly complete extirpation of the tumor in MPM is realistically impossible; thus, EPP by itself is insufficient to result in a reliable cure. Local recurrence is the rule when EPP is the only treatment [23].

The realization that no currently available single modality can improve survival sufficiently for patients with MPM led to the development of a multimodal approach. The main objective of this approach is to provide local and regional control of the disease, with the secondary objective of preventing distant metastasis. Multimodality approaches initially used standard modalities. Radiation therapy has been added after EPP for the purpose of better sterilizing the surgical margins. The removal of the ipsilateral lung allows for a higher dose to be delivered to the entire endothoracic fascial margin from where the pleura was resected and to the incisions in the skin and muscle to prevent drop metastasis, which is common with MPM. Chemotherapy regimens have been added to enhance the efficacy of radiation therapy and with the rationale that the low burden of the remaining tumor is more likely eradicated after surgery. This combination of multimodal therapy of MPM, including surgical resection followed by chemotherapy and radiation therapy, has led to improved clinical experience in disease management and better definition of outcomes in general, and it has allowed us to determine prognostic factors and limitations of trimodality therapy [23].

The application of multimodality therapy led to the appreciation of important lessons about patient selection, staging, complications from therapy, and causes of mortality. One early lesson was that specialized centers with high volume of patients had the lowest mortality and the best results. Equally important were the new concepts that have emerged concerning the biologic behavior of the tumors and current gaps in therapy. In a landmark study, Sugarbaker and colleagues [20] identified positive resection margins and extrapleural lymph nodes as markers of high risk for tumor recurrence after multimodality therapy that included EPP. Although intuitively obvious in retrospect, this was the first proof of the importance of these pathologic markers. This finding about the lymph nodes has led the Brigham group and other groups to mandate preoperative cervical mediastinoscopy before performing EPP.

This and other studies confirmed the suspicion that patients with sarcomatoid and mixed histology fared as a group less well than patients with epithelial histology. The best group of patients—individuals with epithelial histology who had no positive lymph nodes and complete resection with negative margins—derived the greatest benefit from this operation, with a 46% estimated 5-year survival rate [20]. The identification of a subgroup of patients with relatively favorable survival and the demonstration of survival stratification based on lymph node status and disease burden led the Brigham group to develop and propose a new clinical staging schema for MPM.

Another major contribution came when Baldini and colleagues [24] reported the Brigham group's experience with the patterns of disease recurrence after EPP with multimodality therapy. They noted that many patients developed local and regional recurrence in the chest and abdomen despite aggressive therapy. The recurrence in the abdomen was hypothesized to result from the continuity of the chest and peritoneal cavity after the removal of the diaphragm. This new opening presumably allows remaining tumor cells from the chest to seed the abdomen. The obvious conclusion is that whenever the diaphragm is removed, prophylactic therapy of the peritoneum must be considered. The high pattern of chest recurrence suggests that the initial trimodality regimen is inadequate in eliminating all the tumor cells. Additional or improved local therapy is needed. These two gaps in therapy have driven clinical groups to considering different new approaches to therapy.

In the absence of curative intravenous chemotherapy and biologic agents for therapy for MPM, the focus during the past decade has been on improving and innovating local therapeutic modalities. One of the major pushes has been to improve the delivery of radiation therapy to maximize the sterilization of the tumor bed. Standard external beam therapy generally has been used after EPP.

The limitation of radiation therapy after EPP has been related to the incomplete coverage of the tumor bed and minimization of toxicity. From a technical point of view, the reconstruction of the diaphragm after EPP is limited in the sense that the constructed patch is usually placed well above the insertion of the original diaphragm, which is done for two reasons. First, it is technically difficult to place stitches posteriorly where the diaphragmatic attachments reach as low as the kidneys. The liver, spleen, and bowels make such exposure difficult and create substantial tension on the patch. Second, a smaller pleural space is easier to manage postoperatively to reduce infection and mediastinal shifts. The fact that the patch is well above the usual location of the diaphragm leaves some of the bed of the tumor—in the pleural recesses, where tumor balk is usually the largest—untreated by standard radiation methods. Limitation of dose delivery is also related to adjacent organs in the field, including the liver, kidney, bowels, heart, and spine.

There have been several new approaches to improving radiation therapy after EPP [25]. External beam radiation therapy that was previously planned based on chest radiograms is planned in a three-dimensional field with appropriate targeting of the tumor bed based on preoperative CT and markers left by a surgeon to indicate the need for additional boosts [22]. The group at M.D. Anderson Cancer Center in Texas has focused their work on intensity modulated radiation therapy (IMRT). This relatively intensive approach requires careful intraoperative marking of all true margins using the placement of multiple clips and postoperative planning by the radiation oncologist and operating surgeon to ascertain that no involved tumor bed is left outside the field. Unlike standard external beam therapy, IMRT beams differ in intensity to maximize targeting of the tumor bed and avoid toxicity [26–28]. It is still unclear whether substantial benefit is derived from this approach in patients who have MPM.

The pattern of recurrence in the chest after trimodality therapy is consistent with the hypothesis that radiation therapy after EPP is an insufficient method to eradicate microscopic disease. Several novel approaches have been investigated in phase I and II clinical trials, including other methods of radiation delivery, photodynamic therapy, and intraoperative chemotherapy [29,30]. The rationale is that these treatments can extend and sterilize the margin of the resection effectively while allowing for additional radiation therapy. Brachytherapy and intraoperative radiation therapy have been reported for debulking surgery, particularly for pleurectomy. The data reported are not sufficient to conclude on the merit of these approaches, however. Preliminary therapy with photodynamic therapy using several sensitizers demonstrated feasibility and some morbidity for this approach. The general scheme in those studies has been to add intraoperative photodynamic therapy after a debulking procedure, either pleurectomy or EPP.

There has been some positive experience with intrapleural chemotherapy for peritoneal and pleural mesothelioma. The rationale for this therapy has been to provide high dose chemotherapy (usually cisplatin) locally to sterilize the margin after resection. Several groups have used hypothermic chemotherapy to enhance drug absorption and activity in tumor cells [31,32]. Recently, the Brigham group reported phase I and II clinical trials, including surgical debulking followed immediately by intrapleural and intraperitoneal heated (42°C) cisplatin with concomitant intravenous protection, which allowed the delivery of a high dose of the drug. The rationale has been to reduce recurrence in the chest and abdomen. The therapy has been reasonably well tolerated by patients, and the maximal tolerated dose has been determined. Investigation of these types of local eradication approaches will continue until the advent of more effective systemic chemotherapy [33].

Another approach that has been gaining popularity in oncology—specifically in thoracic oncology—is the preoperative or neoadjuvant treatment of patients with chemotherapy or chemotherapy combined with radiation therapy. Several centers have focused on treating many of their patients with neoadjuvant chemotherapy followed by EPP in patients whose disease has not progressed. The feasibility and safety of this approach have been demonstrated in single institutional trials [34]. Currently, a multicenter trial using neoadjuvant chemotherapy with pemetrexed (for injection) and cisplatin followed by EPP is open to accrual in the United States.

A potential confounder of single institution trials for patients who have MPM is that there is some heterogeneity of tumor behavior among patients. Many prognostic indicators have been described over the past decade and include variables from platelet counts to the levels of specific genes and proteins. Genomic studies from our laboratory and others have reported variability in tumor gene expression. Using this information, we have proposed and validated a prognostic scheme based on the ratio combination of four carefully selected genes based on microarray experiments. We reported that this test is more accurate in predicting response to multimodality therapy than the stage of the tumor, the subtype, or lymph node status. This type of molecular staging system eventually will be incorporated in clinical staging and highlights the need to categorize patients carefully in risk groups before multicenter trials are conducted to determine the efficacy of a given therapy [35,36].

MPM continues to be a challenging disease. Most treating physicians in the United States recognize the need for multidisciplinary evaluation and treatment for patients with newly diagnosed mesothelioma. It is also clear that treatment options and outcome are better at specialized high volume medical centers. Our current treatment algorithms at Brigham and Women's Hospital are as follows. Patients are staged with a positron emission tomographic CT, chest MRI, and mediastinoscopy. Cardiorespiratory function is evaluated with pulmonary function tests, quantitative ventilation perfusion scans if indicated, and a Doppler echocardiogram. The goal of therapy is removal of all macroscopic tumors and sterilization of the tumor bed. Patients with good cardiorespiratory function are offered participation in a multimodality protocol that includes EPP with heated intrapleural chemotherapy followed by chemotherapy and radiation therapy. Patients with inadequate cardiopulmonary reserve or minimal disease are offered enrollment in a multimodality protocol that includes pleurectomy with heated intraoperative chemotherapy followed by adjuvant chemotherapy. Patients with positive mediastinoscopy results or more advanced disease are offered enrollment in a neoadjuvant protocol or chemotherapy-only protocols.

Many single institutional protocols have led the way in the treatment of MPM. It is currently acceptable to proceed with multimodal therapy, including aggressive surgery. The next challenge is to define the results of this therapy in multi-institutional studies. The cooperative group Cancer and Leukemia Group B is about to embark on a phase II clinical trial of EPP followed by adjuvant chemotherapy and radiation therapy in patients who have negative lymph nodes to define the morbidity and outcome of this treatment regimen. This study will be the platform for further refinements of all three components of trimodality therapy in patients who have MPM.

References

[1] Peto J, Decarli A, La Vecchia C, et al. The European mesothelioma epidemic. Br J Cancer 1999;79:666–72.

[2] Peto J, Hodgson JT, Matthews FE, et al. Continuing increase in mesothelioma mortality in Britain. Lancet 1995;345:535–9.

[3] Britton M. The epidemiology of mesothelioma. Semin Oncol 2002;29:18–25.

[4] Lange JH. Cough and bronchial responsiveness in firefighters at the World Trade Center site [comment]. N Engl J Med 2003;348:76–7.

[5] Carbone M, Pass HI. Debate on the link between SV40 and human cancer continues [comment]. J Natl Cancer Inst 2002;94:229–30.

[6] Gazdar AF, Butel JS, Carbone M. SV40 and human tumours: myth, association or causality? Nat Rev Cancer 2002;2:957–64.

[7] Sugarbaker DJ, Norberto JJ, Bueno R. Current therapy for mesothelioma. Cancer Control 1997;4:326–34.

[8] Pass H. Malignant pleural mesothelioma: surgical roles and novel therapies. Clin Lung Cancer 2001;3:102–17.

[9] Merritt N, Blewett CJ, Miller JD, et al. Survival after conservative (palliative) management of pleural malignant mesothelioma. J Surg Oncol 2001;78:171–4.

[10] Vogelzang NJ, Rusthoven JJ, Symanowski J, et al. Phase III study of pemetrexed in combination with cisplatin versus cisplatin alone in patients with malignant pleural mesothelioma [comment]. J Clin Oncol 2003;21:2636–44.

[11] Magnani C, Viscomi S, Dalmasso P, et al. Survival after pleural malignant mesothelioma: a population-based study in Italy. Tumori 2002;88:266–9.

[12] van Ruth S, Baas P, Zoetmulder FA. Surgical treatment of malignant pleural mesothelioma: a review. Chest 2003;123:551–61.

[13] Zellos L, Sugarbaker DJ. Current surgical management of malignant pleural mesothelioma. Curr Oncol Rep 2002;4:354–60.

[14] Takagi K, Tsuchiya R, Watanabe Y. Surgical approach to pleural diffuse mesothelioma in Japan. Lung Cancer 2001;31:57–65.

[15] Rusch VW. Indications for pneumonectomy: extrapleural pneumonectomy [review]. Chest Surg Clin North Am 1999;9(2):327–38.

[16] Rusch VW. Pleurectomy/decortication in the setting of multimodality treatment for diffuse malignant pleural mesothelioma [review]. Semin Thorac Cardiovasc Surg 1997;9(4):367–72.

[17] Sugarbaker DJ, Liptay MJ. Therapeutic approaches in malignant mesothelioma. In: Aisner J, Arriagada R, Green MR, et al, editors. Comprehensive textbook of thoracic oncology. Baltimore (MD): Williams and Wilkins; 1996. p. 786–98.

[18] Sugarbaker DJ, Jaklitsch MT, Bueno R, et al. Prevention, early detection, and manage-

ment of complications after 328 consecutive extrapleural pneumonectomies. J Thorac Cardiovasc Surg 2004;128(1):138–46.

[19] Sugarbaker DJ, Garcia JP, Richards WG, et al. Extrapleural pneumonectomy in the multi-modality therapy of malignant pleural mesothelioma: results in 120 consecutive patients. Ann Surg 1996;224:288–94.

[20] Sugarbaker DJ, Flores RM, Jaklitsch MT, et al. Resection margins, extrapleural nodal status, and cell type determine postoperative long-term survival in trimodality therapy of malignant pleural mesothelioma: results in 183 patients. J Thorac Cardiovasc Surg 1999;117: 54–65.

[21] Sugarbaker D, Strauss GM, Lynch TJ, et al. Node status has prognostic significance in the multimodality therapy of diffuse, malignant mesothelioma. J Clin Oncol 1993;11:1172–8.

[22] Rusch VW, Rosenzweig K, Venkatraman E, et al. A phase II trial of surgical resection and adjuvant high-dose hemithoracic radiation for malignant pleural mesothelioma [see comment]. J Thorac Cardiovasc Surg 2001;122(4):788–95.

[23] Jaklitsch M, Wiener D, Bueno R, et al. The development of the Brigham and Women's Hospital multimodality treatment plan for MPM. In: Pass HI, Vogelsang NJ, Carbone M, editors. Malignant mesothelioma. New York: Springer; 2005. p. 696–722.

[24] Baldini EH, DeCamp Jr MM, Katz MS, et al. Patterns of failure after trimodality therapy for malignant pleural mesothelioma. Ann Thorac Surg 1997;63:334–8.

[25] Janne PA, Baldini EH. Patterns of failure following surgical resection for malignant pleural mesothelioma [review]. Thorac Surg Clin 2004;14(4):567–73.

[26] Tobler M, Watson G, Leavitt DD. Intensity-modulated photon arc therapy for treatment of pleural mesothelioma. Med Dosim 2002;27(4):255–9.

[27] Forster KM, Smythe WR, Starkschall G, et al. Intensity-modulated radiotherapy following extrapleural pneumonectomy for the treatment of malignant mesothelioma: clinical implementation. Int J Radiat Oncol Biol Phys 2003;55(3):606–16.

[28] Ahamad A, Stevens CW, Smythe WR, et al. Intensity-modulated radiation therapy: a novel approach to the management of malignant pleural mesothelioma. Int J Radiat Oncol Biol Phys 2003;55(3):768–75.

[29] Rodriguez E, Baas P, Friedberg JS. Innovative therapies: photodynamic therapy [review]. Thorac Surg Clin 2004;14(4):557–66.

[30] Friedberg JS, Mick R, Stevenson JP, et al. Phase II trial of pleural photodynamic therapy and surgery for patients with non-small-cell lung cancer with pleural spread. J Clin Oncol 2004; 22(11):2192–201.

[31] van Ruth S, Verwaal VJ, Hart AA, et al. Heat penetration in locally applied hyperthermia in the abdomen during intra-operative hyperthermic intraperitoneal chemotherapy. Anticancer Res 2003;23(2B):1501–8.

[32] van Ruth S, Mathot RA, Sparidans RW, et al. Population pharmacokinetics and pharmacodynamics of mitomycin during intraoperative hyperthermic intraperitoneal chemotherapy. Clin Pharmacokinet 2004;43(2):131–43.

[33] Piperdi B, Shin DM, Perez-Soler R. Intrapleural chemotherapy with and without surgery in MPM. In: Pass HI, Vogelsang NJ, Carbone M, editors. Malignant mesothelioma. New York: Springer; 2005. p. 631–7.

[34] Vallieres E, Hunt K, Stelzer K. Induction chemotherapy, extrapleural pneumonectomy (EPP), and adjuvant fast neutron radiation therapy (FNRT) for pleural mesothelioma (DMM) [abstract]. Proc Am Soc Clin Oncol 2000;19:578.

[35] Gordon GJ, Rockwell GN, Godfrey PA, et al. Validation of genomics-based prognostic tests in malignant pleural mesothelioma. Clin Cancer Res 2005;11:4406–14.

[36] Gordon GJ, Hsiao L-L, Jensen RV, et al. Using gene expression ratios to predict outcome among patients with mesothelioma. J Natl Cancer Inst 2003;95:598–605.

Hematol Oncol Clin N Am 19 (2005) 1099–1115

HEMATOLOGY/ONCOLOGY CLINICS
OF NORTH AMERICA

Radiotherapy for Mesothelioma

Craig W. Stevens, MD, PhD[a],*, Kenneth M. Forster, PhD[b],
W. Roy Smythe, MD[c], David Rice[d]

[a]Division of Radiation Oncology, H. Lee Moffitt Cancer Center, 12902 Magnolia Drive, Tampa, FL 33612, USA
[b]Department of Radiation Oncology, University of Texas Southwestern Medical Center, Dallas, TX, USA
[c]Department of Surgery, Texas A&M University Medical School, College Station, TX, USA
[d]Department of Thoracic Surgery, University of Texas M.D. Anderson Cancer Center, Houston, TX, USA

Three to four thousand cases of malignant pleural mesothelioma (MPM) will occur in the United States this year. Most patients will be diagnosed with advanced disease and die from local progression. With such a preponderance of locoregional disease, various combinations of locoregional therapies have been attempted. Single-modality therapy with radiation plays a role only for palliation. Radiation can prevent tumor recurrence at drain/instrumentation sites and provide symptomatic relief of pain and other complaints. The large tumor burden, complex tumor shape, respiratory motion, and adjacent radiosensitive normal structures limit the use of high-dose radiotherapy in unresected patients.

Combinations of surgery and radiation also have been attempted. Pleurectomy-decortication combined with radiation resulted in a high incidence of locoregional failure, probably because target motion limited the delivered radiation dose. Outcomes have been achieved best with combinations of extrapleural pneumonectomy (EPP) and radiation. EPP had the advantage that the tumor was completely removed, the diaphragm was removed (and so target motion), and regions at highest risk for recurrence could be marked with radio-opaque clips. Three-year survival rates have ranged from 20% to 55% in selected patients treated with EPP and radiation. Locoregional failure rates range from 6% to 30% with intensity modulated radiotherapy (IMRT) and three-dimensional conformal radiation, respectively.

It is unclear how current systemic regimens will impact on outcome of patients who receive bimodality therapy, but the preponderance of death from distant metastases makes the development of better systemic therapy essential. Better therapy also must be developed for patients who are not candidates for EPP, because only a small minority of such patients can be cured with less aggressive surgery, radiation, or combined modality therapy. Locoregional tumor recurrence essentially can be eliminated with combinations of EPP and radiation

* Corresponding author. E-mail address: stevencw@moffitt.usf.edu (C.W. Stevens).

0889-8588/05/$ – see front matter
doi:10.1016/j.hoc.2005.09.006

therapy, and this treatment is well tolerated. Survival in patients who are in the early stage is excellent. These data justify aggressive screening programs for patients at risk for mesothelioma.

MPM occurs with an incidence of approximately 10 cases per million people per year in the United States [1]. The incidence has been increasing and represents a significant clinical problem in populations of patients exposed to asbestos. The Center for Lung Cancer and Related Disorders estimates approximately 3000 patients per year with malignant mesothelioma, with a peak incidence of approximately 4000 patients per year expected to occur in approximately 2025. Prognosis for MPM has been so poor that survival was equivalent in a trial that compared multimodality treatment to pain management alone [2]. Several recent nonrandomized trials suggested that multimodality therapy may improve outcome for carefully selected patients, however [3–6].

The major clinical problem for patients who have MPM has been local disease progression, with disseminated disease usually reported only late in the course [7,8]. MPM spreads by direct extension and seeding throughout the pleural space, including fissures, diaphragmatic, and pericardial surfaces, through the chest wall, and into the mediastinum, peritoneum, and lymph nodes. Surgery alone, even in carefully selected patients who are in the early stage, has not been shown to improve the 2-year survival rates of 10% to 33% [9] (Butchart et al, 1976; Jaklitsch et al, 2001). This result is not surprising considering the close approximation of the parietal pleura (resected with EPP) and the endothoracic fascia (which remains after EPP), which always leave close surgical margins. Combined modality treatment suggests improved local control and survival rate [10,11] (Calavrezos et al, 1988), although local recurrence is still the most common site of first relapse [3].

Several lines of evidence suggest that radiotherapy should be effective in treating mesothelioma in the postoperative setting. First, mesothelioma cell lines are not particularly radioresistant in vitro. Such cell lines have radio-sensitivities similar to non–small cell lung cancer and other tumor types that demonstrate excellent local control after gross tumor resection [12,13]. Second, there is a dose response for symptom palliation, such that doses more than 40 Gy seem more effective than lower doses [8]. This dose response suggests that clinically significant cell killing can be attained with clinically achievable radiation doses. Third, modest radiation doses can reduce dramatically the local MPM failure rate at thoracotomy or other instrumentation sites. This finding demonstrates that radiation can kill mesothelioma cells effectively in regions in which the tumor burden is low. Because MPM is moderately radiosensitive, it follows that postoperative radiotherapy should be effective in preventing loco-regional recurrence and potentially improve survival.

RADIOTHERAPY FOR PALLIATION
Pain Control
Several lines of evidence suggest that radiation should provide effective palliation for patients with MPM. One small study demonstrated a radiation dose

response after the retrospective review of outcomes of 29 courses of palliative external beam radiotherapy delivered to 17 patients with MPM [8]. Four of six patients treated with more than 40 Gy achieved significant relief of symptoms. The four patients who achieved symptomatic relief were treated for thoracic pain, whereas the patients with poor outcome were treated for superior vena cava obstruction and dyspnea. Only one patient treated with lower doses achieved significant palliation of any symptom, and this was for a painful chest wall mass.

In another study [13a], 26 radiotherapy courses were reviewed for any symptomatic improvement. Pain relief was a common finding, with 13 of 18 cases having improvement. In contrast with the previous study, the response was similar regardless of dose/fractionation (20 Gy/5 fractionation or 30 Gy/10 fractionation), although radiobiologically they are similar doses. Treatment also was effective for "mass," Pancoast's syndrome, and SVC (superior vena cava) syndrome. Although the sample size was small, palliation was achieved in approximately 50% of cases in this diverse patient group. The duration of response was not assessed in either study. These data suggested that symptoms from mesothelioma usually can be palliated effectively with brief courses of radiotherapy. Where possible, doses more than 40 Gy should be delivered. The standard palliative dose at the University of Texas M.D. Anderson Cancer Center is 45 Gy delivered in 3 weeks—the same dose fractionation regimen used to palliate non–small cell lung cancer patients with good performance status.

Preventing Recurrence at Drain Sites

Unlike most malignancies, MPM has a tendency to recur predictably along tracks of previous chest wall instrumentation [14]. One group hypothesized that local radiotherapy might prevent this type of painful tumor growth pattern [15]. Forty consecutive patients with pathologically proven MPM were randomized to immediate prophylactic radiotherapy to each site of instrumentation, or to observation. Prophylactic treatment was 21 Gy in three fractions delivered using an appositional electron field. Tissue equivalent bolus material was placed over each target to improve dose delivery to the skin. The prescription point or electron energy was not further described. The authors found no subcutaneous MPM progression in the irradiated patients, whereas such nodules developed in 8 of 20 (40%) of the untreated patients, with a median time to recurrence of 6 months. Subcutaneous recurrence was not correlated with a positive cytologic study, histologic type, disease stage, subsequent treatment, or the size of the tracts. They concluded that because such recurrences are typically painful, prophylactic irradiation was a safe and effective means of maintaining patient quality of life.

Discussion of Palliative Therapy

Palliative therapy must be individualized. Pain is fairly well controlled with radiotherapy doses more than 40 Gy, and prophylactic treatment is effective with 21 Gy delivered in three fractions (although this approach has not been widely used in the United States). Our approach has been to use 45 Gy in

15 fractions for patients with good performance status, because this regimen has shown better palliative effects for patients with other thoracic malignancies [16]. This approach also combines a relatively short treatment course with a dose more than 40 Gy. Superior vena cava obstruction, dyspnea, and Pancoast's syndrome are more difficult to palliate, with only approximately 50% of patients demonstrating benefit. Investigation is warranted to determine the role of prophylactic radiotherapy to the mediastinum and drain sites.

POTENTIALLY CURATIVE RADIOTHERAPY

Radiotherapy Alone

Radiotherapy alone is clearly not the treatment of choice for this disease. The lung is sensitive to radiotherapy, and the volume of lung irradiated at more than 20 Gy (V20) has been linked to pulmonary toxicity. A 41% pneumonitis rate has been reported if the V20 was more than 40%, with more than half of these being severe (≥grade 3) [17]. Delivery of a potentially curative dose (eg, >60 Gy) would irradiate the entire ipsilateral lung (or 50% of the total lung volume) more than 20 Gy unless parts of the lung can be spared.

Such sparing is difficult if the lung and diaphragm remain in place because of two problems with the target volumes. The first problem involves intrapulmonary fissures. The fissures are bathed in pleural fluid and so with mesothelioma cells. The fissures should be included as part of the target volume. Unfortunately, the intrapulmonary fissures are complex three-dimensional structures surrounded by lung (Fig. 1). Three-dimensional conformal radiotherapy cannot irradiate the fissures and spare any significant lung volume. IMRT also cannot treat these structures because they move with respiration if the diaphragm is intact.

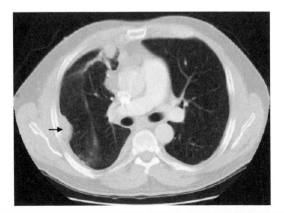

Fig. 1. The interlobar fissures are complex three-dimensional structures. The interlobar fissures are covered with pleural and pleural fluid, which often contains mesothelioma cells. The fissures have complex shapes and move/distort with respiration, which makes them difficult targets for radiotherapy. Note the subpleural nodule (*arrow*) and the S-shaped fissure that contains effusion.

Respiratory motion is the second and most important problem for radiotherapy as a sole modality. When the diaphragm is in place, there can be 2 to 3 cm of superior-inferior motion, 1 to 2 cm of mediolateral motion along the mediastinum, and 1 to 1.5 cm of anterior chest wall motion. Expanding the pulmonary target volume to account for this motion results in destruction of the liver in right-sided MPM, the most common side, and delivers high cardiac and bowel doses in left-sided cases. Radiotherapy without surgery is best considered as a palliative treatment, with doses and volumes appropriately limited.

These concerns led to limited data from small studies. In one of the largest studies, 12 patients were irradiated with curative intent between 1981 and 1985 at the Peter MacCallum Cancer Institute. The results were described as part of a larger retrospective study [13a]. Patients were treated with anterior/posterior (AP/PA) beam geometry, including the mediastinum to 40 Gy. The mediastinum/spinal cord was then shielded and an additional 10 Gy delivered. No attempt was made to shield the lung or the liver. The target volume included any surgical scars, but the inferior borders were not described. The median survival time for the 12 patients was 17 months, compared with 7 months for 20 patients treated palliatively, but both curves converged by 24 months. Two patients died from treatment. The first patient died from liver failure 7 weeks after completing treatment because the entire liver was irradiated to 50 Gy. The second patient died from progressive neurologic deterioration approximately 11 months after irradiation. Autopsy revealed radiation myelopathy despite spinal cord shielding after 40 Gy.

Radiotherapy Combined with Chemotherapy

No prospective or retrospective trials could be found in which radiotherapy and chemotherapy were combined without surgery. Because of the difficulties in radiating the target volumes, a bimodal approach with chemotherapy and radiation should be considered only palliative.

Radiotherapy Combined with Surgery

Several groups recently reported promising outcome for patients who have MPM and are treated with surgery and radiotherapy, with or without chemotherapy. Operative approaches have used either pleurectomy/decortication or EPP.

Radiotherapy After Pleurectomy and Decortication

Thirty-four patients with pathologically proven MPM were treated between 1982 and 1988 at the Helsinki University Central Hospital [18,19]. Twenty-nine patients underwent partial pleurectomy, whereas the others had only biopsy. Patients were irradiated with one of three schedules that delivered between 55 Gy and 70 Gy to the hemithorax. The extent of disease and the field borders were not described, but no lung or liver shielding was used. Their median survival was approximately 12 months [20], with approximately one third having in-field progression and the remainder having "stable" disease. This approach also led to progressive deterioration of pulmonary function. Within

12 months, all patients had complete destruction of all visible alveoli, which paralleled a decrease in DLCO (diffusing capacity of the lung for carbon monoxide) that was consistent with complete pneumonectomy. FVC (forced vital capacity) also decreased, which is consistent with the complete pulmonary fibrosis described. The PaO_2 decreased transiently between 2 and 4 months after irradiation but then returned to baseline, which suggested that there is minimal left-right shunting after whole lung irradiation for MPM. The authors did not describe any effects on renal or hepatic function.

A similar study was performed at the Memorial Sloan Kettering Cancer Center [21]. They reported the results of 41 patients treated with partial pleurectomy, although all had residual gross disease that was boosted with permanent ^{125}I implantation at surgery. Photon and electron fields were combined to treat the superficial chest wall and spare the underlying lung. Radiation doses were 45 Gy to the pleural surface, and most of the lung was kept at less than 20 Gy. Local recurrence developed in 29 of 41 patients, with 22 having distant failure. Median time to local failure was 9 months. Radiation-related toxicity occurred in 4 patients (one each of radiation pneumonitis, pulmonary fibrosis, pericardial effusion, and esophagitis), but the severity of toxicity was not described.

These data were updated briefly, and results from 105 patients treated with pleurectomy/decortication from 1976 to 1988 were described [7,9]. Forty-one patients received external beam treatment only, whereas 53 patients received external beam with an intraoperatively placed ^{125}I boost to gross disease. Median survival was 12.6 months, but 12 patients developed radiation pneumonitis and 8 patients developed radiation pericarditis. The severity of these reactions and local control in this larger patient group were not described.

A more recent paper described the results of 24 patients treated with pleurectomy/decortication, intraoperative radiotherapy, and postoperative external beam radiotherapy [22]. Fourteen patients were irradiated using three-dimensional conformal radiotherapy, and IMRT was used to treat 10 patients. Intraoperative radiotherapy was targeted mainly to the intrapulmonary fissures, pericardium, and diaphragm, with doses ranging from 5 to 15 Gy. The target volumes for the external beam treatments were not described, but the doses ranged from 30.1 to 48.8 Gy (median, 41.4 Gy). Twelve patients also received chemotherapy (cyclophosphamide, doxorubicin, and cisplatin) at the discretion of the treating physician. Surgical staging demonstrated AJCC (American Joint Committee on Cancer) T stage 1, 2, and 3 in 1, 18, and 7 patients, respectively. Three patients also had lymph node metastases. Despite the relatively early stage, outcome was relatively poor, with median OS (overall survival) of 18 months and PFS (progression-free survival) of 12 months. Major complications included radiation pneumonitis in 4 patients, pericarditis in 1 patient, and esophageal stricture in 1 patient who had received previous radiotherapy to the esophagus. Only the esophageal stricture required more than conservative management (balloon dilation for the esophageal stricture). There was no difference in the toxicity between three-dimensional CRT (conformal radiation therapy) and IMRT, although the patient numbers were small. Tumor recurrence was mostly locoregional at sites of previous gross tumor. Only the number of intraoperative radiotherapy sites was predictive of overall survival, which suggested that higher external beam doses might be required for this approach to be used widely.

Pleurectomy/decortication followed by radiotherapy can reduce locoregional failure compared with historic controls. Local failure is common, however, and survival is disappointing even when modern IMRT techniques are applied. Although overall median survivals in these pleurectomy/decortication studies tend to be approximately 2 years, carefully selected early-stage patients treated with EPP can expect median survivals of more than 4 years [10]. Unfortunately, there are no prospective randomized trials to guide therapy. Pleurectomy seems to prolong life longer than biopsy alone [23] and is preferable to no treatment. In light of the recent finding that EPP promotes longer disease-free intervals than pleurectomy [24] and that EPP is better preparation for radiotherapy, EPP should be considered the surgical treatment of choice for MPM.

Radiotherapy After Extrapleural Pneumonectomy

Radiotherapy after EPP was first described in 1997 [3]. In 35 of 49 patients, four to six cycles of chemotherapy were given postoperatively followed by radiation. Radiation details, such as target volumes, margins, and treatment technique, were not described. The prescribed dose was 30.6 Gy to the hemithorax followed by a boost to bring the target dose to approximately 50 Gy. The criteria for boost, the locations, volumes, and techniques were not described. Sixteen irradiated patients developed a local recurrence; however, of those patients with abdominal failure, 5 had a chest mass that extended into the abdomen, 2 had ascites, and 4 had a retroperitoneal mass. This last complication is potentially important because of the tendency of surgeons to reconstruct the diaphragm much higher than the preoperative insertion of the diaphragm, which "abdominalizes" the posterior recess of the diaphragm. Failure to irradiate this region, which can be below the ipsilateral kidney, can result in apparent retroperitoneal recurrences. The true rate of locoregional failure was at least 21 of 49 and possibly as high as 25 of 49. Despite the high incidence of locoregional failure, the 3-year overall survival rate was 34%. Radiation-induced toxicity was tolerable and included esophagitis and thrombocytopenia. No radiation pneumonitis was described, but five patients experienced respiratory compromise, one of whom died of pneumonia. Our experience also suggests that infectious pneumonia is not a rare complication of pneumonectomy. These data provide the first substantial experience demonstrating that postoperative radiotherapy could reduce local recurrence and result in long-term survival in well-selected patients.

Encouraging results also were reported from Memorial Sloan Kettering Cancer Center [5]. From 1995 to 1998, 54 patients (mostly stage III) underwent EPP followed by radiotherapy using their previously published techniques [25]. The inferior field rarely included the ipsilateral kidney. The treatment technique involved photon radiation to a dose of 54 Gy in 30 fractions. The spinal cord was shielded after 41.4 Gy. Liver and heart were shielded at lower doses. The chest wall in the shielded regions was irradiated with matched electron fields so that the goal dose of 54 Gy could be achieved more safely. The median survival was approximately 18 months. Only 7 patients had local recurrence (2 local only). Another 22 patients had peritoneal or ipsilateral visceral recurrence.

Memorial Sloan Kettering Cancer Center recently updated their experience and provided a detailed description of the radiotherapy technique and outcome [26]. Thirty-five patients underwent radiotherapy after EPP, with the goal of delivering 54 Gy in 30 fractions. The target volume was the ipsilateral hemithorax from the top of T1, ideally the bottom of L2, and laterally to flash the skin. All drain sites were included. The medial field edge was the contralateral edge of the vertebral bodies if mediastinal lymph nodes were negative; otherwise the field was extended 1.5 to 2 cm beyond the contralateral edge of the vertebral bodies. For right-sided lesions, the liver and ipsilateral kidney were blocked. For left-sided lesions, the heart was blocked after 19.8 Gy. The blocked regions were boosted superficially with electrons. After 41.4 cGy, the medial field edge was moved to the ipsilateral edge of the vertebral bodies. Patients tolerate this therapy well, with the main toxicities being nausea and vomiting and dysphagia.

The results of this study, however, were difficult to interpret. Local failure was documented in 13 of 35 patients, but in-field failures were not separated from marginal misses. It is not clear if the pattern of failure results from close margins, match line dosimetry issues at the junction of electron and photon fields, or inadequate dose. Of the remaining 22 patients with local control, only 5 are disease free, however.

An alternative treatment approach using IMRT after EPP was reported [6,27,28]. Twenty-six of 28 patients were stage III, most had involved lymph nodes, and all patients required partial chest wall resection. During the EPP, radio-opaque surgical clips were placed at the insertion of the diaphragm, including the crus, and the anterior-medial pleural extension, which often crosses midline over the heart. The target volume included the entire hemithorax and all surgical clips, all sites of instrumentation, and the ipsilateral mediastinum. Boosts were given to any close or positive resection margins. All volumes were reviewed with the treating surgeon at the treatment planning workstation. The goal was a minimum dose of 45 to 50 Gy to the hemithorax and 60 Gy to the boost volume. All irradiation was completed in 25 fractions. The 2-year overall survival rate was 62%. There were no in-field failures. Two marginal misses occurred: one near the crus and one across midline anterior to the heart. Major toxicities included nausea and vomiting, fatigue, and skin irritation. This series has been extended to 62 patients with EPP followed by IMRT to 45 or 50 Gy. Three marginal failures have been reported: one at the crus of the diaphragm before clipping was routine, one at the anterior medial pleural reflection anterior to the heart, and one in the contralateral mediastinum. One patient with epithelioid histology failed in multiple locations within and outside the radiated volume. One fatal case of radiation pneumonitis occurred several weeks after completion of IMRT. More than half of these patients failed distantly, but the 3-year DFS (disease-free survival) for patients with epithelioid histology and negative nodes was 45%.

When we began our IMRT trials, most radiotherapy treatment planning systems were incapable of calculating IMRT doses to such large volumes. Several planning systems were tested recently, and it was found that Corvus, Pinnacle, and Eclipse planning systems were MPM capable. Dose volume histograms were similar across platforms; however, Corvus-based plans required more monitor units and more segments than either Pinnacle or Eclipse [28a]. These data suggested that IMRT should be deliverable in many institutions around the world. We recently completed a phase I/II trial that compared 45 to 50 Gy with IMRT in 30 patients. The toxicity and local control were identical, which suggested that a minimum CTV (clinical target volume) dose of 45 Gy is adequate.

Another approach was described by Weder and colleagues [29]. Induction chemotherapy with gemcitabine and cisplatin preceded EPP. Radiotherapy was delivered to selected volumes. Of the 13 patients treated in this way, 8 experienced recurrence within the ipsilateral hemithorax. Pleurectomy and chemotherapy were performed without radiation [30], and all 40 patients developed ipsilateral chest failure. These data demonstrated that induction chemotherapy cannot make up for inadequate radiotherapy.

The data described previously and summarized in Table 1 demonstrated several important points that are critical to future MPM trial development:

1. High-dose postoperative radiotherapy can reduce ipsilateral thoracic failures dramatically, which is consistent with the radiosensitivity of MPM cell lines and suggests that postoperative radiotherapy should be a component of all future trials.
2. Radiotherapy after pleural decortication results in a much higher rate of locoregional failure than does radiotherapy after EPP. It is not clear whether this is caused by lower radiation doses, motion of the target volume, or inadequate delineation of target volumes. EPP with postoperative radiotherapy seems preferable to less morbid but much less effective approaches.
3. A detailed description of the target volumes only recently was published [27]. Because earlier reports did not precisely define the target, it is difficult to determine a local failure versus a marginal miss. True in-field failure must be well documented so that it can be explained.
4. Radiotherapy after EPP is well tolerated.
5. Postoperative radiotherapy changes the pattern of relapse so that distant metastases become more prevalent, which suggests the potential need for systemic therapy.
6. Current chemotherapy regimens cannot replace adequate radiotherapy.

Radiotherapy Technique

Postoperative three-dimensional conformal radiation techniques have been well described [26], as have techniques for IMRT [27,28]. These references should be

Table 1
Largest studies combining surgery with post-operative radiotherapy

Study [reference]	Surgery	No. of patients	Radiotherapy dose	Local failure	Survival
Maasilta, 1991 [19]	Pleurectomy	34	55 Gy–70 Gy	33% progression, but remainder with "stable"	12 mo median
Hilaris et al, 1984 [21]	Pleurectomy	41	45 Gy + implant	29/41	12.6 mo median
Lee et al, 2002 [22]	Pleurectomy	24	41.4 Gy median 5–15 Gy IORT	"Most"	18 mo median
Baldini et al, 1997 [3]	EPP	49	30.6 Gy 20 Gy boost	21/49	22 mo
Rusch et al, 2001 [5]	EPP	55	54 Gy	7/55	Stage I–II: 34 mo Stage III–IV: 10 mo
Ahamad et al, 2004 [6]	EPP	28	45–50 Gy	0 2 marginal miss	Not yet reached (2 y overall survival 62%)
Yajnik et al, 2003 [26]	EPP	35	54 Gy	13/35	Not reported
Weder et al, 2003 [29]	Chemotherapy + EPP	19	Selected volumes	8/13	16.5 mo

reviewed in detail before treating patients with either technique. Both approaches require reproducible daily setup. Treatment planning CTs should be acquired in the treatment position. Because of the large targets, we find 5-mm slice thickness to be adequate. Most planning systems fail if 3-mm slice thickness (our standard for lung treatment planning) are used because of system memory.

Target Volume Delineation

There is general consensus that the ipsilateral mediastinum should be included in the target volume [5,27,30a]. The superior border is at the thoracic inlet. The medial border includes the ipsilateral nodal regions, trachea, and subcarinal regions [28] or the vertebral body [26]. The posterior mediastinal structures behind the heart need not be included, because no failures in this region have been recorded as a result [30b].

In our experience, the anterior medial pleural reflection also can be a potential problem for target volume delineation, because the medial pleural space sometimes can cross midline. This anatomic relationship can be lost after surgery. When possible, this region should be marked intraoperatively with radio-opaque clips. Alternatively, the medial extent of the pleura could be identified on preoperative CT scans and this extent estimated on the treatment planning CT.

The inferior border should be the insertion of the diaphragm, the location of which varies and ranges from L1 to L4. Because of the variability, the diaphragm insertion should be marked either by intraoperative placement of radio-opaque clips [6] or by suturing the neodiaphragm in this location [26]. When the border of intrathoracic contents and abdominal contents is well marked, the radiotherapy margins can be reduced maximally. Another potential source of contouring error is the medial extent of the crus of the diaphragm, especially at its most inferior extent. The ipsilateral crus is difficult to identify without clips. The best way to individualize the inferior edge of the target volume is with extensive intraoperative placement of radio-opaque clips, with particular attention paid to the crus (Fig. 2).

All chest tube or biopsy sites should be included in the target volume because of the risk of tumor tracking along the instrumentation track. These sites should be contoured to the skin, as should any regions of subcutaneous tissue disruption. Typically, the skin incision does not directly overlie the regions where the ribs are entered. Because there is tunneling under the subcutaneous fat, the entire disturbed region should be irradiated, including the subscapular tissues. Disrupted tissue planes often can be identified at postoperative CT simulation and should be included in the CTV.

Ideally the surgeon, radiation oncologist, and radiation treatment planning physicist should discuss the target volumes at the planning workstation. This consultation is particularly important for the first few cases irradiated by a physician group. This level of involvement allows for unambiguous target volume identification and helps a radiation oncologist to better understand the anatomy and extent of disease. Likewise, a surgeon gains an appreciation of the limits of target volume identification and clipping. The treatment planner gains

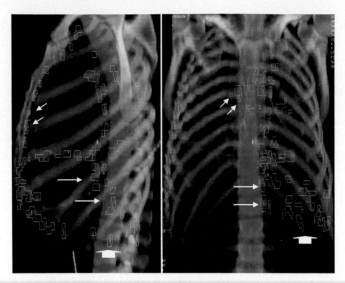

Fig. 2. Targets that require special care. Three regions of the target volume are potentially difficult to appreciate without great care. These regions (*small arrows*) are the anterior-medial pleural, which can be clipped during EPP or estimate on the preoperative CT (*large arrows*), the inferior, and medial extents of the crus of the diaphragm, which should be clipped at EPP, and the inferior insertion of the diaphragm (*arrowheads*), which also should be marked at EPP.

insight into which regions of this large CTV are critical, and the physicist gains insight into the planning constraints for each case.

TREATMENT PLANNING
Three-dimensional Conformal Radiation Therapy
The three-dimensional CRT approach has been described best in two reports from the Memorial Sloan Kettering Cancer Center [25,26]. The technique applies AP/PA beam geometry to the hemithorax using the volumes described previously as CTV. For right-sided cases, an abdominal block is present throughout treatment, and the region is boosted with electrons at 1.53 Gy per day, which accounts for scatter under the block. For left-sided cases, the kidney and heart are blocked. The kidney block is present throughout treatment, and the heart block is added after 19.8 Gy. The spinal cord is shielded after 41.4 Gy in all cases. The goal dose to the target volume is 54 Gy in 30 fractions, with dose calculated at midplane with equally weighted beams. Patients were treated with arms akimbo.

Treatment by this simple approach results in good coverage of most of the volumes at risk to the target dose of 54 Gy. Doses are homogeneous within the regions at risk, although some regions (eg, the crus, pericardium, and neodia-phragm) may be difficult to treat. The match lines between the electron and photon fields also can be problematic. The radiosensitive structures, such as the

Table 2
Target doses to the targets and dose-volume constraints of the organs at risk

Target or organ	Goal dose or constraint dose
CTV	45 Gy in 25 fractions
bCTV	60 Gy in 25 fractions
Lung	<20% to receive >20 Gy and mean less than 9.5Gy
Liver	<30% to receive >30 Gy
Contralateral kidney	<20% to receive >15 Gy
Heart	<50% to receive >45 Gy
Spinal cord	<10% to receive >45 Gy and no portion to receive >50 Gy
Esophagus	<30% to receive >55 Gy

liver and heart, can be spared well. Protection of the ipsilateral kidney is clearly better than with IMRT.

Intensity Modulated Radiotherapy

The target doses and the dose volume limits for the critical structures are listed in Table 2. Treatment is delivered with 13 to 27 intensity modulated fields using 8 to 11 gantry angles, typically with 100 segments per intensity-modulated field. The dose limits for critical structures are the standard values used in clinical practice at the M.D. Anderson Cancer Center, with the exception of the contralateral lung dose. Because patients have only one lung after EPP, the volumes of contralateral lung irradiated should be limited such that the mean lung dose is less than 9.5 Gy. This level is consistent with results of whole lung irradiation delivered during preparation for bone marrow transplant [31]. All patients can be set up and treated within a 45-minute period.

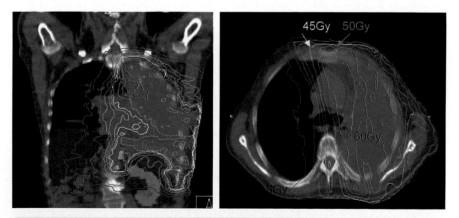

Fig. 3. Dose distributions from IMRT. The dose distribution demonstrates good coverage of the CTV and the high dose gradients achievable with this technique. The goal was 50 Gy to the CTV. The 50-, 45-, 30-, and 5-Gy isodose lines are shown in orange, yellow, green, and blue, respectively.

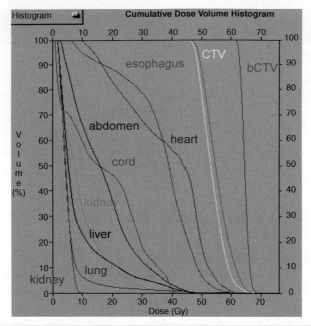

Fig. 4. Dose volume histogram from the case shown in Fig. 3. Coverage of the target volumes is adequate. The contralateral kidney was well below the goal dose, as was approximately 80% of the ipsilateral kidney. The mean lung dose was 5.3 Gy. Although this example was left sided, the heart constraints were met.

IMRT is more complicated to deliver and requires more machine time than three-dimensional CRT; however, good coverage of the target can be achieved. As shown in Fig. 3, the 50-Gy isodose line encompasses most of the CTV. Review of the dose volume histogram for this case (Fig. 4) demonstrates that the target volume is well covered and the normal tissue constraints are met. The liver and contralateral lung are spared with this technique. In this patient it was possible to spare the ipsilateral kidney because the organ was particularly low, which is unusual. The ipsilateral kidney usually receives high dose because the CTV typically abuts its posterior edge. Adequate contralateral renal function is assured by pretreatment renal ultrasounds. For left-sided lesions, the spleen is also likely to receive a high radiation dose. Therefore, pneumococcal prophylaxis is recommended.

SUMMARY AND FUTURE DIRECTIONS

A review of many small, nonrandomized studies (see Table 1) of combined modality therapy for MPM suggests that EPP followed by irradiation gives better local control than pleurectomy followed by radiation. Postoperative radiotherapy should include the entire volume immediately adjacent to the pleural space that is at highest risk for microscopic residual disease. This volume should include all sites of pleural reflection, the ipsilateral mediastinum, and the insertion of the diaphragm, because chemotherapy cannot yet make up for inadequate radiotherapy. The technique by which radiation is delivered (three-dimensional conformal versus IMRT) is probably not as important as the target volume delineation and coverage. IMRT usually has a better dose distribution but is more time consuming to deliver.

From a radiation oncology point of view, the most important aspect of future trials is firmly documented sites of regional relapse. True in-field failures must be documented and explained, which will help to determine the adequacy of target volume delineation and determine if more–or possibly less–dose is needed to prevent recurrence. EPP followed by radiation changes the pattern of recurrence such that distant metastases become the most common cause of death. This has several implications. First, it is important to include systemic therapy in the treatment program. The optimal sequencing of systemic therapy currently is unclear, because induction chemotherapy seems to make surgical resection slightly more risky [32]. Unlike non–small cell lung cancer, however, concurrent chemoradiotherapy does not seem necessary currently because of excellent locoregional control. Second, the current staging system requires modification, because it was designed at a time when locoregional recurrence was the most common cause of death, and it requires an operation for adequate staging. Because survival depends more on distant metastases, a more robust preoperative staging system must be developed. Although some risk factors for metastases, perhaps nodal metastases, likely will continue to be important predictors of survival, others (eg, parietal versus pleural involvement) might become less important. Third, because locoregional failure can be reduced dramatically, more emphasis should be placed on screening programs to identify patients with earlier disease. In summary, this is a time for cautious optimism in MPM.

References

[1] Connelly RR, Spirtas R, Myers MH, et al. Demographic patterns for mesothelioma in the United States. J Natl Cancer Inst 1997;8:1053–60.

[2] Law MR, Hodson ME, Warwick-Turner M. Malignant mesothelioma of the pleura: clinical aspects and symptomatic treatment. Eur J Respir Dis 1984;65:162–8.

[3] Baldini EH, Recht A, Strauss GM, et al. Patterns of failure after trimodality therapy for malignant pleural mesothelioma. Ann Thorac Surg 1997;63(2):334–8.

[4] Sugarbaker DJ, Flores RM, Jaklitsch MT, et al. Resection margins, extrapleural nodal status, and cell type determine postoperative long-term survival in trimodality therapy of malignant pleural mesothelioma: results in 183 patients. J Thorac Cardiovasc Surg 1999;177:34–63.

[5] Rusch VW, Rosenzweig K, Venkatraman E, et al. A phase II trial of surgical resection and adjuvant high-dose hemithoracic radiation for malignant pleural mesothelioma. J Thorac Cardiovasc Surg 2001;122(4):788–95.

[6] Ahamad A, Stevens CW, Smythe WR, et al. Promising early local control of malignant pleural mesothelioma following postoperative intensity modulated radiotherapy (IMRT) to the chest. Cancer J 2004;9(6):476–84.

[7] Rusch VW. Pleurectomy/decortication and adjuvant therapy for malignant mesothelioma. Chest 1993;103(4 Suppl):382S–4S.

[8] Gordon Jr W, Antman KH, Greenberger JS, et al. Radiation therapy in the management of patients with mesothelioma. Int J Radiat Oncol Biol Phys 1982;8(1):19–25.

 [9] Rusch VW, Piantadosi S, Holmes EC. The role of extrapleural pneumonectomy in malignant pleural mesothelioma: a lung cancer study group trial. J Thorac Cardiovasc Surg 1991;102(1):1–9.
[10] Sugarbaker DJ, Flores RM, Jaklitsch MT, et al. Resection margins, extrapleural nodal status, and cell type determine postoperative long-term survival in trimodality therapy of malignant pleural mesothelioma: results in 183 patients. J Thorac Cardiovasc Surg 1999; 117(1):54–63.
[11] Huncharek M, Kelsey K, Mark EJ, et al. Treatment and survival in diffuse malignant pleural mesothelioma: a study of 83 cases from the Massachusetts General Hospital. Anticancer Res 1996;16(3A):1265–8.
[12] Hakkinen AM, Laasonen A, Linnainmaa K, et al. Radiosensitivity of mesothelioma cell lines. Acta Oncol (Madr) 1996;35(4):451–6.
[13] Carmichael J, Degraff WG, Gamson J, et al. Radiation sensitivity of human lung cancer cell lines. Eur J Cancer Clin Oncol 1989;25(3):527–34.
[13a] Ball DL, Cruickshank DG. The treatment of malignant mesothelioma of the pleura: review of a 5-year experience, with special reference to radiotherapy. Am J Clin Oncol 1990; 13(1):4–9.
[14] Van Ooijen B, Eggermont AMM, Wiggers T. Subcutaneous tumor growth complicating the positioning of Denver shunt and intrapleural port-a-cath in mesothelioma patients. Eur J Surg Oncol 1992;18:638–40.
[15] Boutin C, Rey F, Viallat JR. Prevention of malignant seeding after invasive diagnostic procedures in patients with pleural mesothelioma: a randomized trial of local radiotherapy. Chest 1995;108:754–75.
[16] Nguyen LN, Komaki R, Allen P, et al. Effectiveness of accelerated radiotherapy for patients with inoperable nonsmall cell lung cancer (NSCLC) and borderline prognostic factors without distant metastasis: a retrospective review. Int J Radiat Oncol Biol Phys 1999;44:1053–6.
[17] Graham MV, Purdy JA, Emami B, et al. Clinical dose-volume histogram analysis for pneumonitis after 3D treatment for non-small cell lung cancer (NSCLC). Int J Radiat Oncol Biol Phys 1999;45(2):323–9.
[18] Maasilta P, Kivisaari L, Holsti LR, et al. Radiographic chest assessment of lung injury following hemithorax irradiation for pleural mesothelioma. Eur Respir J 1991;4(1): 76–83.
[19] Maasilta P. Deterioration in lung function following hemithorax irradiation for pleural mesothelioma. Int J Radiat Oncol Biol Phys 1991;20(3):433–8.
[20] Mattson K, Holsti LR, Tammilehto L, et al. Multimodality treatment programs for malignant pleural mesothelioma using high-dose hemithorax irradiation. Int J Radiat Oncol Biol Phys 1992;24(4):643–50.
[21] Hilaris BS, Nori D, Kwong E, et al. Pleurectomy and intraoperative brachytherapy and postoperative radiation in the treatment of malignant pleural mesothelioma. Int J Radiat Oncol Biol Phys 1984;10(3):325–31.
[22] Lee TT, Everett DL, Shu HG, et al. Radical pleurectomy/decortication and intraoperative radiotherapy followed by conformal radiation with or without chemotherapy for malignant pleural mesothelioma. J Thorac Cardiovasc Surg 2002;124:1183–9.
[23] Halstead JC, Lim E, Venkateswaran RM, et al. Improved survival with VATS pleurectomy-decortication in advanced malignant mesothelioma. Eur J Surg Oncol 2005;31(3):314–20.
[24] Stewart DJ, Martin-Ucar A, Pilling JE, et al. The effect of extent of local resection on patterns of disease progression in malignant pleural mesothelioma. Ann Thorac Surg 2004;78(1):245–52.
[25] Kutcher GJ, Kestler C, Greenblatt D, et al. Technique for external beam treatment for mesothelioma. Int J Radiat Oncol Biol Phys 1987;13(11):1747–52.
[26] Yajnik S, Rosenzweig KE, Mychalczak B, et al. Hemithoracic radiation after extrapleural pneumonectomy for malignant pleural mesothelioma. Int J Radiat Oncol Biol Phys 2003; 56(5):1319–26.

[27] Ahamad A, Stevens CW, Smythe WR, et al. Intensity-modulated radiation therapy: a novel approach to the management of malignant pleural mesothelioma. Int J Radiat Oncol Biol Phys 2003;55(3):768–75.

[28] Forster KM, Smythe WR, Starkschall G, et al. Intensity-modulated radiotherapy following extrapleural pneumonectomy for the treatment of malignant mesothelioma: clinical implementation. Int J Radiat Oncol Biol Phys 2003;55(3):606–16.

[28a] Stevens CW, Wong PF, Rice D, et al. Treatment planning system evaluation for mesothelioma IMRT. Lung Cancer 2005;49(Suppl 1):S75–81.

[29] Weder W, Ketstenholz P, Taverna C, et al. Neoadjuvant chemotherapy followed by extrapleural pneumonectomy in malignant pleural mesothelioma. J Clin Oncol 2004; 22:3451–7.

[30] Colaut F, Toniolo L, Vicario G, et al. Pleurectomy/decortication plus chemotherapy: outcomes of 40 cases of malignant pleural mesothelioma. Chir Ital 2004;56(6):781–6.

[30a] Baldini EH, Recht A, Strauss GM, et al. Patterns of failure after trimodality therapy for malignant pleural mesothelioma. Ann Thorac Surg 1997;63(2):334–8.

[30b] Ahamad A, Stevens CW, Smythe WR, et al. Promising early local control of malignant pleural mesothelioma following postoperative intensity modulated radiotherapy (IMRT) to the chest. Cancer J 2004;9(6):476–84.

[31] Della Volpe A, Ferreri AJ, Annaloro C, et al. Lethal pulmonary complications significantly correlate with individually assessed mean lung dose in patients with hematologic malignancies treated with total body irradiation. Int J Radiat Oncol Biol Phys 2002;52(2):483–8.

[32] Stewart DJ, Martin-Ucar AE, Edwards JG, et al. Extra-pleural pneumonectomy for malignant pleural mesothelioma: the risks of induction chemotherapy, right-sided procedures and prolonged operations. Eur J Cardiothor Surg 2005;27(3):373–8.

Hematol Oncol Clin N Am 19 (2005) 1117–1136

HEMATOLOGY/ONCOLOGY CLINICS
OF NORTH AMERICA

An Overview of Chemotherapy for Mesothelioma

Lee M. Krug, MD

Thoracic Oncology Service, Department of Medicine, Memorial Sloan-Kettering Cancer Center, 1275 York Avenue, New York, NY 10021, USA

Among the thoracic tumors, malignant pleural mesothelioma notoriously has been one of the most difficult to treat. Because mesothelioma is relatively rare, with an incidence of only 2000 to 3000 cases annually in the United States [1], research interest historically has been meager and large studies were difficult to conduct. Mostly, however, the lack of efficacy for any modality of therapy dampened enthusiasm for treating patients stricken with this disease. Because the tumor essentially encases the entire lung and often invades the chest wall or mediastinum, even radical surgical resection typically leaves disease behind. Treating the pleura with radiation offers a major challenge in delivering adequate doses without damaging the underlying lung. Despite innumerable studies with varied chemotherapeutic agents, no regimen previously showed superiority.

Fortunately, over the last several years, these sentiments have begun to change as improvements have been made in the treatment options for mesothelioma. This change has been most evident in the realm of chemotherapy and was heralded by the US Food and Drug Administration's approval in 2004 of the first chemotherapy regimen for this disease, pemetrexed and cisplatin. The emergence of effective chemotherapy has sparked a greater interest not only in treating patients but also in a surge of studies of new approaches and novel therapeutics that likely will further improve our treatments in the near future.

This article reviews the emerging data regarding the development of effective chemotherapy. The data on specific classes of chemotherapeutic agents are described, and seminal clinical trials are highlighted. Next, the goals of chemotherapy treatment are analyzed in various disease settings. Finally, new agents currently under study are discussed. Other excellent reviews that have been published recently offer the reader further information on this topic [2,3].

CHEMOTHERAPY

Nearly every chemotherapy agent has been tried for the treatment of mesothelioma, with generally unfavorable results (Table 1). Most trials have had a

E-mail address: krugl@mskcc.org

Table 1
Trials that tested single-agent chemotherapy in mesothelioma

Agent [reference]	Dose/schedule	No. of patients	Response rate (%)	Median survival (mo)
Anthracyclines				
Doxorubicin [4]	Several	51	14	7.5
Doxorubicin [5]	60 mg/m² every 3 wk	21	0	NR
Doxorubicin [6]	60 mg/m² every 3 wk	70	NR	8
Doxorubicin [7]	120 mg/m² every 3 wk (with dexrazoxane and GM-CSF)	10	0	4.8
Liposomal daunorubicin [8]	120 mg/m² every 4 wk	14	0	6
Liposomal doxorubicin [9]	50 mg/m² every 4 wk	24	0	9
Liposomal doxorubicin [10]	45 mg/m² every 4 wk	33	6	13
Liposomal doxorubicin [99]	55 mg/m² every 4 wk	15	7	NR
Alkylating agents				
Cyclophosphamide [5]	1500 mg/m² every 3 wk	21	0	NR
Ifosfamide [100]	2 g/m² × 4 d every 3 wk	26	8	6.5
Ifosfamide [101]	1.2–1.5 g/m² × 5 d every 3 wk	17	24	9
Ifosfamide [102]	1.5 g/m² × 5 d every 3 wk	40	3	6.9
Mitomycin C [103]	10 mg/m² every 4 wk	19	21	NR
Temozolamide [104]	200 mg/m²/d × 5 d every 4 wk	27	4	8.2
Platinums				
Cisplatin [18]	120 mg/m² every 4 wk	24	13	5
Cisplatin [19]	100 mg/m² every 3 wk	35	14	7.5
Cisplatin [20]	75 mg/m² every 3 wk	222	17	9.3
Cisplatin [21]	80 mg/m² every 3 wk	124	14	8.8
Carboplatin [23]	300–400 mg/m² every 4 wk	17	12	NR
Carboplatin [25]	150 mg/m² × 3 d	31	16	8
Carboplatin [24]	400 mg/m² every 4 wk	40	5	7.1

Agent	Dose/schedule			
Antimicrotubule agents				
Vinblastine [31]	1.4 mg/m² continuous infusion × 5 d every 3 wk	20	0	3
Vincristine [33]	1.3 mg/m²/wk	23	0	7
Vindesine [32]	3 mg/m²/wk	17	6	NR
Vinorelbine [34]	30 mg/m²/wk	29	24	10.6
Paclitaxel [36]	200 mg/m² over 3 h every 3 wk	25	0	9
Paclitaxel [37]	250 mg/m² over 24 h every 3 wk plus G-CSF	35	9	5
Docetaxel [38]	100 mg/m² every 3 wk	30	10	12
Docetaxel [39]	100 mg/m² every 3 wk	19	5	4
Topoisomerase inhibitors				
Etoposide (IV) [105]	150 mg/m² d 1, 3, 5 every 3 wk	49	4	7.3
Etoposide (oral) [105]	100 mg/m²/d × 21 d every 5 wk	45	7	9.5
Topotecan [40]	1.5 mg/m²/d × 5 every 3 wk	22	0	8
Irinotecan [41]	125 mg/m²/wk × 4 every 6 wk	28	0	7.9
Antimetabolites				
Gemcitabine [44]	1500 mg/m² d 1, 8, 15 every 4 wk	17	0	4.7
Gemcitabine [45]	1250 mg/m² d 1, 8, 15 every 4 wk	27	7	8
Capecitabine [106]	2500 mg/m²/d × 14 d every 3 wk	27	4	4.9
Methotrexate [50]	3 g (with citrovorum factor rescue) every 10 d	63	37	11
Trimetrexate [49]	6 or 10 mg/m²/d × 5 every 3 wk	52	12	5.0 and 8.9
Edatrexate [52]	80 mg/m²/wk	20	25	9.6
Edatrexate [52]	80 mg/m²/wk with leucovorin	38	16	6.6
Pemetrexed [55]	500 mg/m² every 3 wk	21	10	8.0
Pemetrexed [55]	500 mg/m² every 3 wk with B_{12} and folic acid	43	16	13.0

Abbreviations: NR, not reported.

Table 2
A comparison of two randomized phase III trials that combined antifolates with cisplatin

Trial [reference]	No. of patients	Response rate	Median time to progression	Median survival	1-year survival
Pemetrexed + cisplatin vs.	226	41%	5.7 mo	12.1 mo	50%
cisplatin [20]	222	17%	3.9 mo	9.3 mo	38%
(intent to treat)		P<.001	P=.001	P=.02	P=.012
Pemetrexed + cisplatin vs.	168	46%	6.1 mo	13.3 mo	57%
cisplatin [20]	163	20%	3.9 mo	10.0 mo	42%
(vitamin supplemented)		P<.001	P=.001	P=.05	P=.01
Raltitrexed + cisplatin vs.	126	24%	NR	11.4 mo	46%
cisplatin [21]	124	14%		8.8 mo	40%
		P=.056			P=.048

phase II design with a relatively small sample size. Various combinations also have been tested, with some modest improvement noted in response rates though generally unclear survival benefits. Only a few randomized trials have been powered appropriately to compare treatments properly (Table 2).

Anthracyclines and Alkylating Agents

Doxorubicin was one of the earliest drugs used in the treatment of mesothelioma. Between 1972 and 1980, the Eastern Cooperative Oncology Group conducted studies in which 7 of 51 (14%) of patients treated with single agent doxorubicin and 2 of 24 (8%) treated with doxorubicin combinations demonstrated responses [4]. Follow-up studies have produced much less satisfactory results. Single-agent doxorubicin has served as the control arm in two randomized trials. In one trial, patients were treated with doxorubicin, 60 mg/m^2, or cyclophosphamide, 1500 mg/m^2, every 3 weeks and then were crossed over to the other arm at progression [5]. None of the 30 evaluable patients responded to either drug. In the other randomized trial, doxorubicin was compared with ranpirnase, an agent that degrades RNA [6]. Preliminary results showed similar survival for the two treatments in intent to treat analysis (median survival 7.7 versus 8.2 months). Even high-dose doxorubicin (90–120 mg/m^2) administered with the cardioprotectant dexrazoxane and with prophylactic GM-CSF (granulocyte macrophage colony stimulating factor) did not produce any responses, yet it did cause excessive toxicity, which resulted in early trial closure [7]. Liposomal doxorubicin and daunorubicin have been tested as single agents but also have shown poor efficacy [8–10].

Doxorubicin combined with alkylating agents, such as cyclophosphamide or ifosfamide, platinums, or other agents, have yielded somewhat better response rates, although in most cases, no improvement in survival [11–16]. As the control arm of a small randomized study, doxorubicin plus cyclophosphamide had a response rate of 11% and a median survival of 7 months. The addition of imidazole and carboxamide did not provide any benefit. More promising results were reported in a study from M.D. Anderson that combined doxorubicin, cisplatin, and cyclophosphamide and had with a response rate of 30%, including one pathologic complete response, and a median survival of 14 months [16]. The Italian "MMM" regimen of mitoxantrone, methotrexate, and mitomycin had a 32% response rate and considerable symptomatic benefit, but grade 3 or 4 neutropenia (82%), anemia (14%), and thrombocytopenia (23%) were problematic [17].

Platinums

Cisplatin has yielded a consistent level of single-agent activity across several studies. The response rate of 13% to 14% observed in phase II studies [18,19] was nearly duplicated in two phase III trials that used cisplatin as the control treatment [20,21]. In a systematic meta-analysis that encompassed 83 phase II trials, cisplatin had the greatest single-agent activity, and doxorubicin plus cisplatin was the best combination [22]. Justifiably, cisplatin has supplied the backbone of several different regimens. Trials with other platinum analogs, namely single-agent carboplatin or combinations that incorporate carboplatin or oxaliplatin, have shown comparable results in smaller trials [23–29].

Antimicrotubule Agents

Older vinca alkaloids, namely vinblastine, vincristine, and vindesine, have shown minimal to no single-agent activity [30–33]. Vinorelbine, on the other hand, seems somewhat more effective. In Steele and colleagues' [34] phase II study of vinorelbine given at 30 mg/m^2 weekly, 7 of 29 patients (24%) responded, including 2 patients with sarcomatoid histology and 1 with mixed histology. The median survival was 10.6 months, and 1-year survival rate was 41%. The same group subsequently combined vinorelbine with oxaliplatin, but the response rate (23%), median survival (8.8 months), and 1-year survival rate (27%) were no better [35].

Taxanes have had a poor track record in mesothelioma. Paclitaxel was studied in two cooperative group studies, first by EORTC at a dose of 200 mg/m^2 over 3 hours, and then by Cancer and Leukemia Group B (CALGB) at 250 mg/m^2 over 24 hours [36,37]. The response rates were 0% and 9%, and the median survival was 9 months and 5 months in those two trials, respectively. Similarly, little efficacy was observed with docetaxel, dosed at 100 mg/m^2 every 3 weeks, in two phase II trials [38,39].

Topoisomerase Inhibitors

As a class, topoisomerase inhibitors have fared poorly against mesothelioma. Neither intravenous nor oral etoposide had any significant antitumor activity. Phase II trials of topotecan conducted by the North Central Cancer Treatment Group and of irinotecan conducted by CALGB had no responses [40,41]. A Japanese study of irinotecan, 60 mg/m^2 days 1, 8, and 15, with cisplatin, 60 mg/m^2 day 1, saw responses in 4 of 15 (40%) of patients [42]. A British study added mitomycin C to the irinotecan, cisplatin combination and reported a 50% response rate in 18 evaluable patients and a 71% response in the 7 patients with non-epithelioid histology [43].

Antimetabolites

Although single-agent gemcitabine yields few responses, the trials that combined gemcitabine with cisplatin ushered in a new era of optimism for chemotherapy in mesothelioma. Two published phase II trials of gemcitabine from CALGB and EORTC reported response rates of 0% and 7%, respectively [44,45]. Perhaps because of additive effects noted in murine mesothelioma models [46], gemcitabine combined with platinums has more impressive activity. The first report of this was from a single institution study in Australia, in which patients were treated with gemcitabine, 1000 mg/m^2 days 1, 8, and 15, with cisplatin, 100 mg/m^2 on day 1, every 4 weeks [47]. Forty-eight percent of patients were deemed to have a partial response, and the median survival was 10 months. Subsequently, the Australians conducted a multicenter trial of this same regimen; the response rate dropped to 33%, although the median survival remained at 11 months [48]. A Dutch group used a slightly different dosing schedule that involved gemcitabine, 1250 mg/m^2 days 1 and 8, with cisplatin, 80 mg/m^2 on day 1, and reported a response rate of 16% and median survival of 10 months [49]. Gemcitabine was combined with carboplatin in one phase II trial with 50 patients: the response rate was 26% and the median survival was 15 months [26]. Gemcitabine combined with oxaliplatin yielded a 40% response rate and a 13-month median survival [29].

Antifolates have garnered some of the most favorable results as single agents and in combinations, particularly with platinums. Solheim and colleagues [50] reported a respectable 37% response rate and 11-month median survival using high-dose methotrexate, 3 g intravenously, with citrovorum rescue. Trimetrexate and edatrexate were tested by CALGB [51,52]. Twelve percent of the 17 patients treated with trimetrexate responded, and the effect did not differ whether treated at low or high dose. Edatrexate had slightly more activity, with a 25% response rate, including one complete response, which yielded a median survival of 10 months. When leucovorin was added in an attempt to ameliorate toxicity, however, the response rate and median survival lowered to 16% and 7 months, respectively [52]. This change raised the concern that vitamin supplementation interfered with the drug's therapeutic efficacy.

Pemetrexed is the antifolate with the largest body of data supporting its role as the standard chemotherapy for first-line treatment of unresectable mesothelioma. In distinction from other antifolates, pemetrexed inhibits multiple enzymes in purine and pyrimidine synthesis, including thymidylate synthase, dihydrofolate reductase, and glycinamide ribonucleotide formyltransferase [53]. The activity in mesothelioma was identified serendipitously in a phase I trial that established the recommended doses as pemetrexed, 500 mg/m^2, with cisplatin, 75 mg/m^2, every 3 weeks. Thirteen patients who have mesothelioma were enrolled on that trial, and 5 had a partial response. These encouraging results led to a large international randomized trial (see Table 2). Four hundred fifty-six patients were enrolled and assigned treatment with pemetrexed plus cisplatin or cisplatin alone. Overall, patient characteristics were balanced across the two treatment arms, as designed by the randomization, and were typical, with approximately 70% epithelial histology, 80% male gender, generally good performance status, and advanced stage. Treatment with pemetrexed plus cisplatin improved survival over treatment with cisplatin alone. The overall median survival improved from 9.3 months to 12.1 months ($P=.20$) and the 1-year survival rate improved from 38% to 50% (Fig. 1). Time to progression increased from 3.9 to 5.7 months ($P=.001$). The response rate in the cisplatin arm, 17%, corresponded to the reports from previous studies. With the addition of pemetrexed, the response rate increased to 41%, which is relatively high for an historically "chemoresistant" disease.

While this trial was ongoing, a multivariate analysis of the characteristics for patients enrolled in pemetrexed trials identified homocysteine and methylmalonic acid levels (markers of folate and vitamin B_{12} status, respectively) as predictors of excess toxicity. At that point, all patients treated with pemetrexed were managed with vitamin supplementation. This change occurred after the first 70 patients had been enrolled on the phase III trial, and so

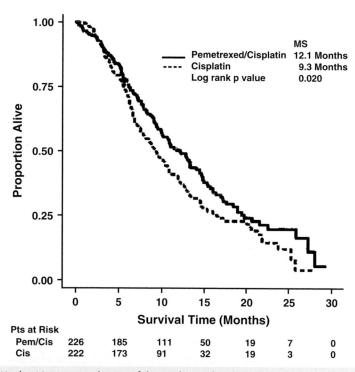

Fig. 1. Kaplan-Meier survival curve of the randomized trial comparing pemetrexed + cisplatin to cisplatin alone. Cis, cisplatin; MS, median survival; Pem/Cis, pemetrexed/cisplatin; Pts, patients. (*From* Vogelzang NJ, Rusthoven JJ, Symanowski J, et al. Phase III study of pemetrexed in combination with cisplatin versus cisplatin alone in patients with malignant pleural mesothelioma. J Clin Oncol 2003;21(14):2640; with permission.)

the accrual was expanded to adjust for this modification. As opposed to the edatrexate studies, in which the addition of leucovorin seemed to affect the treatment efficacy adversely [52], all outcome parameters in the pemetrexed/ cisplatin study improved with the use of folate and B_{12} supplementation. Median survival for fully supplemented patients was 10 months for the cisplatin arm and 13.3 months for the pemetrexed/cisplatin arm. Response rates were 20% and 46%, respectively. Vitamin supplementation clearly lessened toxicity, particularly febrile neutropenia and gastrointestinal complaints, which allowed for better drug delivery and likely accounted for the improved outcomes.

A large, randomized trial with a comparable design evaluated another antifolate/platinum combination (see Table 2) [21]. Raltitrexed, a specific inhibitor of thymidylate synthase with single-agent activity in mesothelioma [54], demonstrated promising results when combined with oxaliplatin [27], which prompted the phase III study. The trial design involved stratifying patients who had unresectable mesothelioma by performance status, white blood count, and institution, and then randomizing them to receive raltitrexed, 3 mg/m^2, plus cisplatin, 80 mg/m^2, or cisplatin alone, every 3 weeks. The baseline characteristics of the 250 patients enrolled were similar in the two arms except for histology. More patients in the combination arm had epithelial subtype than in the cisplatin arm (75% versus 61%). The response rates (24% versus 14%), median overall survival (11.4 versus 8.8 months), and 1-year survival rate (46% versus 40%) all favored the raltitrexed plus cisplatin arm ($P=.48$ for 1-year survival). This study confirms that treatment with an antifolate plus cisplatin is superior to treatment with cisplatin alone in mesothelioma.

With this information, pemetrexed and cisplatin emerges as the standard first-line chemotherapy regimen for patients who have unresectable mesothelioma. Substituting cisplatin with carboplatin was tested in one phase I trial with 27 patients [28]. Pemetrexed, 500 mg/m^2, plus carboplatin AUC (area under the curve) 5 every 3 weeks was the recommended dosing schedule. In this phase I trial that selectively enrolled patients who had mesothelioma, the response rate was 32% and the median survival was 15 months. Single-agent pemetrexed was tested in a phase II trial that enrolled 64 patients, of which 43 received folic acid and vitamin B_{12} supplementation [55]. The overall response rate was 14%, and the median survival was 10.7 months. Less toxicity occurred in the supplemented patients, however, which allowed better drug delivery and a median survival of 13 months in this group. Jänne and colleagues [56] reported their preliminary results that combined pemetrexed with gemcitabine. Fifty-three chemo-naive patients were treated with gemcitabine, 1250 mg/m^2 days 1 and 8, and pemetrexed, 500 mg/m^2 on day 8. In this group of patients, of whom 67% had epithelial histology and 76% had stage IV disease, the response rate was 20% and the stable disease rate was 58%. Grade 3/4 neutropenia occurred in 24% of cycles, but febrile neutropenia occurred in only 2%. Pemetrexed alone or in combination with carboplatin or gemcitabine may be a reasonable alternative for patients who cannot tolerate cisplatin.

GOALS OF THERAPY
Advanced Disease
As with other oncologic diseases, the goals of therapy for patients who have mesothelioma must be established at the onset of treatment. Most patients diagnosed with mesothelioma have advanced disease and symptom palliation has utmost priority. These patients may suffer from debilitating chest pain caused by the pleural tumor invading into the surrounding chest wall or into mediastinal structures. Encasement of the lung by the inflexible tumor causes poor lung expansion with inspiration, which results in shortness of breath and predisposes patients to pneumonia. Metastases to the peritoneum cause abdominal pain, ascites, and bowel obstruction. Constitutional symptoms, such as fatigue and weight loss, are also common.

Several trials have demonstrated that chemotherapy can improve symptoms from mesothelioma. In an analysis of 150 patients treated with mitomycin, vinblastine, and cisplatin [57], 69% reported an improvement in symptoms that were graded by the treating physician. Specifically, improvements in pain (71%), cough (62%), and dyspnea (50%) were noted. These improvements occurred despite a response rate of only 15% and a median survival of 7 months. In a phase II trial of single-agent vinorelbine [34], quality of life, as measured by the Rotterdam Symptom Checklist, improved in most patients. Patients with treatment response and stable disease had improved psychological, physical, and lung-related symptoms, although overall physical activity levels were less. The randomized trial of pemetrexed plus cisplatin versus cisplatin used a modification of the Lung Cancer Symptom Scale to measure symptom and quality-of-life parameters, and a statistically significant improvement was observed with the combination therapy [58,59].

Several factors predict which patients are most likely to gain benefit from chemotherapy. The strongest of these factors is histologic subtype: epithelioid tumors generally respond more frequently, sarcomatoid tumors rarely respond, and biphasic tumors have an intermediate response rate. These factors should be taken into account whenever one reviews the results from chemotherapy trials, because variations in the percent of patients with different histologic subtypes can impact significantly the outcomes. Others have found age, performance status, gender, asbestos exposure, symptomatology (eg, chest pain or weight loss), white blood cell count, and platelet count to have prognostic significance [60]. The CALGB proposed separating patients who had mesothelioma into six prognostic groups as determined by performance status, age, hemoglobin, white blood cell count, presence of chest pain, and weight loss [60]. Based on the data from a series of CALGB phase II trials, patients with a performance status of 0 and age younger than 49 or, alternately, a performance status of 0, age older than 49, and hemoglobin ≥14.6 had the best median survival (13.9 months). Patients with a performance status of 1 or 2 and white blood cell count ≥15.6 had the worst median survival (4 months). This information emphasizes the range of outcomes that can be observed.

Traditionally, most phase II trials of chemotherapeutic agents define the primary endpoint as response rate. This is particularly problematic in mesothelioma because radiologically, it appears as a rind of tumor surrounding the lung, which is in contrast with other tumors that appear as a separate mass more easily measured in two dimensions. For this reason, bidimensional tumor measurement is not reliable in mesothelioma. The newer RECIST (Response Evaluation Criteria In Solid Tumors) criteria may be better, since this uses a unidimensional measurement which can be applied to tumor thickness along the pleura. When designing the phase III trial of pemetrexed plus cisplatin versus cisplatin [20], the investigators paid careful attention to this issue. They measured pleural thickness at up to three different areas on at least three different sections at least 2 cm apart. A ≥30% decrease in the sum of the unidimensional measurements constituted a partial response. This modified RECIST technique has been validated and should be taken as the standard for future trial design [61].

The ultimate question remains whether chemotherapy improves survival in mesothelioma. In other diseases, such as non–small cell lung cancer, several randomized trials confirmed that chemotherapy does improve survival, but similar data are lacking in mesothelioma. Most chemotherapy clinical trials in mesothelioma have had a phase II design that makes it impossible to determine whether the treatment had any impact on survival. The phase III trial of pemetrexed plus cisplatin versus cisplatin alone supports the fact that combination chemotherapy can improve survival, because patients treated with pemetrexed plus cisplatin lived longer (median survival improved from 9–12 months). The first large, randomized trial in mesothelioma that compared chemotherapy treatment to supportive care is ongoing. Sponsored by the Medical Research Council, this ambitious trial intends to randomize 840 patients with unresectable mesothelioma to treatment with mitomycin, vinblastine, and cisplatin, or vinorelbine or best supportive care alone [62,63]. The two treatment arms were chosen based on the results of the studies described previously. Unfortunately, a pemetrexed/cisplatin treatment arm is not included in the Medical Research Council trial.

Second-line Chemotherapy

For patients with progression of disease after first-line chemotherapy, the role for second-line chemotherapy is essentially unknown. Only one trial, that of ZD0473, a platinum analog, selectively enrolled previously treated patients [64]. Although there were no partial responses, 12% had a minor response, but the median time to progression was a brief 2.5 months. Two other trials included a portion of previously treated patients [27,65]. In one trial, treatment with oxaliplatin and raltitrexed resulted in a 20% response rate and 10-month median survival in patients pretreated with platinums, although the response rate and survival were better than in the group of chemo-naive patients [27]. The results of these three studies are impossible to compare because of the variability in patient characteristics and range of efficacy of these agents. The best course for patients in this situation who are fit enough for more therapy would be enrollment on clinical trials. Should randomized studies that evaluate newer therapies be pursued in this setting, best supportive care would be a valid comparator arm, as it was in trials conducted in second-line non–small cell lung cancer [66].

Perioperative Therapy

With the advent of effective chemotherapy, the question of whether it could be used in conjunction with surgery has been posed. A small proportion of patients who have mesothelioma may have early-stage disease and are fit enough to be managed surgically. This management could involve either a pleurectomy/decortication, which is a debulking procedure aimed at removing gross disease, or an extrapleural pneumonectomy, which involves en bloc resection of the pleura, lung, hemidiaphragm and a portion of the pericardium. In either case, local and distant recurrence is a major problem.

Several groups have used intracavitary chemotherapy (usually cisplatin) in the perioperative setting in an attempt to improve relapse along the chest wall, the site at highest risk [67–69]. In sum, these trials generally have shown excess toxicity, with no improvement in survival or even local control. Photodynamic therapy also has yielded disappointing results to this end [70]. External beam radiation therapy, especially after extrapleural pneumonectomy, may provide better local disease control, but most patients still relapse distantly [71]. This observation led groups to add systemic chemotherapy to the multimodality approach.

Investigators at Brigham and Women's Hospital have favored using chemotherapy and chemoradiation after extrapleural pneumonectomy. The chemotherapy regimens have evolved over time and have included doxorubicin and cyclophosphamide, paclitaxel and carboplatin, and gemcitabine plus cisplatin or carboplatin. In a series of 183 patients, these investigators have reported 2- and 5-year survival rates of 38% and 15%, respectively [72]. Building on this approach but using more modern chemotherapy, the CALGB is developing a multicenter, multimodality study in which patients receive extrapleural pneumonectomy followed by pemetrexed/cisplatin and intensity-modulated radiation therapy.

Other groups have reported their experience with the administration of chemotherapy before extrapleural pneumonectomy and radiation. Pilot studies conducted in Switzerland [73] and at Memorial Sloan-Kettering Cancer Center [74] showed this approach to be safe using the regimen of gemcitabine and cisplatin. A follow-up multicenter trial from Switzerland tested this approach in 61 patients [75]. Fifty-eight patients completed the planned three cycles of chemotherapy. Sixty-one percent of patients underwent complete resection with a remarkable 2% operative mortality rate, and 78% completed the prescribed course of radiation. The median survival for all patients was 18 months, and for patients who had resection it was 26 months. The median time to recurrence was 14 months. A US multicenter trial of pemetrexed and cisplatin followed by extrapleural pneumonectomy and hemithoracic radiation is ongoing [76].

NOVEL THERAPEUTICS

As with other malignancies, oncologists hope that advances in understanding the biology of certain tumors will lead to the development of agents that target these mechanisms, allowing us to move beyond cytotoxic agents as the primary form of therapy. In that regard, several agents have been tested recently in patients who had mesothelioma. The agents, the targets, and the status of various clinical trials are described in Table 3.

Ranpirnase

Ranpirnase is an enzyme that degrades cytosolic tRNA. Administered intravenously, its toxicities are generally mild and include fatigue and edema but not myelosuppression. Several relatively large clinical trials with this agent have been conducted in patients who have mesothelioma. First, a single-agent study enrolled 105 patients (37% previously treated) who received ranpirnase, 480 µg/m^2, weekly [65]. The primary endpoint was survival. Based on intent to treat, the median survival was 6 months and the 1- and 2-year survival rates were 34% and 22%, respectively. In a retrospective subgroup analysis based on the CALGB stratification in which the patients with the worst prognosis were excluded, the median survival was 8.3 months, and 1- and 2-year survival rates were 42% and 27%, respectively. Four of 81 evaluable patients had a partial response, 2 had minor responses, and 35 had stable disease. Preliminary results of a randomized study that compared ranpirnase to doxorubicin also

Table 3
Targeted agents studied in mesothelioma

Agent	Relevant target/ mechanism of action	Trial design	Status [reference]
Ranpirnase	Degrades tRNA	Phase II single agent	Completed [65]
		Phase III ranpirnase vs. doxorubicin	Completed
		Phase III ranpirnase plus doxorubicin vs. doxorubicin	Ongoing
Imatinib	Inhibits PDGFR	Phase II single agent	Completed [78–80]
Gefitinib	EGFR-TKI	Phase II single agent	Completed [85]
Erlotinib	EGFR-TKI	Phase II single agent	Completed [75]
BAY 43-9006	Raf kinase inhibitor	Phase II single agent	Ongoing
SU5416	VEGFR-TKI	Phase II single agent	Completed [92]
Bevacizumab	Monoclonal antibody binding VEGF	Randomized phase II gemcitabine/cisplatin ± bevacizumab	Ongoing [93]
PTK787	Inhibits KDR, Flt-1, and PDGFR	Phase II single agent	Completed [94]
Suberoylanilide hydroxamic acid	Histone deacetylase inhibitor	Phase I / Phase III	Completed [97,98] / Ongoing

Abbreviations: EGFR-TKI, epidermal growth factor receptor tyrosine kinase inhibitor; KDR, kinase insert domain-containing receptor; PDGFR, platelet-derived growth factor receptor; VEGFR-TKI, vascular endothelial growth factor receptor tyrosine kinase inhibitor.

have been reported. One hundred fifty-four patients were enrolled and stratified by histology and performance status. Survival was the same in both arms (8 months), although using CALGB subgroup analysis, the investigators claim that ranpirnase may be superior to doxorubicin in some patients. No response rates were reported. Another phase III trial that compares doxorubicin plus ranpirnase to doxorubicin is ongoing.

Tyrosine Kinase Inhibitors

Tyrosine kinase inhibitors with proven efficacy in other diseases have had less success in mesothelioma despite excellent rationale for their testing. Imatinib, an oral inhibitor with astounding activity in chronic myelogenous leukemia because of inhibition of bcr-abl and gastrointestinal stromal tumors because of inhibition of c-kit, also inhibits the platelet-derived growth factor receptor. In culture, mesothelioma cell lines express platelet-derived growth factor α and β receptors and platelet-derived growth factor ligand, which implicate an autocrine growth loop and suggest that inhibitors of this pathway warrant study [77]. Phase II trials of imatinib from several groups failed to show any responses, however, and treatment was poorly tolerated [78–80].

Similarly, the epidermal growth factor receptor inhibitors gefitinib and erlotinib are small molecule inhibitors that have well-established activity in patients with non–small cell lung cancer [81]. The high rate of epidermal growth factor receptor expression in mesothelioma tumor samples [82,83] and the growth inhibition observed in mesothelioma cell lines exposed to gefitinib [84] provided the rationale for study. In a CALGB phase II trial that enrolled 43 patients, however, only one response was seen despite 96% of tumors having 2+ to 3+ epidermal growth factor receptor expression [85]. Similarly no responses were observed out of 31 evaluable patients in a SWOG (Southwest Oncology Group) trial of erlotinib [86]. Tumor sensitivity to imatinib and gefitinib/erlotinib in most cases corresponds to the presence of activating mutations in the genes for the relevant receptors [87,88]. The absence of these mutations in mesothelioma may explain the lack of activity. A phase II study of an raf kinase inhibitor, BAY 43-9006, is currently ongoing in the CALGB.

Angiogenesis Inhibitors

Angiogenesis inhibitors have garnered intense enthusiasm for the treatment of mesothelioma. Angiogenesis is in part regulated by the vascular endothelial growth factor (VEGF), which serves as ligand to fms-like tyrosine kinase-1 and the kinase insert domain-containing receptor. Several lines of evidence support targeting VEGF in mesothelioma. VEGF induces proliferation of mesothelial cells in culture, and the addition of VEGF neutralizing antibodies inhibits this effect [89]. Mesothelioma tumor specimens express VEGF and its receptors [89,90]. High levels of VEGF also have been detected in the serum and pleural effusions of patients who have mesothelioma and correlate with poorer survival [89,91].

In a completed trial, the kinase insert domain-containing receptor tyrosine kinase inhibitor, SU5416, showed some evidence of clinical activity [92], although development of this agent has been halted. Other studies with angiogenesis inhibitors are ongoing. Bevacizumab, a monoclonal antibody that binds VEGF, or placebo is combined with gemcitabine and cisplatin in a randomized phase II trial [93]. While the final results of that trial as broken down by treatment arm await an adequate number of events to be realized, the overall survival of 15.7 months and the progression free survival of 6.4 months are encouraging. An interesting correlative to this study was that higher serum VEGF levels corresponded with poorer survival, further justifying VEGFR as a relevant target in the treatment of mesothelioma. PTK787, an inhibitor of kinase insert domain-containing receptor, fms-like tyrosine kinase-1, and platelet-derived growth factor receptor, has also been tested in a CALGB phase II trial. Forty-seven patients with a median age of 75 years were enrolled over an 18-month period and received vatalanib as first-line therapy. The response rate was 8% and another 72% had stable disease. Despite this, the median progression free survival of 5 months and median overall survival of 6.6 months were disappointing [94].

Histone Deacetylase Inhibitors

Histone deacetylase inhibitors are a class of therapeutics that permits DNA uncoiling and regulates the transcription of gene subsets [95]. Phase I trials of intravenous and oral formulations of suberoylanilide hydroxamic acid have shown that it inhibits histone acetylation in peripheral blood mononuclear cells and that it has a broad range of antitumor activity in hematologic and solid malignancies [96,97]. After an index patient who had mesothelioma who was enrolled on the phase I trial with oral suberoylanilide hydroxamic acid demonstrated a response, the cohort was expanded to enroll additional patients who had mesothelioma. In all, 13 patients who had mesothelioma were included in the phase I trial of oral suberoylanilide hydroxamic acid [98]. All but one had previously been treated with chemotherapy. Four patients completed six or more cycles of therapy. Two patients demonstrated partial responses. A multicenter phase III international study of oral suberoylanilide hydroxamic acid versus placebo is ongoing for patients with mesothelioma who have failed treatment with pemetrexed.

SUMMARY

Effective chemotherapy for mesothelioma is currently available. Hopefully, it will provide a springboard for further advances, such as in the areas of targeted therapies and combined modality treatment because there remains a lot of room for improvement.

References

[1] Price B, Ware A. Mesothelioma trends in the United States: an update based on Surveillance, Epidemiology, and End Results Program data for 1973 through 2003. Am J Epidemiol 2004;159(2):107–12.

[2] Janne PA. Chemotherapy for malignant pleural mesothelioma. Clin Lung Cancer 2003; 5(2):98–106.

[3] Tomek S, Manegold C. Chemotherapy for malignant pleural mesothelioma: past results and recent developments. Lung Cancer 2004;45(Suppl 1):S103–19.

[4] Lerner HJ, Schoenfeld DA, Martin A, et al. Malignant mesothelioma: the Eastern Cooperative Oncology Group (ECOG) experience. Cancer 1983;52(11):1981–5.

[5] Sorensen PG, Bach F, Bork E, et al. Randomized trial of doxorubicin versus cyclophosphamide in diffuse malignant pleural mesothelioma. Cancer Treat Rep 1985;69(12): 1431–2.

[6] Vogelzang NJ, Taub R, Shin D, et al. Phase III randomized trial of onconase vs. doxorubicin in patients with unresectable malignant mesothelioma: analysis of survival [abstract 2274]. Proc Am Soc Clin Oncol 2000;19:577a.

[7] Kosty MP, Herndon II JE, Vogelzang NJ, et al. High-dose doxorubicin, dexrazoxane, and GM-CSF in malignant mesothelioma: a phase II study. Cancer and Leukemia Group B 9631. Lung Cancer 2001;34(2):289–95.

[8] Steele JP, O'Doherty CA, Shamash J, et al. Phase II trial of liposomal daunorubicin in malignant pleural mesothelioma. Ann Oncol 2001;12(4):497–9.

[9] Oh Y, Perez-Soler R, Fossella FV, et al. Phase II study of intravenous doxil in malignant pleural mesothelioma. Invest New Drugs 2000;18(3):243–5.

[10] Baas P, van Meerbeeck J, Groen H, et al. Caelyx in malignant mesothelioma: a phase II EORTC study. Ann Oncol 2000;11(6):697–700.

[11] Dirix LY, van Meerbeeck J, Schrijvers D, et al. A phase II trial of dose-escalated doxorubicin and ifosfamide/mesna in patients with malignant mesothelioma. Ann Oncol 1994;5(7):653–5.

[12] Carmichael J, Cantwell BM, Harris AL. A phase II trial of ifosfamide/mesna with doxorubicin for malignant mesothelioma. Eur J Cancer Clin Oncol 1989;25(5):911–2.

[13] Samson MK, Wasser LP, Borden EC, et al. Randomized comparison of cyclophosphamide, imidazole carboxamide, and adriamycin versus cyclophosphamide and adriamycin in patients with advanced stage malignant mesothelioma: a Sarcoma Intergroup Study. J Clin Oncol 1987;5(1):86–91.

[14] Ardizzoni A, Rosso R, Salvati F, et al. Activity of doxorubicin and cisplatin combination chemotherapy in patients with diffuse malignant pleural mesothelioma: an Italian Lung Cancer Task Force (FONICAP) phase II study. Cancer 1991;67(12):2984–7.

[15] Pennucci MC, Ardizzoni A, Pronzato P, et al. Combined cisplatin, doxorubicin, and mitomycin for the treatment of advanced pleural mesothelioma: a phase II FONICAP trial. Italian Lung Cancer Task Force. Cancer 1997;79(10):1897–902.

[16] Shin DM, Fossella FV, Umsawasdi T, et al. Prospective study of combination chemotherapy with cyclophosphamide, doxorubicin, and cisplatin for unresectable or metastatic malignant pleural mesothelioma. Cancer 1995;76(11):2230–6.

[17] Pinto C, Marino A, Guaraldi M, et al. Combination chemotherapy with mitoxantrone, methotrexate, and mitomycin (MMM Regimen) in malignant pleural mesothelioma. Am J Clin Oncol 2001;24(1):143–7.

[18] Mintzer DM, Kelsen D, Frimmer D, et al. Phase II trial of high-dose cisplatin in patients with malignant mesothelioma. Cancer Treat Rep 1985;69(6):711–2.

[19] Zidar BL, Green S, Pierce HI, et al. A phase II evaluation of cisplatin in unresectable diffuse malignant mesothelioma: a Southwest Oncology Group study. Invest New Drugs 1988;6(3):223–6.

[20] Vogelzang NJ, Rusthoven JJ, Symanowski J, et al. Phase III study of pemetrexed in combination with cisplatin versus cisplatin alone in patients with malignant pleural mesothelioma. J Clin Oncol 2003;21(14):2636–44.

[21] van Meerbeeck J, Gaafar R, Manegold C, et al. Randomized phase III study of cisplatin with or without raltitrexed in patients with malignant pleural mesothelioma: an intergroup study of the European Organisation for Research and Treatment of Cancer Lung Cancer Group and the National Cancer Institute of Canada. J Clin Oncol 2005;23(28): 6881–9.

[22] Berghmans T, Paesmans M, Lalami Y, et al. Activity of chemotherapy and immunotherapy

on malignant mesothelioma: a systematic review of the literature with meta-analysis. Lung Cancer 2002;38(2):111–21.

[23] Mbidde EK, Harland SJ, Calvert AH, et al. Phase II trial of carboplatin (JM8) in treatment of patients with malignant mesothelioma. Cancer Chemother Pharmacol 1986;18(3): 284–5.

[24] Vogelzang NJ, Goutsou M, Corson JM, et al. Carboplatin in malignant mesothelioma: a phase II study of the Cancer and Leukemia Group B. Cancer Chemother Pharmacol 1990;27(3):239–42.

[25] Raghavan D, Gianoutsos P, Bishop J, et al. Phase II trial of carboplatin in the management of malignant mesothelioma. J Clin Oncol 1990;8(1):151–4.

[26] Favaretto AG, Aversa SM, Paccagnella A, et al. Gemcitabine combined with carboplatin in patients with malignant pleural mesothelioma: a multicentric phase II study. Cancer 2003;97(11):2791–7.

[27] Fizazi K, Doubre H, Le Chevalier T, et al. Combination of raltitrexed and oxaliplatin is an active regimen in malignant mesothelioma: results of a phase II study. J Clin Oncol 2003; 21(2):349–54.

[28] Hughes A, Calvert P, Azzabi A, et al. Phase I clinical and pharmacokinetic study of pemetrexed and carboplatin in patients with malignant pleural mesothelioma. J Clin Oncol 2002;20(16):3533–44.

[29] Schutte W, Blankenburg T, Lauerwald K, et al. A multicenter phase II study of gemcitabine and oxaliplatin for malignant pleural mesothelioma. Clin Lung Cancer 2003;4(5):294–7.

[30] Kelsen D, Gralla R, Cheng E, et al. Vindesine in the treatment of malignant mesothelioma: a phase II study. Cancer Treat Rep 1983;67(9):821–2.

[31] Cowan JD, Green S, Lucas J, et al. Phase II trial of five day intravenous infusion vinblastine sulfate in patients with diffuse malignant mesothelioma: a Southwest Oncology Group study. Invest New Drugs 1988;6(3):247–8.

[32] Boutin C, Irisson M, Guerin JC, et al. Phase II trial of vindesine in malignant pleural mesothelioma. Cancer Treat Rep 1987;71(2):205–6.

[33] Martensson G, Sorenson S. A phase II study of vincristine in malignant mesothelioma: a negative report. Cancer Chemother Pharmacol 1989;24(2):133–4.

[34] Steele JP, Shamash J, Evans MT, et al. Phase II study of vinorelbine in patients with malignant pleural mesothelioma. J Clin Oncol 2000;18(23):3912–7.

[35] Fennell DA, Steele JP, Shamash J, et al. Phase II trial of vinorelbine and oxaliplatin as first-line therapy in malignant pleural mesothelioma. Lung Cancer 2005;47(2):277–81.

[36] van Meerbeeck J, Debruyne C, van Zandwijk N, et al. Paclitaxel for malignant pleural mesothelioma: a phase II study of the EORTC Lung Cancer Cooperative Group. Br J Cancer 1996;74(6):961–3.

[37] Vogelzang NJ, Herndon II JE, Miller A, et al. High-dose paclitaxel plus G-CSF for malignant mesothelioma: CALGB phase II study 9234. Ann Oncol 1999;10(5):597–600.

[38] Vorobiof DA, Rapoport BL, Chasen MR, et al. Malignant pleural mesothelioma: a phase II trial with docetaxel. Ann Oncol 2002;13(3):412–5.

[39] Belani CP, Adak S, Aisner S, et al. Docetaxel for malignant mesothelioma: phase II study of the Eastern Cooperative Oncology Group. Clin Lung Cancer 2004;6(1):43–7.

[40] Maksymiuk AW, Marschke Jr RF, Tazelaar HD, et al. Phase II trial of topotecan for the treatment of mesothelioma. Am J Clin Oncol 1998;21(6):610–3.

[41] Kindler HL, Herndon JE, Zhang C, et al. CPT-11 in malignant mesothelioma: a phase II trial by the Cancer and Leukemia Group B. Lung Cancer 2005;48(3):423–8.

[42] Nakano T, Chahinian AP, Shinjo M, et al. Cisplatin in combination with irinotecan in the treatment of patients with malignant pleural mesothelioma: a pilot phase II clinical trial and pharmacokinetic profile. Cancer 1999;85(11):2375–84.

[43] Steele JP, Shamash J, Barlow CS, et al. Phase II trial of irinotecan, cisplatin and mitomycin C (IPM) in malignant pleural mesothelioma [abstract 1227]. Proc Am Soc Clin Oncol 2002;21:307a.

[44] Kindler HL, Millard F, Herndon II JE, et al. Gemcitabine for malignant mesotheli-

oma: a phase II trial by the Cancer and Leukemia Group B. Lung Cancer 2001; 31(2–3):311–7.

[45] van Meerbeeck JP, Baas P, Debruyne C, et al. A phase II study of gemcitabine in patients with malignant pleural mesothelioma. Cancer 1999;85(12):2577–82.

[46] Davidson JA, Robinson BWS. Gemcitabine activity on murine and human malignant mesothelioma cell lines show additive activity in combination with cisplatin. Aust N Z J Med 1997;27:213.

[47] Byrne MJ, Davidson JA, Musk AW, et al. Cisplatin and gemcitabine treatment for malignant mesothelioma: a phase II study. J Clin Oncol 1999;17:25–30.

[48] Nowak AK, Byrne MJ, Williamson R, et al. A multicentre phase II study of cisplatin and gemcitabine for malignant mesothelioma. Br J Cancer 2002;87(5):491–6.

[49] van Haarst JM, Baas P, Manegold C, et al. Multicentre phase II study of gemcitabine and cisplatin in malignant pleural mesothelioma. Br J Cancer 2002;86(3):342–5.

[50] Solheim OP, Saeter G, Finnanger AM, et al. High-dose methotrexate in the treatment of malignant mesothelioma of the pleura: a phase II study. Br J Cancer 1992;65: 956–60.

[51] Vogelzang NJ, Weissman LB, Herndon II JE, et al. Trimetrexate in malignant mesothelioma: a Cancer and Leukemia Group B Phase II study. J Clin Oncol 1994;12(7): 1436–42.

[52] Kindler HL, Belani CP, Herndon JE, et al. Edatrexate (10-ethyl-deaza-aminopterin) (NSC #626715) with or without leucovorin rescue for malignant mesothelioma. Cancer 1999; 86:1985–91.

[53] Shih C, Habeck LL, Mendelsohn LG, et al. Multiple folate enzyme inhibition: mechanism of a novel pyrrolopyrimidine-based antifolate LY231514 (MTA). Adv Enzyme Regul 1998;38:135–52.

[54] Baas P, Ardizzoni A, Grossi F, et al. The activity of raltitrexed (Tomudex) in malignant pleural mesothelioma: an EORTC phase II study (08992). Eur J Cancer 2003;39(3): 353–7.

[55] Scagliotti GV, Shin DM, Kindler HL, et al. Phase II study of pemetrexed with and without folic acid and vitamin B12 as front-line therapy in malignant pleural mesothelioma. J Clin Oncol 2003;21(8):1556–61.

[56] Janne PA, Obasaju C, Simon G, et al. A phase 2 clinical trial of pemetrexed plus gemcitabine as front-line chemotherapy for patients with malignant pleural mesothelioma [abstract 7053]. J Clin Oncol 2004;23:626.

[57] Andreopoulou E, Ross PJ, O'Brien ME, et al. The palliative benefits of MVP (mitomycin C, vinblastine and cisplatin) chemotherapy in patients with malignant mesothelioma. Ann Oncol 2004;15(9):1406–12.

[58] Hollen PJ, Gralla RJ, Liepa AM, et al. Adapting the lung cancer symptom scale (LCSS) to mesothelioma: using the LCSS-Meso conceptual model for validation. Cancer 2004; 101(3):587–95.

[59] Gralla RJ, Hollen PJ, Liepa AM, et al. Improving quality of life in patients with malignant pleural mesothelioma: results of the randomized pemetrexed + cisplatin vs. cisplatin trial using the LCSS-meso instrument [abstract 2496]. Proc Am Soc Clin Oncol 2003;22:621.

[60] Herndon JE, Green MR, Chahinian AP, et al. Factors predictive of survival among 337 patients with mesothelioma treated between 1984 and 1994 by the Cancer and Leukemia Group B. Chest 1998;113(3):723–31.

[61] Byrne MJ, Nowak AK. Modified RECIST criteria for assessment of response in malignant pleural mesothelioma. Ann Oncol 2004;15(2):257–60.

[62] Muers MF, Rudd RM, O'Brien ME, et al. BTS randomised feasibility study of active symptom control with or without chemotherapy in malignant pleural mesothelioma: ISRCTN 54469112. Thorax 2004;59(2):144–8.

[63] Girling DJ, Muers MF, Qian W, et al. Multicenter randomized controlled trial of the management of unresectable malignant mesothelioma proposed by the British Thoracic Society and the British Medical Research Council. Semin Oncol 2002;29(1):97–101.

[64] Giaccone G, O'Brien ME, Byrne MJ, et al. Phase II trial of ZD0473 as second-line therapy in mesothelioma. Eur J Cancer 2002;38(Suppl 8):S19–24.

[65] Mikulski SM, Costanzi JJ, Vogelzang NJ, et al. Phase II trial of a single weekly intravenous dose of ranpirnase in patients with unresectable malignant mesothelioma. J Clin Oncol 2002;20(1):274–81.

[66] Shepherd FA, Dancey J, Ramlau R, et al. Prospective randomized trial of docetaxel versus best supportive care in patients with non-small-cell lung cancer previously treated with platinum-based chemotherapy. J Clin Oncol 2000;18:2095–103.

[67] Rusch V, Saltz L, Venkatraman E, et al. A phase II trial of pleurectomy/decortication followed by intrapleural and systemic chemotherapy for malignant pleural mesothelioma. J Clin Oncol 1994;12(6):1156–63.

[68] Chang MY, Sugarbaker DJ. Innovative therapies: intraoperative intracavitary chemotherapy. Thorac Surg Clin 2004;14(4):549–56.

[69] de Bree E, van Ruth S, Baas P, et al. Cytoreductive surgery and intraoperative hyperthermic intrathoracic chemotherapy in patients with malignant pleural mesothelioma or pleural metastases of thymoma. Chest 2002;121(2):480–7.

[70] Pass HI, Temeck BK, Kranda K, et al. Phase III randomized trial of surgery with or without intraoperative photodynamic therapy and postoperative immunochemotherapy for malignant pleural mesothelioma. Ann Surg Oncol 1997;4(8):628–33.

[71] Yajnik S, Rosenzweig KE, Mychalczak B, et al. Hemithoracic radiation after extrapleural pneumonectomy for malignant pleural mesothelioma. Int J Radiat Oncol Biol Phys 2003;56(5):1319–26.

[72] Sugarbaker DJ, Flores RM, Jaklitsch MT, et al. Resection margins, extrapleural node status, and cell type determine post-operative long term survival in trimodality therapy of malignant pleural mesothelioma. J Thorac Cardiovasc Surg 1999;117(1):54–63.

[73] Weder W, Kestenholz P, Taverna C, et al. Neoadjuvant chemotherapy followed by extrapleural pneumonectomy in malignant pleural mesothelioma. J Clin Oncol 2004;22(17):3451–7.

[74] Flores R, Krug L, Rosenzweig K, et al. Induction chemotherapy, extrapleural pneumonectomy, and adjuvant hemithoracic radiation are feasible and effective for locally advanced malignant pleural mesothelioma [abstract 7193]. J Clin Oncol 2004;23:661.

[75] Stahel RA, Weder W, Ballabeni P, et al. Neoadjuvant chemotherapy followed by extrapleural pneumonectomy for malignant pleural mesothelioma: a multicenter phase II trial of the SAKK [abstract 7052]. J Clin Oncol 2004;22:14S.

[76] Krug L, Pass H, Rusch V, et al. A multicenter phase II trial of neo-adjuvant pemetrexed plus cisplatin followed by extrapleural pneumonectomy (EPP) and radiation (RT) for malignant pleural mesothelioma [abstract P-407]. Lung Cancer 2005;49(Suppl 2):S223.

[77] Versnel MA, Claesson-Welsh L, Hammacher A, et al. Human malignant mesothelioma cell lines express PDGF beta-receptors whereas cultured normal mesothelial cells express predominantly PDGF alpha-receptors. Oncogene 1991;6(11):2005–11.

[78] Mathy A, Baas P, Dalesio O, et al. Limited efficacy of imatinib mesylate in malignant mesothelioma: A phase II trial. Lung Cancer 2005;50:83–6.

[79] Millward M, Parnis F, Byrne MJ, et al. Phase II trial of imatinib mesylate in patients with advanced pleural mesothelioma [abstract 912]. Proc Am Soc Clin Oncol 2003;22:228.

[80] Villano JL, Husain AN, Stadler WM, et al. A phase II trial of imatinib mesylate in patients with malignant mesothelioma [abstract 7200]. J Clin Oncol 2004;23:663.

[81] Kris MG, Natale RB, Herbst RS, et al. Efficacy of gefitinib, an inhibitor of the epidermal growth factor receptor tyrosine kinase, in symptomatic patients with non-small cell lung cancer: a randomized trial. JAMA 2003;290(16):2149–58.

[82] Dazzi H, Hasleton PS, Thatcher N, et al. Malignant pleural mesothelioma and epidermal growth factor receptor (EGF-R): relationship of EGF-R with histology and survival using fixed paraffin embedded tissue and the F4, monoclonal antibody. Br J Cancer 1990;61(6):924–6.

[83] Govindan R, Ritter J, Suppiah R. EGFR and HER-2 overexpression in malignant mesothelioma [abstract 3106]. Proc Am Soc Clin Oncol 2001;20:339b.

[84] Janne PA, Taffaro ML, Salgia R, et al. Inhibition of epidermal growth factor receptor signaling in malignant pleural mesothelioma. Cancer Res 2002;62(18):5242–7.

[85] Govindan R, Kratzke RA, Herndon JE, et al. Gefitinib in patients with malignant mesothelioma: a phase II study by the Cancer and Leukemia Group B. Clin Cancer Res 2005; 11(6):2300–4.

[86] Garland L, Rankin C, Scott K, et al. Molecular correlates of the EGFR signaling pathway in association with SWOG S0218: a phase II study of oral EGFR tyrosine kinase inhibitor OSI-774 in patients with malignant pleural mesothelioma [abstract 3007]. J Clin Oncol 2004;22:14S.

[87] Heinrich MC, Corless CL, Demetri GD, et al. Kinase mutations and imatinib response in patients with metastatic gastrointestinal stromal tumor. J Clin Oncol 2003;21(23): 4342–9.

[88] Paez JG, Janne PA, Lee JC, et al. EGFR mutations in lung cancer: correlation with clinical response to gefitinib therapy. Science 2004;304:1497–500.

[89] Strizzi L, Catalano A, Vianale G, et al. Vascular endothelial growth factor is an autocrine growth factor in human malignant mesothelioma. J Pathol 2001;193(4):468–75.

[90] Konig J, Tolnay E, Wiethege T, et al. Co-expression of vascular endothelial growth factor and its receptor flt-1 in malignant pleural mesothelioma. Respiration (Herrlisheim) 2000; 67(1):36–40.

[91] Linder C, Linder S, Munck-Wikland E, et al. Independent expression of serum vascular endothelial growth factor (VEGF) and basic fibroblast growth factor (bFGF) in patients with carcinoma and sarcoma. Anticancer Res 1998;18(3B):2063–8.

[92] Kindler HL, Vogelzang NJ, Chien K, et al. SU5416 in malignant mesothelioma: a University of Chicago phase II consortium study [abstract 1359]. Proc Am Soc Clin Oncol 2001;20:341a.

[93] Kindler HL, Karrison T, Lu C, et al. A multi-center, double-blind, placebo-controlled randomized phase II trial of gemcitabine/cisplatin plus bevacizumab or placebo in patients with malignant mesothelioma [abstract]. Proc Am Soc Clin Oncol 2005;23(16S):625s.

[94] Jahan T, Gu L, Wang X, et al. Vatalanib in patients with previously untreated advanced malignant mesothelioma: preliminary analysis of a phase II study by the cancer and Leukemia Group B (CALGB 30107) [abstract P-403]. Lung Cancer 2005;49(Suppl 2):S222.

[95] Marks P, Rifkind RA, Richon VM, et al. Histone deacetylases and cancer: causes and therapies. Nat Rev Cancer 2001;1(3):194–202.

[96] Kelly WK, Richon VM, O'Connor O, et al. Phase I clinical trial of histone deacetylase inhibitor: suberoylanilide hydroxamic acid administered intravenously. Clin Cancer Res 2003;9(10 Pt 1):3578–88.

[97] Kelly WK, O'Connor OA, Krug LM. Phase I study of an oral histone deacetylase inhibitor, suberoylanilide hydroxamic acid, in patients with advanced cancer. J Clin Oncol 2005; 23(17):3923–31.

[98] Krug LM, Kelly WK, Curley T, et al. Clinical experience of the histone deacetylase inhibitor suberoylanilide hydroxamic acid (SAHA) in patients with malignant pleural mesothelioma. Presented at the 7th Meeting of the International Mesothelioma Interest Group (IMIG). Brescia (Italy), June 24–26, 2004.

[99] Skubitz KM. Phase II trial of pegylated-liposomal doxorubicin (Doxil) in mesothelioma. Cancer Invest 2002;20(5–6):693–9.

[100] Zidar BL, Metch B, Balcerzak SP, et al. A phase II evaluation of ifosfamide and mesna in unresectable diffuse malignant mesothelioma: a Southwest Oncology Group study. Cancer 1992;70(10):2547–51.

[101] Alberts AS, Falkson G, Van Zyl L. Malignant pleural mesothelioma: phase II pilot study of ifosfamide and mesna. J Natl Cancer Inst 1988;80(9):698–700.

[102] Falkson G, Hunt M, Borden EC, et al. An extended phase II trial of ifosfamide plus mesna in malignant mesothelioma. Invest New Drugs 1992;10(4):337–43.

[103] Bajorin D, Kelsen D, Mintzer DM. Phase II trial of mitomycin in malignant mesothelioma. Cancer Treat Rep 1987;71(9):857–8.

[104] van Meerbeeck JP, Baas P, Debruyne C, et al. A phase II EORTC study of temozolomide in patients with malignant pleural mesothelioma. Eur J Cancer 2002;38(6):779–83.

[105] Sahmoud T, Postmus PE, van Pottelsberghe C, et al. Etoposide in malignant pleural mesothelioma: two phase II trials of the EORTC Lung Cancer Cooperative Group. Eur J Cancer 1997;33(13):2211–5.

[106] Otterson GA, Herndon II JE, Watson D, et al. Capecitabine in malignant mesothelioma: a phase II trial by the Cancer and Leukemia Group B (39807). Lung Cancer 2004;44(2): 251–9.

Hematol Oncol Clin N Am 19 (2005)1137–1145

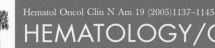

HEMATOLOGY/ONCOLOGY CLINICS
OF NORTH AMERICA

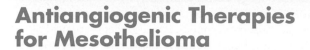

Antiangiogenic Therapies for Mesothelioma

Jonathan E. Dowell, MD[a,b,*], Hedy Lee Kindler, MD[c]

[a]University of Texas–Southwestern Medical Center, 5323 Harry Hines Boulevard, Dallas, TX 75390-8852, USA
[b]Division of Hematology & Oncology, Dallas Veterans Affairs Medical Center, Dallas, TX, USA
[c]Section of Hematology/Oncology, University of Chicago, Chicago, IL, USA

Malignant mesothelioma is an aggressive tumor of the pleura and peritoneum that has been linked to occupational exposure to asbestos. Although it remains an uncommon malignancy, approximately 2500 new cases are diagnosed in the United States each year, and projections suggest that the incidence will continue to rise. Curative surgical resection is rarely possible for these patients, and less than 15% of patients survive 5 years [1–3].

Historically, chemotherapy has shown limited efficacy in the treatment of advanced mesothelioma. Response rates with single-agent chemotherapy are typically less than 20%, and the resultant median survivals are only 6 to 10 months [4]. A small number of chemotherapy combinations also have been evaluated, but until recently, none has been shown to be clearly beneficial. Vogelzang and colleagues [5] reported the results of a randomized phase III trial of pemetrexed and cisplatin versus cisplatin alone in untreated patients who have mesothelioma. The trial showed that the combination had a significantly superior response rate (41.3% versus 16.7%), progression-free survival (5.7 months versus 3.9 months), and overall survival (12.1 months versus 9.3 months) than that seen with cisplatin alone. Although this regimen is the first to be approved by the US Food and Drug Administration for use in patients who have mesothelioma, the unfortunate reality is that even with treatment, few patients survive 2 years. This relative resistance to chemotherapy makes mesothelioma an ideal tumor in which to evaluate novel therapeutic targets and approaches.

Angiogenesis is the formation of new vasculature from existing blood vessels. The development of new blood vessels allows an adequate supply of nutrients to be provided to cancer cells and is necessary for tumors to grow beyond 1 to 2 mm in diameter. The disruption of angiogenesis has emerged as an important

* Corresponding author. University of Texas–Southwestern Medical Center, 5323 Harry Hines Boulevard, Dallas, TX 75390-8852. *E-mail address:* jonathan.dowell@utsouthwestern.edu (J.E. Dowell).

0889-8588/05/$ – see front matter
doi:10.1016/j.hoc.2005.09.008

Published by Elsevier Inc.
hemonc.theclinics.com

therapeutic strategy in cancer. Angiogenesis is controlled by several mediators, including vascular endothelial growth factor (VEGF) and basic fibroblast growth factor [6]. Several antiangiogenic compounds that target these mediators and others are currently being developed, and a few of these agents, such as bevacizumab and thalidomide, are available as cancer therapies.

A large body of preclinical and clinical evidence suggests that angiogenesis may be a critical step in the pathogenesis of mesothelioma. One of the first reports that linked mesothelioma and angiogenesis came from Branchaud and colleagues [7] in 1989. They found that weekly intraperitoneal injections of crocidolite asbestos fibers produced mesotheliomas in mice after 30 to 50 weeks. One of the earliest pathologic changes noted was the development of neovascularization around the injected fibers, which occurred as early as 14 days after the first injection.

Several investigators also have shown that mesothelioma cell lines produce large amounts of the angiogenic factors VEGF [8–11] and fibroblast growth factor [10], often significantly more than that produced by normal mesothelial cells or fibroblasts [9,10]. These groups also have shown that mesothelioma cells express the VEGF receptors flk-1 and flt-1 [8,9,11]. In these cells, VEGF seems to cause cellular proliferation that is mediated through its receptors, and monoclonal antibodies directed against either VEGF or its receptors and VEGF antisense prevent this proliferation [9,11]. In similar fashion, investigators evaluated human mesotheliomas for the presence of the angiogenic factors hepatocyte growth factor/scatter factor and platelet-derived growth factor (PDGF) and their receptors and found expression of both in a large number of tumors [12,13]. This finding provides strong evidence that these angiogenic mediators and their receptors constitute autocrine growth loops in mesothelioma and that in addition to their effects on new blood vessel formation, they directly influence cellular proliferation.

Several groups have evaluated human mesothelioma specimens for the presence of VEGF and other mediators of angiogenesis. Kumar-Singh and colleagues [10] reported that immunoreactivity for fibroblast growth factors 1 and 2 was seen in 67% and 92% of mesotheliomas, respectively, and in 50% and 40% of nonneoplastic mesothelium, respectively. Tumor expression of the VEGF protein is seen in 45% to 81% of cases, whereas benign pleural tissue shows expression in only 0% to 20% of specimens [10,11,14,15]. Twenty percent to 71% of mesotheliomas express at least one of the VEGF receptors [11,15]. VEGF expression also has been shown to correlate directly with the microvessel density of the tumor, and several groups have demonstrated that increased microvessel density is an independent predictor of poor prognosis in mesothelioma [16–20].

Recent data also suggest a link between the polyomavirus simian virus 40 (SV40) and VEGF in mesothelioma. Although the true significance of this association remains controversial, several reports describe the presence of SV40 in malignant mesotheliomas, and a large body of evidence currently suggests that it may be a causative agent for this tumor. Although geographic variation is observed, SV40 is present in approximately 50% of all human malignant mesotheliomas. The virus consistently transforms human mesothelial cells in vitro and induces mesothelioma development in hamsters. The pathogenesis of SV40-induced mesotheliomas is likely mediated by the large T antigen (Tag), which is an oncogenic protein that binds and inactivates the p53 and retinoblastoma tumor suppressor proteins [21]. In primary malignant mesothelioma cell cultures, mean VEGF levels were significantly higher in cell lines that were SV40 positive. Normal human mesothelial cells transfected with full-length SV40 or only SV40 Tag released significantly greater amounts of VEGF than either SV40-negative malignant mesothelioma or normal human mesothelial cells [22]. A second group also found that transfection of human mesothelioma cell lines with SV40 Tag lead to significant increases in VEGF protein and mRNA and human mesothelioma cell line proliferation. This proliferation was abolished by inactivation of the VEGF signal transduction pathway with a soluble form of the VEGF receptor flt-1 [23]. These data suggest that mesotheliomas that express SV40 may be particularly sensitive to therapy directed against VEGF.

Angiogenesis inhibitors have been shown to be effective in several preclinical models of mesothelioma. Catalano and colleagues [24] observed that mesothelioma cell lines express significantly greater amounts of methionine aminopeptidase-2 than normal mesothelial cells. Methionine aminopeptidase-2 is the molecular target of the angiogenesis inhibitors fumagillin and ovalacin. This group also demonstrated that treatment with fumagillin consistently induced apoptosis in malignant mesothelial cells but not in their benign counterparts. In a separate experiment, the VEGF inhibitor SU1498 was found to reduce proliferation in mesothelioma cells in vitro, and these effects were enhanced synergistically by the cyclo-oxygenase-2 inhibitor celecoxib [25]. Using a syngeneic murine mesothelioma model and an orthotopic model, Meritt and colleagues [26] demonstrated that intratumoral administration of adenoviral vectors known to inhibit VEGF and the angiogenesis mediator pigment epithelium-derived factor prevented mesothelioma growth, prolonged survival, and decreased microvessel density.

The available data suggest a critical role for angiogenesis in mesothelioma biology and that patients who have mesothelioma are appropriate candidates for trials of angiogenesis inhibitors. Several of these agents are currently under evaluation in this population [27].

SU5416

One of the first angiogenesis inhibitors to be evaluated in patients who have mesothelioma was SU5416 (semaxanib), a selective inhibitor of the tyrosine kinase activity of the VEGF receptor flk-1. Investigators at the University of Chicago assessed the activity of single-agent SU5416 in malignant mesothelioma in 23 previously treated patients. A partial response rate of 11% was observed; median survival was 12.4 months. No correlation was noted among pretreatment VEGF levels, basic fibroblast growth factor, VCAM-1 (vascular cell adhesion molecule–1), and response or survival [28,29]. This drug is not being developed further by the manufacturer.

THALIDOMIDE

Thalidomide is believed to inhibit angiogenesis mediated by VEGF, basic fibroblast growth factor, and transforming growth factor-alpha. Investigators at the Netherlands Cancer Institute recently reported the results of a phase II trial of thalidomide in 40 patients who have mesothelioma, of whom 50% had received prior chemotherapy. The primary endpoint was time to progression. Patients received increasing doses of 100, 200, or 400 mg as tolerated; 200 mg was the recommended dose for further studies. Disease stabilization for longer than 6 months was observed in 27.5% of the patients [30]. A similar trial at the University of Maryland used tumor response as the primary endpoint. Response will be correlated with SV40 Tag expression and with standardized uptake value on pretreatment positron emission tomography scan.

On the basis of the Dutch data, which suggest a disease-stabilizing effect of thalidomide, these investigators recently launched the NVALT (Nederlandse Vereniging voor Artsen Longziekten en Tuberculose) study, in which thalidomide is being evaluated as a maintenance treatment after initial chemotherapy in 216 patients who have advanced mesothelioma. All patients receive four cycles of pemetrexed with either cis- or carboplatin. Patients who have a response or stable disease at the completion of four cycles are randomized to either daily thalidomide or observation. The study is powered to detect a 50% improvement in time to progression (from 5–7.5 months).

Pavlakis and colleagues [31] evaluated thalidomide alone or in combination with gemcitabine/cisplatin in two parallel nonrandomized phase II studies. Single-agent thalidomide, 100 to 500 mg, was administered to 22 patients who were not considered suitable for chemotherapy or who had progressed on chemotherapy, whereas gemcitabine plus cisplatin was given with thalidomide to 16 chemotherapy-naïve patients. Similar to the Dutch study, they observed that 25% of the patients who received single-agent thalidomide achieved disease stabilization for longer than 6 months. In the combination arm, a partial response rate of 14% was reported, and 32% of these patients achieved disease stabilization for longer than 6 months. Although it did not reach statistical significance, a trend suggested that higher baseline levels of VEGF correlated with a shorter survival in both arms [31].

BEVACIZUMAB

Bevacizumab is a recombinant humanized monoclonal antibody that blocks the binding of VEGF to its receptor. Investigators at the University of Chicago are leading a multicenter, randomized, double-blind, placebo-controlled phase II trial of gemcitabine and cisplatin with bevacizumab or placebo in 106 patients who have untreated malignant mesothelioma. The primary endpoint is time to progression. An interim analysis on the first 101 evaluable patients recently was presented at the American Society of Clinical Oncology meeting in

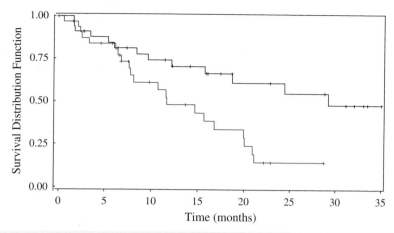

Fig. 1. Overall survival, both treatment arms combined, stratified by baseline VEGF, in a randomized phase II trial of gemcitabine, cisplatin plus bevacizumab, or placebo. Black line is below median. Red line is above median. Logrank $P = .008$. (*From* Kindler HL, Karrison T, Lu C, et al. A multi-center, double-blind, placebo-controlled randomized phase II trial of gemcitabine/cisplatin plus bevacizumab or placebo in patients with malignant mesothelioma [abstract]. Proc Am Soc Clin Oncol 2005;23(16S):625S; with permission.)

June 2005; the study was not unblinded. The median pooled progression-free survival for both arms was 6.4 months, the median overall survival was 15.7 months, and 1-year survival rate was 60%. There was a statistically significant correlation between baseline VEGF and overall survival ($P = .008$) (Fig. 1) [32].

Building on the activity of pemetrexed plus cisplatin in this disease, a multi-center phase II trial of the combination of cisplatin, pemetrexed, and bevacizumab will open shortly at the University of Texas–Southwestern and the University of Chicago. The primary endpoint is time to progression. Correlative studies in pretreatment biopsy specimens will measure expression of the VEGF/KDR complex and SV40 Tag.

Janne and colleagues (unpublished data, 2005) are evaluating the combination of bevacizumab with the epidermal growth factor receptor tyrosine kinase inhibitor erlotinib in previously treated patients who have mesothelioma. Substantial preclinical evidence supports targeting these pathways simultaneously, and this combination has shown activity and been well tolerated in a phase II trial in non–small cell lung cancer [33]. The primary endpoint is objective response rate. Several correlative markers also are being assessed, including serum VEGF levels, tumor expression of VEGF, epidermal growth factor receptor, flt-1, and measurement of circulating endothelial cells.

PTK787

PTK787 is an oral tyrosine kinase inhibitor of the VEGF receptors flt-1 and flk-1 and the PDGF receptor β. The Cancer and Leukemia Group B is conducting a phase II study of PTK787 in chemotherapy-naïve patients who have malignant mesothelioma. The primary endpoint is 3-month progression-free survival based on the extensive Cancer and Leukemia Group B database. Preliminary data suggest some activity in this disease. Partial responses were observed in 6% of patients, and stable disease was observed in 58%. Correlative studies will determine if pretreatment serum levels of VEGF/PDGF and levels of VEGF mRNA isoforms isolated from circulating tumor cells correlate with response [34].

IMATINIB MESYLATE
Imatinib mesylate was developed to target the bcr-abl tyrosine kinase associated with chronic myelogenous leukemia. It also inhibits the tyrosine kinases associated with the receptors for stem cell factor (c-kit) and the angiogenic factor PDGF. Three separate phase II trials have evaluated the activity of this agent in patients who have mesothelioma. Millward and colleagues [35] administered single-agent imatinib at a dose of 800 mg/d to 29 patients who had advanced mesothelioma and who had received no more than one prior chemotherapy regimen. One minor response was seen (25% reduction in pleural thickness), and on serial positron emission tomography scanning, no significant reductions in FDG uptake were observed. In a trial at the University of Chicago, 17 patients who had unresectable mesothelioma received imatinib at a dose of 600 mg/d. No objective responses were observed [36]. Neither tumor expression of c-kit or PDGFR nor baseline plasma levels of PDGF isoforms correlated with progression-free or overall survival. Investigators at the Netherlands Cancer Institute administered 400 mg of imatinib daily and similarly observed no responses in 25 patients [37].

TETRATHIOMOLYBDATE
Tetrathiomolybdate is an oral copper-depleting agent that inhibits angiogenesis and decreases VEGF levels when ceruloplasmin is reduced. Pass and colleagues [38] reported preliminary results of a phase II trial of tetrathiomolybdate after cytoreductive surgery in 34 patients who had malignant mesothelioma. The hypothesis is that an antiangiogenic compound such as tetrathiomolybdate may be particularly effective in the setting of microscopic residual disease by preventing the development of the vascular network that allows tumor growth and metastasis. In stage I and II patients treated with tetrathiomolybdate, 69% remained progression free at 24 months. All patients reached target ceruloplasmin levels at an average of 34 days, and serum VEGF levels were reduced significantly once the target ceruloplasmin level was achieved [38].

OTHER AGENTS IN EARLY STUDIES
BAY43-9006 is an inhibitor of multiple kinases, including VEGF receptor-2, PDGF-β, and raf kinase. The Cancer and Leukemia Group B is currently evaluating BAY43-9006 in patients who have mesothelioma who have had no

more than one prior chemotherapy regimen. The primary endpoint is objective response. Correlative studies will determine if changes in serum VEGF or PDGF levels from baseline, tumor expression of phosphorylated ERK 1/2 as assessed by immunohistochemistry, or the presence of a mutation in exons 11 to 15 of the B-raf gene correlate with response to treatment.

AZD2171 is an oral agent that inhibits the kinase activity associated with the VEGF receptors KDR and flt-1. Two studies in mesothelioma are in development, as led by the University of Chicago and the Southwest Oncology Group, respectively.

SUMMARY

Although treatment with standard chemotherapy for mesothelioma produces a modest survival benefit, most patients still die from their cancer. It is clear that the activity of conventional chemotherapy alone will never be sufficient to eradicate advanced disease. An improved understanding of the biology of mesothelioma has allowed the identification of rational molecular targets for therapeutic endeavors. Inhibition of angiogenesis is a particularly promising avenue that is being pursued actively in this disease. If activity is demonstrated in the current studies, the next step involves more trials of these targeted agents in combination with chemotherapy or other targeted agents. The hope is that with continued thoughtful development of these novel compounds, significant advances in the treatment of mesothelioma can be achieved.

References

[1] Britton M. The epidemiology of mesothelioma. Semin Oncol 2002;29(1):18–25.

[2] Peto J, Decarli A, La Vecchia C, et al. The European mesothelioma epidemic. Br J Cancer 1999;79(3–4):666–72.

[3] Peto J, Hodgson JT, Matthews FE, et al. Continuing increase in mesothelioma mortality in Britain. Lancet 1995;345(8949):535–9.

[4] Janne PA. Chemotherapy for malignant pleural mesothelioma. Clin Lung Cancer 2003; 5(2):98–106.

[5] Vogelzang NJ, Rusthoven JJ, Symanowski J, et al. Phase III study of pemetrexed in combination with cisplatin versus cisplatin alone in patients with malignant pleural mesothelioma. J Clin Oncol 2003;21(14):2636–44.

[6] Cao Y. Antiangiogenic cancer therapy. Semin Cancer Biol 2004;14(2):139–45.

[7] Branchaud RM, MacDonald JL, Kane AB. Induction of angiogenesis by intraperitoneal injection of asbestos fibers. FASEB J 1989;3(6):1747–52.

[8] Strizzi L, Catalano A, Vianale G, et al. Vascular endothelial growth factor is an autocrine growth factor in human malignant mesothelioma. J Pathol 2001;93(4):468–75.

[9] Masood R, Kundra A, Zhu S, et al. Malignant mesothelioma growth inhibition by agents that target the VEGF and VEGF-C autocrine loops. Int J Cancer 2003;104(5):603–10.

[10] Kumar-Singh S, Weyler J, Martin MJ, et al. Angiogenic cytokines in mesothelioma: a study of VEGF, FGF-1 and -2, and TGF beta expression. J Pathol 1999;189(1):72–8.

[11] Ohta Y, Shridhar V, Bright RK, et al. VEGF and VEGF type C play an important role in angiogenesis and lymphangiogenesis in human malignant mesothelioma tumours. Br J Cancer 1999;81(1):54–61.

[12] Tolnay E, Kuhnen C, Wiethege T, et al. Hepatocyte growth factor/scatter factor and its receptor c-Met are overexpressed and associated with an increased microvessel density in malignant pleural mesothelioma. J Cancer Res Clin Oncol 1998;124(6):291–6.

[13] Langerak AW, De Laat PA, Van Der Linden-Van Beurden CA, et al. Expression of platelet-derived growth factor (PDGF) and PDGF receptors in human malignant mesothelioma in vitro and in vivo. J Pathol 1996;178(2):151–60.

[14] Konig JE, Tolnay E, Wiethege T, et al. Expression of vascular endothelial growth factor in diffuse malignant pleural mesothelioma. Virchows Arch 1999;435(1):8–12.

[15] Soini Y, Puhakka A, Kahlos K, et al. Endothelial nitric oxide synthase is strongly expressed in malignant mesothelioma but does not associate with vascular density or the expression of VEGF, FLK1 or FLT1. Histopathology 2001;39(2):179–86.

[16] Edwards JG, Swinson DE, Jones JL, et al. Tumor necrosis correlates with angiogenesis and is a predictor of poor prognosis in malignant mesothelioma. Chest 2003;124(5):1916–23.

[17] Edwards JG, Cox G, Andi A, et al. Angiogenesis is an independent prognostic factor in malignant mesothelioma. Br J Cancer 2001;85(6):863–8.

[18] Kumar-Singh S, Vermeulen PB, Weyler J, et al. Evaluation of tumour angiogenesis as a prognostic marker in malignant mesothelioma. J Pathol 1997;182(2):211–6.

[19] O'Byrne KJ, Edwards JG, Waller DA. Clinico-pathological and biological prognostic factors in pleural malignant mesothelioma. Lung Cancer 2004;45(Suppl 1):S45–8.

[20] Weyn B, Tjalma WA, Vermeylen P, et al. Determination of tumour prognosis based on angiogenesis-related vascular patterns measured by fractal and syntactic structure analysis. Clin Oncol (R Coll Radiol) 2004;16(4):307–16.

[21] Gazdar AF, Butel JS, Carbone M. SV40 and human tumours: myth, association or causality? Nat Rev Cancer 2002;2(12):957–64.

[22] Cacciotti P, Strizzi L, Vianale G, et al. The presence of simian-virus 40 sequences in mesothelioma and mesothelial cells is associated with high levels of vascular endothelial growth factor. Am J Respir Cell Mol Biol 2002;26(2):189–93.

[23] Catalano A, Romano M, Martinotti S, et al. Enhanced expression of vascular endothelial growth factor (VEGF) plays a critical role in the tumor progression potential induced by simian virus 40 large T antigen. Oncogene 2002;21(18):2896–900.

[24] Catalano A, Romano M, Robuffo I, et al. Methionine aminopeptidase-2 regulates human mesothelioma cell survival: role of Bcl-2 expression and telomerase activity. Am J Pathol 2001;159(2):721–31.

[25] Catalano A, Graciotti L, Rinaldi L, et al. Preclinical evaluation of the nonsteroidal anti-inflammatory agent celecoxib on malignant mesothelioma chemoprevention. Int J Cancer 2004;109(3):322–8.

[26] Merritt RE, Yamada RE, Wasif N, et al. Effect of inhibition of multiple steps of angiogenesis in syngeneic murine pleural mesothelioma. Ann Thorac Surg 2004;78(3):1042–51 [discussion: 1042–51].

[27] Kindler HL. Moving beyond chemotherapy: novel cytostatic agents for malignant mesothelioma. Lung Cancer 2004;45(Suppl 1):S125–7.

[28] Kindler H, Vogelzang NJ, Chien K, et al. SU5416 in malignant mesothelioma: a University of Chicago consortium study. Proc Am Soc Clin Oncol 2001;20:341a.

[29] Medved M, Karczmar G, Yang C, et al. Semiquantitative analysis of dynamic contrast enhanced MRI in cancer patients: variability and changes in tumor tissue over time. J Magn Reson Imaging 2004;20(1):122–8.

[30] Baas P, Boogerd W, Dalesio O, et al. Thalidomide in patients with malignant pleural mesothelioma. Lung Cancer 2005;48(2):291–6.

[31] Pavlakis N, Abraham R, Harvie R, et al. Thalidomide alone or in combination with cisplatin/gemcitabine in malignant pleural mesothelioma: interim results from two parallel non randomized phase II studies [abstract]. Lung Cancer 2003;41(Suppl 2):S11.

[32] Kindler HL, Karrison T, Lu C, et al. A multi-center, double-blind, placebo-controlled randomized phase II trial of gemcitabine/cisplatin plus bevacizumab or placebo in patients with malignant mesothelioma [abstract]. Proc Am Soc Clin Oncol 2005;23(16S):625S.

[33] Sandler AB, Blumenschein GR, Henderson T, et al. Phase I/II trial evaluating the anti-VEGF Mab bevacizumab in combination with erlotinib, a HER1/EGFR-TK inhibitor, for patients with recurrent non-small cell lung cancer. Proc Am Soc Clin Oncol 2004;23:127.

[34] Jahan T, Gu L, Wang X, et al. Vatalanib in patients with previously untreated advanced malignant mesothelioma: preliminary analysis of a phase II study by the Cancer and Leukemia Group B (CALGB 30107) [abstract]. Lung Cancer 2005;49(Suppl 2):S222.

[35] Millward M, Parnis F, Byrne M, et al. Phase II trial of imatinib mesylate in patients with advanced pleural mesothelioma. Proc Am Soc Clin Oncol 2003;22:228.

[36] Villano JL, Husain AN, Stadler WM, et al. A phase II trial of imatinib mesylate in patients with malignant mesothelioma. Proc Am Soc Clin Oncol 2004;23:663.

[37] Mathy A, Baas P, Dalesio O, et al. Limited efficacy of imatinib mesylate in malignant mesothelioma: a phase II trial. Lung Cancer 2005;50(1):83–6.

[38] Pass HI, Brewer G, Stevens T, et al. A phase II trial of tetrathiomolybdate after cytoreductive surgery for malignant pleural mesothelioma. Proc Am Soc Clin Oncol 2004;23:626.

Hematol Oncol Clin N Am 19 (2005) 1147–1173

HEMATOLOGY/ONCOLOGY CLINICS
OF NORTH AMERICA

ELSEVIER
SAUNDERS

Gene Therapy for Malignant Pleural Mesothelioma

Daniel H. Sterman, MD

Thoracic Oncology Research Laboratory, Pulmonary, Allergy, and Critical Care Division, Department of Medicine, University of Pennsylvania Medical Center, Philadelphia, PA 19104-4283, USA

T he molecular revolution in biology in general, and in oncology in particular, has facilitated the development of genetic manipulation (gene therapy) as a new therapeutic modality. Investigations into the role of gene therapy in cancer have involved the insertion of therapeutic genes via various delivery systems (vectors) into tumor cells for the purpose of inducing apoptosis, necrosis, and anti-tumoral immune responses.

Malignant pleural mesothelioma (MPM) has several characteristics that make it an attractive target for gene therapy: (1) paucity of effective therapies, (2) accessibility of the pleural space for biopsy and localized delivery of experimental agents, and (3) morbidity and mortality primarily related to regional disease extension. Unlike other malignancies that metastasize earlier in their course, mesothelioma exerts its morbidity and mortality through local spread to adjacent vital intrathoracic structures. New treatment modalities that decrease local tumor burden can translate into significant palliative benefits (and potentially prolonged survival). Gene therapy clinical trials for MPM also could serve as a paradigm for treatment of other malignancies localized to body cavities, such as ovarian or bladder carcinoma.

GENE THERAPY: PRINCIPLES AND VECTORS

Gene therapy was originally conceived as a putative treatment for inherited recessive disorders in which transfer of a normal copy of a defective gene could forestall disease onset or reverse phenotypic expression [1]. It soon became clear, however, that cancer would be one of the most important targets for gene

The HSV TK and Interferon-Beta studies were supported by National Cancer Institute grant P01 CA66726 and grant MO1-RR00040 to the General Clinical Research Center of the University of Pennsylvania Medical Center, as well as BiogenIDEC Corporation, the National Gene Vector Laboratories, the Nicolette Asbestos Trust, the Benjamin Shein Foundation for Humanity, the Edward J. Walton, Jr, Fund, the Joseph Amento Fund for Mesothelioma Research, and the Samuel H. Lunenfeld Charitable Foundation. Institutional support was provided by the Abramson Cancer Center of the University of Pennsylvania.
E-mail address: sterman@mail.med.upenn.edu

0889-8588/05/$ – see front matter
doi:10.1016/j.hoc.2005.09.004

therapy. Cancer gene therapy is defined as the transfer of genetic material, including full-length genes, complementary DNA, RNA, or oligonucleotides into cancer or host cells, for the ultimate purpose of killing autologous tumor.

Vectors Used in Gene Therapy: Adenovirus

The transport mechanism for delivery and expression of this genetic material is termed the "vector." Various viral and nonviral gene transfer vectors are currently available, ranging from replicating and nonreplicating viruses to bacteria and liposomes. Each of these vectors has certain advantages with regard to DNA carrying capacity, types of targeted cells, in vivo gene transfer efficiency, duration of expression, and degree of induced inflammation (Table 1). It has become clear that no single gene delivery system is suitable for all candidate disorders.

Recombinant adenoviruses (rAd) have been the most widely used vector system for in vivo cancer gene therapy. Most rAd vectors used for in vivo gene therapy study were derived by genomic deletion of early replicatory viral genes (ie, the E1A/B regions) and provision of these functions in trans via a packaging cell line [2–6]. Genomic deletion of the early Ad viral genes renders these vectors replication incompetent. The deleted gene regions can be replaced with expression cassettes that contain the desired gene under the control of general or tumor-specific promoters. rAd vector systems offer numerous advantages compared with other vector systems (see Table 1): efficient transduction of a wide range of target cells, transduction of dividing and nondividing cells, and resultant high target tissue expression of the therapeutic transgene [7,8]. Importantly, these vectors are stable in vivo, which permits direct gene delivery to many tissue sites, including the mesothelium of the pleural space. Recombinant adenoviral vectors carry distinct disadvantages associated with vector toxicity and delivery limitation: transient gene expression and virion-induced local and systemic inflammatory responses. The latter includes an early innate immune response that culminates in proinflammatory cytokine release and a late acquired immune response that results in the generation of neutralizing anti-adenoviral antibodies and cytotoxic T lymphocytes [9–14].

Adenoviral-mediated Gene Therapy Strategies in Mesothelioma

Several different cancer gene therapy approaches have been studied in MPM, including use of so-called "suicide genes," delivery of tumor suppressor genes, and transfer of immunomodulatory genes. Several of these approaches have been applied in phase I clinical trials of MPM using various vector systems, including rAd, recombinant vaccinia virus (VV), and modified ovarian carcinoma cells [7,15,16]. Others remain in the preclinical stage but with plans for future clinical trials (see Table 1).

Suicide gene therapy

Suicide gene therapy was an early approach in mesothelioma gene therapy experimentation. This method involves the transduction of tumor cells with complementary DNA encoding for an enzyme that converts a benign prodrug to

Table 1
Gene therapy approaches for mesothelioma

Strategy	Vector	Therapeutic gene	Molecular mechanism	Location
Suicide gene	Recombinant, replication deficient, adenovirus	HSVtk	Delivery of gene encoding for enzyme that generates toxic metabolites after exposure to acyclic nucleotides (ie, GCV)	University of Pennsylvania Medical Center, Philadelphia, Pennsylvania, USA (1995–1999)
Genetic immunopotentiation	Replication-restricted vaccinia virus	Human IL-2	Augmentation of immune response to tumor	Queen Elizabeth II Medical Center, Perth, Western Australia, Australia (1990s)
	Vaccinia virus	Modified SV40 T-antigen	Stimulation of immune response against SV40+ mesothelioma cells	University of Michigan Medical Center and Wayne State University Medical Center, Detroit, Michigan, USA (Pending)
	Replication deficient, adenovirus	Interferon-beta	Induction of antitumor immune response	University of Pennsylvania Medical Center, Philadelphia, Pennsylvania, USA (Ongoing)
	Cationic liposome	Prokaryotic DNA (CpG motifs)	Nonspecific induction of innate and acquired immunity	(No active clinical protocols)
Combination suicide gene and tumor vaccine	Irradiated, allogeneic ovarian carcinoma cells (PA1-STK)	HSVtk	Generation of toxic metabolite and antitumor immune responses	Louisiana State University Medical Center, New Orleans, Louisiana, USA (Completed)
Mutation compensation	Oligonucleotides	Antisense oligonucleotides versus SV40 Tag mRNA	Inhibition of dominant oncogenes	(No active clinical protocols)
	Adenovirus	Wild-type p14(ARF)/p16	Restoration of tumor suppressors	University of Minnesota Medical Center, Minneapolis, Minnesota, USA (Planned)
	Adenovirus	Wild-type p53/Bak	Induction of apoptosis	(No active clinical protocols)
Replication-competent viral lytic therapy	Replication-restricted adenovirus (ONYX-01555)	None	Tumor-restricted viral replication and cytotoxicity	(No active clinical protocols)

a toxic metabolite [8]. Subsequent administration of the prodrug engenders selective accumulation of the toxic metabolite within the tumor cells, which results in tumor cell death ("suicide"). The enzymes encoded by the suicide gene are often of nonhuman origin (ie, the *Escherichia coli* cytosine deaminase gene [9] or the herpes simplex virus-1 thymidine kinase [HSV*tk*] gene), which limits toxicity in normal human tissues [10]. For example, HSV*tk* differs sufficiently from mammalian cellular kinases that transfected malignant cells, but not normal nontransduced cells, convert the nucleoside analog ganciclovir (GCV) to its toxic metabolite.

As mentioned, GCV (9-[1,3 dihydroxy-2-propoxy)methyl]-guanine) is an acyclic nucleoside that is poorly metabolized by mammalian cells and is generally nontoxic. After enzymatic conversion to GCV-monophosphate by HSV*tk*, however, it is rapidly metabolized to GCV-triphosphate by endogenous mammalian kinases. Intracellular production of these GCV metabolites induces tumor cell death [8,11]. GCV-triphosphate is toxic to the cell because it is a potent inhibitor of DNA polymerase and competes with normal mammalian nucleosides for DNA replication [11]. Incorporation of GCV-monophosphate into the cellular DNA template can induce significant cytotoxicity [12]. This suicide process is magnified by the presence of bystander effects, which facilitate the death of neighboring nontransduced tumor cells for achievement of maximal tumor response [13].

Bystander effects of herpes simplex virus-1 thymidine kinase suicide gene therapy
Given the limited efficiency of various gene transfer vector systems in vivo, direct killing of significant numbers of malignant cells within a solid tumor may be difficult to achieve. Thus the presence of a bystander effect, whereby non-transduced cells are killed by an indirect mechanism, is extremely important. The bystander effect concept originated with the observation that tumor regression in in vivo HSV*tk* experiments occurred in the absence of ubiquitous transgene expression. This effect was further demonstrated by in vitro mixing experiments, as well as in vivo experiments involving tumors with only 10–20% HSV*tk* expression: complete tumor regression was noted in tumor bearing animals treated with HSVtk after GCV treatment[14,17–20]. The nature of this bystander effect is complex and involves passage of toxic GCV metabolites (GCV-monophosphate and GCV-triphosphate) from transduced to non-transduced cells via gap junctions or apoptotic vesicles [21,22], as well as induction of anti-tumor immune responses capable of killing non-HSV*tk* expressing tumor cells ("cross tolerance") [13].

Herpes Simplex Virus-1 Thymidine Kinase/Ganciclovir Gene Therapy for Malignant Pleural Mesothelioma

Preclinical data: animal and toxicity studies
Initial experiments in our laboratory demonstrated that replication-deficient adenoviral HSV*tk* (Ad.HSV*tk*) vectors transduced mesothelioma cells in tissue culture and animal models and facilitated HSV*tk*-mediated killing of human

mesothelioma cells in the presence of low concentrations of GCV [23,24]. Subsequently, Ad.HSV*tk*/GCV gene therapy was used to treat established human mesothelioma and lung cancer xenografts in the peritoneal cavities of immunodeficient mice, which resulted in significant tumor reduction and prolongation of survival [25–27]. Other investigators independently confirmed the in vitro and in vivo sensitivities of human mesothelioma cells to HSV*tk*/GCV gene therapy [28].

Experiments in syngeneic immunocompetent murine and rat models of malignant mesothelioma
Based on the efficacy data in animals, we conducted preclinical toxicity studies in preparation for the initiation of human clinical trials. Rats were given high doses of Ad.*tk* virus intrapleurally followed by systemic administration of GCV at the same dose proposed for initial use in the clinical trial (10 mg/kg/d). The predominant adverse effects seen in this preclinical toxicology study were localized pleural and pericardial inflammatory changes. Formal toxicology studies also were conducted in three nonhuman primates given high intrapleural doses of Ad.HSV*tk* (10^{12} plaque-forming units [pfu]) and GCV [29]. No adverse clinical effects were documented, nor were there any significant hematologic or biochemical abnormalities. Necropsy findings confirmed the presence of inflammatory changes in the chest wall and intrathoracic serosa but no major organ damage.

Initial phase I clinical trial
We initiated a phase I clinical trial of Ad.*tk*/GCV gene therapy in patients with advanced pleural mesothelioma in 1995 at the University of Pennsylvania Medical Center in conjunction with Penn's Institute for Human Gene Therapy. The goals of this dose escalation trial were to determine the toxicity, gene transfer efficacy, and induced immune responses generated related to the intrapleural instillation of Ad.HSV*tk*, starting with a vector dose of 1×10^9 pfu and increasing in half-log increments to the maximal dose level of 1×10^{12} pfu. Mesothelioma patients who met inclusion criteria, including the presence of an accessible pleural cavity, received a single intrapleural dose of Ad.HSV*tk* vector followed by 2 weeks of intravenous GCV at standard doses of 5 mg/kg twice daily [30,31].

   The adenoviral vector initially used in this trial was a first-generation recombinant replication-deficient virus, deleted in the early genes E1A and E3 with the HSV*tk* gene cassette inserted in the vacated E1A region. Participants were evaluated for evidence of toxicity, viral shedding, immune responses to the virus, and radiographic evidence of tumor response. Twenty-six patients (21 men, 5 women) who ranged in age from 37 to 81 years were enrolled in this 2-year study (1995–1997) (Fig. 1) [31]. Intratumoral HSV*tk* gene transfer was documented in 17 of 25 evaluable patients in a dose-related fashion. All patients treated at a dose of 3.2×10^{11} pfu or more demonstrated evidence of intratumoral HSV*tk* protein expression via immunohistochemistry using a murine monoclonal antibody directed against HSV*tk* [31]. The Ad.*tk*/GCV combination was generally well tolerated, and a maximal tolerated dose was not achieved. Toxicities included reversible transaminase elevations, anemia, fever, and bullous skin eruption at the instillation site. At the highest dose level of 1×10^{12} pfu, 2 patients developed brief periods of hypotension and hypoxemia within hours after vector instillation that resolved rapidly with supplemental oxygen and intravenous fluids [31].

Evaluation of patients' serum and peripheral blood mononuclear cells (and pleural fluid, when available) detected strong antiadenoviral humoral and cellular immune responses, including generation of high serum and pleural fluid titers of antiadenoviral neutralizing antibodies, generation of serum antibodies against adenoviral structural proteins, and increased peripheral blood mononuclear cell proliferative responses to adenoviral proteins [32].

We conducted a small pilot study designed to assess preliminarily the effects of immunosuppression on the degree of intratumoral gene transfer and antiadenoviral immune responses in which five patients (patients 19–23) received peri-

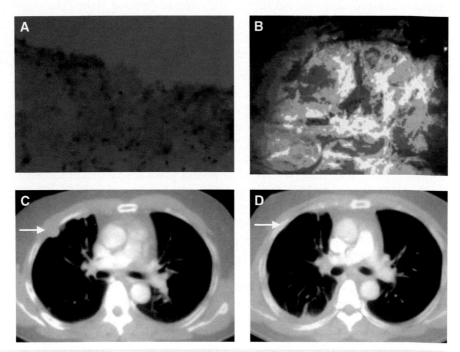

Fig. 1. (A) Patient 26. Immunohistochemical staining of a section of sarcomatoid mesothelioma with a monoclonal antibody directed against the HSV*tk* protein. Impressive, albeit superficial, gene transfer was seen at this highest dose level of the first generation Ad.HSV*tk* vector (1×10^{12} pfu). (B) The significant pleural inflammation induced by high-dose adenoviral vector infusion into the pleural cavity. (C, D) Radiographic evidence of tumor response to intrapleural suicide gene therapy is documented on these pre- and postgene transfer chest CT scans, which reveal regression of parietal pleural nodules (*arrows*) after a single dose of HSV*tk* followed by 2 weeks of ganciclovir.

instillational intravenous corticosteroids. General decreases in induced fever and hypoxemia were noted, but there was also an increased incidence of reversible mental status changes at the highest steroid dose levels. No diminution in antiadenoviral immune responses was demonstrated among the patients who received corticosteroids, nor were there any appreciable differences in the degree of intratumoral gene transfer [33].

Of the 26 patients who had mesothelioma who were enrolled in the initial phase I trials from 1995 to 1997, 25 have since died, with a median posttreatment survival of approximately 11 months (see Fig. 1). One patient (patient 20) in the corticosteroid pilot study who had stage IV mesothelioma at the time of enrollment died 2 weeks after completion of the protocol from rapid progression of his mesothelioma with malignant involvement of the contralateral hemithorax. Several patients with stage IA/IB epithelioid mesothelioma had posttreatment survival of more than 3 years, with one patient surviving more than 4 years. The initial patient enrolled in the trial (patient 001) remains alive with minimal residual disease almost 10 years after completion of the Ad.*tk*/GCV protocol. He did, however, have evidence of local tumor recurrence approximately 3 years after enrollment and underwent treatment with pleurectomy and intraoperative photodynamic therapy. Of the trial participants who are deceased, all had progressive mesothelioma as their primary cause of death. Only 1 of the 26 patients (patient 26) had radiographic evidence of intrathoracic tumor regression after Ad.*tk*/GCV on follow-up chest CT scan (see Fig. 1). This patient eventually died 26 months after completion of the protocol from intraperitoneal disease progression. At autopsy there was extensive intra-abdominal tumor but minimal residual disease in the treated thoracic cavity.

Additional phase I trials of adenoviral herpes simplex virus-1 thymidine kinase gene therapy for mesothelioma

We demonstrated in our first phase I trial that intrapleural Ad.HSV*tk*/GCV gene therapy carried minimal toxicity, effectively delivered transgene to superficial tumor regions, and induced significant humoral and cellular responses to the Ad vector [31,32]. One option for improving intratumoral gene transfer efficacy was to increase the vector dose, but doing so with the first-generation vector was problematic because of potential vector lot contamination with high levels of replication-competent adenovirus.

For these reasons, in 1998 a new phase I clinical trial was initiated that used an advanced-generation adenoviral vector that contained deletions in the early viral genes E1 and E4 with preservation of the E3 region. The presence of an intact E4 region, unlike E3, is critical to the late phase of the viral life cycle; therefore, E4 deletions decrease viral DNA synthesis and late gene expression. Adenoviral vectors with lethal deletions in E1 and E4 offered theoretical advantages over first-generation vectors by virtue of diminished cytopathic effects and reduced cellular immune responses [34]. Because two crucial early genes were deleted, simple recombination could not produce replication-competent virus in the vector production process.

The primary goals of the second phase I clinical trial were to determine the toxicity, gene transfer efficiency, and immune responses associated with the intrapleural injection of high titers of the E1/E4-deleted Ad.HSVtk vector combined with systemic GCV. Five patients were treated under this initial protocol, starting at a dose one log lower than the highest dose used with the E1/E3-deleted Ad vector (1.5×10^{13} viral particles). In the two patients treated at this lower dose, there was minimal toxicity, primarily transitory fever (grade 1). The next three patients were treated with a dose of 5.0×10^{13} viral particles with evidenced of increased toxicity, which was non–dose limiting. All three patients at the higher dose level experienced acute febrile responses (grade 1) after vector instillation, with rapid defervescence. One patient (patient 29) developed hypotension and hypoxemia (grade 2) within hours after vector administration that resolved with supplemental oxygen and intravenous fluids. This patient also developed transitory elevations in serum transaminases (National Cancer Institute grade 2) after vector delivery, with no associated elevations in serum bilirubin or prothrombin time and no clinical evidence of hepatic dysfunction. The third patient treated at the higher dose level (patient 31) developed low-grade fever (grade 1) after intrapleural vector instillation and contralateral pleural inflammation. Overall, there seemed to be less hepatotoxicity in the patients treated with the E1/E4-deleted vector compared with patients treated with equivalent doses of the E1/E3-deleted rAd, but with a similar pattern of increased systemic side effects at higher dose levels [35].

Dose-related gene transfer was detected in all patients at both dose levels via immunohistochemistry. As in the initial phase I trial, significant humoral responses to the rAd virus were seen in all five patients, with the development of high serum titers of total and neutralizing antiadenoviral antibodies within 15 to 20 days of vector instillation [36].

Of the five patients treated in this second phase I trial in 1998, there are two surviving (patients 29 and 30), each treated at the higher dose level of 5.0×10^{13} particles of Ad.HSVtk (see Fig. 1). Both patients had stage I epithelioid mesothelioma at diagnosis, and both have had minimal residual disease without additional antineoplastic therapy more than 6 years after completion of the Ad.tk/GCV protocol. Patient 29, for example, demonstrated diminution of tumor metabolic activity on serial 18-fluorodeoxyglucose positron emission tomography ([18]-FDG PET) scans over a period of several months (Fig. 2). This delayed decrease in tumor metabolic activity after completion of the suicide gene therapy protocol suggests the induction of a secondary immune bystander effect by Ad.HSVtk/GCV, because toxic GCV metabolites would not persist intratumorally for this length of time [35]. Patient 29 had evidence of possible focal tumor recurrence at a new anatomic location along the midportion of the right hemidiaphragm on repeat PET scan performed in October 2003. She has, however, deferred any biopsy or resection of this lesion because she remains generally asymptomatic. Patient 30 recently had evidence of focal tumor recurrence at a prior thoracostomy site, treated only with excisional biopsy. She also

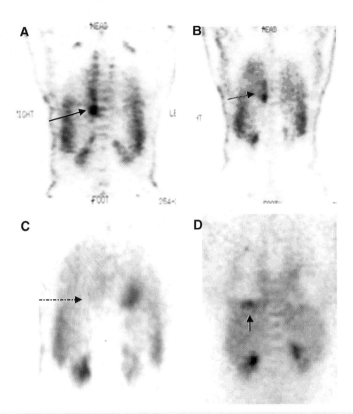

Fig. 2. (A, B) Patient 29, one of eight patients enrolled in trials with the third-generation E1/E4-deleted Ad.HSV*tk* vector, showed evidence of decreased tumor metabolic activity on pre- and 6 week postgene therapy 18-FDG PET imaging, with complete absence of FDG uptake on an 18-FDG PET scan performed 3 years after completion of the protocol (C). This objective metabolic response correlated with stability on serial chest CT scans. Repeat 18-FDG PET performed 5 years after undergoing gene transfer with no other antineoplastic therapy showed a new area of uptake on the midportion of the right hemidiaphragm (D).

eschewed additional therapy (chemotherapy or radiation) because she was otherwise without symptoms or signs of active disease.

Based on in vitro and animal experiments in mesothelioma models that demonstrated a direct correlation between GCV dose and tumor response after *tk* transduction, we initiated an amended phase I trial that combined GCV dose escalation with intrapleural E1/E4-deleted Ad.*tk* [26,31,36–38]. We completed the first patient cohort at dose levels of 3.0×10^{13} particles of Ad.RSV*tk* (E1/E4-deleted) and 15 mg/kg/d of GCV. All three patients tolerated the treatment well. Toxicities were non–dose limiting and included fever, lymphopenia, transaminase elevations, hyponatremia, and hypokalemia. No durable clinical responses were noted in any of the three patients treated in this protocol, although the initial patient who was treated (patient 101) demonstrated reduced [18]FDG uptake in the mediastinal and parietal pleural regions on his posttreatment PET scan. Subsequent ^{18}FDG PET scanning at day 170, however, showed significant increase in tracer uptake consistent with increased tumor metabolic activity. This finding correlated with the patient's increasing clinical symptoms and progression on repeat chest CT scan. Patients 102 and 103 demonstrated increased ^{18}FDG uptake on their day 80 PET studies and concomitant clear evidence of progression on chest CT.

Challenges and future directions

Based on our clinical trial experiences of minimal toxicity, superficial gene transfer, and anecdotal tumor responses, we believed that Ad.HSV*tk*/GCV suicide gene therapy bore promise for future treatment of malignant mesothelioma and other localized malignancies. Unfortunately, these phase I trials were halted in midstream because of the death of a participant in an unrelated adenoviral gene transfer clinical trial for ornithine transcarbamylase deficiency at the University of Pennsylvania Medical Center that involved direct intrahepatic artery rAd vector infusion [2].

The initial Ad.HSV*tk*/GCV strategy, however, carried significant limitations, particularly the expectation of therapeutic efficacy only in patients with small tumor burdens. One alternative approach would be to maximize the vector: tumor cell ratio by surgical debulking to minimize tumor mass, followed by adjuvant administration of Ad.HSV*tk*/GCV. Another potential method of improving efficiency of intratumoral gene transfer would involve repeated administration of vector and GCV. Studies in immunocompetent mice with established peritoneal tumors by our group [3] and others [4] demonstrated marked increase in tumor response after multiple intraperitoneal injections of Ad.HSV*tk*. Data from our initial clinical trials suggested that rAd gene transfer is possible even in patients with significant titers of anti-Ad neutralizing antibodies of up to 1:500, as would be expected with repeated Ad vector administration.

Another proposed approach to maximize gene transfer involved enhancing the efficacy of the expressed HSV*tk* enzyme itself. One intriguing aspect of the HSV*tk* suicide gene schema is that compared with mammalian cellular kinases, the HSV*tk*-1 enzyme has a relaxed specificity that allows it to phosphorylate not only thymidine but other nucleoside analogs, such as GCV and acyclovir. Unfortunately, HSV*tk* has a high affinity for thymidine ($K_m = 0.5$ uM), with lower affinities for GCV ($K_m = 45$ uM) and acyclovir ($K_m \geq 400$ uM) [5]. Molecular remodeling of the HSV*tk* gene enabled the production of novel *tk* enzymes with increased specificity for GCV and acyclovir [5]. These HSV*tk* mutants demonstrated increased acyclovir- and GCV-mediated cytotoxicity and enhanced bystander effects in mixing experiments [6,39]. Our laboratory has produced novel adenoviral vectors that contain similar mutated HSV*tk*s and confirmed enhanced cell killing and augmented bystander effect in in vitro and in vivo models of mesothelioma [40].

An additional mechanism of maximizing intratumoral gene transfer involves the use of HSV*tk*-bearing adenoviral vectors capable of selective replication in mesothelioma cells. In this system, tumor killing could occur via two mechanisms: direct tumor lysis caused by viral replication and HSV*tk*-mediated killing after administration of GCV. Widespread dissemination would be precluded by an intact host immune response [41]. Our laboratory developed tumor-selective replicating Ad.HSV*tk* vectors by substituting the adenoviral E1 promoter with promoters for tumor-related proteins, such as manganese superoxide dismutase, calretinin, and mesothelin [42]. Investigations by Kinnula's laboratory in Finland elucidated the fact that manganese superoxide dismutase is highly expressed in human malignant mesothelioma explants and cell lines [43]. Calretinin is a 29-kD calcium-binding protein that is expressed primarily in the nervous system, but high levels of expression also have been noted in cells of mesothelial origin [44,45]. Mesothelin is a 40-kD surface protein of unknown function that is expressed only on the mesodermal-derived tissues that form the pleural, pericardial, and peritoneal membranes [46]. Other more general tumor-selective promoters, such as those that respond to the transcription factor E2F [42] or the survivin gene [47], also would be potential candidates to drive semi-mesothelioma–selective adenoviral vectors.

Along these same lines of achieving specific expression of the transfected HSVtk suicide gene in malignant mesothelioma cells, investigators from Tokyo Medical and Dental University conducted in vitro and in vivo studies with a vector bearing the keratin 19 enhancer/promoter [48]. They initially performed Northern blot analysis of three mesothelioma cell lines and demonstrated that K19 mRNA was expressed abundantly in the H2052 mesothelioma cell line. Luciferase reporter assays showed that K19 enhancer/promoter (260 bp) exhibited higher promoter activity in H2052 cells than in the other two cell lines. After transfecting an expression vector that contained the K19 enhancer/promoter-bound thymidine kinase gene (pK19-TK) into the H2052 cells, the pK19-TK transfected cells demonstrated enhanced sensitivity to GCV compared with nontransfected cells. In a murine intraperitoneal model of malignant mesothelioma, cationic liposome-mediated in vivo transfection with pK19-TK followed by systemic administration of GCV inhibited the growth of peritoneal tumors [48].

Another novel approach to potentially maximizing efficacy would involve using a different viral vector for *tk* delivery that would allow more frequent dosing without abrogation of gene expression. The recombinant adeno-associated virus 2, a nonimmunogenic virus with more prolonged transgene expression than Ad vectors, could be given in repeated fashion with minimal induction of anti-vector humoral or cellular immune responses. Berlinghoff and colleagues [49] described a series of in vitro experiments that used a novel recombinant adeno-associated virus vector that contained a fusion gene consisting of the HSV*tk* gene and the marker gene green fluorescent protein, driven by various constituitive promoters. Transduction with the recombinant adeno-associated virus-2-*tk* green fluorescent protein vector achieved high green fluorescent protein expression levels in three mesothelioma cell lines (H-Meso-1, MSTO-211H, NCI-H28). The vector driven by the elongation factor-1 alpha promoter showed the highest expression rates. When GCV was added in vitro to the transduced mesothelioma cells, near-complete tumor cell eradication was achieved. Further in vivo testing in immunocompetent animal models of mesothelioma is necessary to evaluate the beneficial effects of repeated dosing with this recombinant adeno-associated virus-2-*tk* vector.

SUICIDE GENE VACCINES

A growing body of evidence supports the hypothesis that HSV*tk*/GCV gene therapy engenders an immunologic bystander effect that enhances antitumoral cytotoxicity at the site of vector delivery and at distant, nontransduced tumor sites [13,20,50–52]. This putative antitumoral immune reaction may result from nonapoptotic HSV*tk*/GCV-mediated tumor necrosis, a variant of cell death that releases immunologic danger signals that then activate cellular immune responses against the tumor cells [52,53]. Generation of these danger signals may be enhanced by transduction of tumor cells with the HSV*tk* gene in combination with a cytokine gene, such as the gene for interleukin-2 (IL-2). Augmented tumor cytotoxicty has been reported with administration of HSV*tk* plus IL-2 in murine models of colon carcinoma, squamous cell carcinoma, and melanoma [54–57].

This concept of enhancing mesothelioma tumor destruction via the immuno-logic bystander effects of HSVtk/GCV gene therapy, a presumptive suicide gene vaccine, was tested in a phase I clinical trial conducted by Schwarzenberger and colleagues [16] at the Louisiana State University Medical Center in New Orleans in the mid-1990s (see Table 1). The protocol designed by the Louisiana State University investigators involved intrapleural instillation, via an indwelling pleural catheter, of an irradiated allogeneic ovarian carcinoma cell line (PA-1) retrovirally transfected with HSVtk (PA1-STK cells), followed by systemic administration of GCV. Schwarzenberger and colleagues [16] hypothesized that the PA1-STK cells would migrate to areas of intrapleural tumor after instillation, undergo necrotic cell death after exposure to GCV, and generate immune responses that would facilitate killing of adjacent mesothelioma cells. Antimesothelioma immune responses in this system were believed to be related to the local generation of proinflammatory cytokines, which, in turn, summon an influx of cytotoxic lymphocytes to the area that produces hemorrhagic tumor necrosis [16,58].

The Louisiana State University group initially performed in vitro mixing experiments that demonstrated that PA1-STK cells, in combination with GCV, killed mouse and human mesothelioma cells in a dose-dependent manner. In syngeneic murine models of mesothelioma, PA1-STK cells administration (with GCV) prolonged survival when the percentage of transduced tumor cells was high (70%), but there was no survival benefit when the percentage of PA1-STK cells was low (30%) [59].

The group then conducted a phase I clinical trial to assess the safety, toxicity profile, and therapeutic efficacy of PA1-STK cells and GCV in the treatment of malignant mesothelioma. Patients received PA1-STK cells administered intra-pleurally and then received GCV (5 mg/kg/d) twice daily for 7 days. Minimal side effects of this treatment were seen. In four of the patients who had mesothelioma in this study, PA1-STK cells radiolabeled with ^{99}Tc were infused into the pleural space. The patients were then scanned to determine the distribution of the cells. PA1-STK cells recognized and adhered preferentially to tumor lining the chest wall, which demonstrated that PA1-STK cells home to mesothelioma deposits in patients after intrapleural instillation [60]. Posttreatment immune analysis of patients in this phase I trial showed significant increases in the percentage of CD8 T lymphocytes in the pleural fluid [58].

To determine if the cytokine profiles of a patient's pleural fluid and blood were altered after PA1-STK/GCV treatment, blood and pleural fluid samples were drawn twice daily after PA1-STK administration, and the levels of several cytokines and soluble Fas ligand were measured. Results of the cytokine analysis showed that IL-2, IL-4, IL-10, IL-12p70, and IL-15 levels increased in a patient's pleural fluid and serum samples in a PA1-STK dose-dependent manner. These results confirmed that the PA1-STK/GCV suicide gene vaccine modulates the immunologic environment of the pleural cavity [61].

CYTOKINE GENE THERAPY FOR MESOTHELIOMA

Based on prior experience with intrapleural cytokine delivery in MPM and the putative immune responses seen in the Ad.HSV*tk*/GCV clinical trials, our group has developed a significant interest in the delivery of genes that encode for proinflammatory cytokines to the pleural space of patients with malignant mesothelioma. One important basis for cytokine gene therapy in MPM is the demonstrated capability of exogenous cytokines for direct antiproliferative effects on mesothelioma cells and the ability of certain cytokines to activate systemic, intrapleural, and intratumoral immune effector cells. Expression of cytokine genes by mesothelioma cells generates high intratumoral cytokine levels in an autocrine and paracrine fashion, which induces powerful local immunologic effects without significant systemic toxicity. Prolonged local cytokine expression facilitates activation of tumor-associated dendritic cells to express major histocompatibility complex tumor antigen heterodimers in conjunction with costimulatory molecules. These activated dendritic cells can migrate to regional lymph nodes, where they stimulate proliferation of tumor-specific CD8 and CD4 lymphocytes, inducing antitumoral cytotoxicity at distant tumor sites. Some proinflammatory cytokines, such as IL-2, directly activate CD8$^+$ tumor-infiltrating lymphocytes and overcome local tolerance signals to produce tumor-specific cytotoxic T lymphocytes (CTLs). Increased intratumoral IL-2 also may activate natural killer (NK) cells and lymphokine-activated killer cells. Experiments with syngeneic murine tumor models have shown that injection of IL-2–transduced tumor cells increases specific antitumoral activity, generates systemic responses to the parental tumor, augments the immune response against autologous tumor, and causes rejection of rechallenged tumor cells [62,63].

Several published phase I and phase II clinical trials in mesothelioma have documented impressive clinical responses to intrapleural infusion of IL-2, interferon-beta (IFN-β), and interferon-gamma (IFN-γ) [64–70]. In particular,

Boutin and colleagues [67,68] at the Hôpital de la Conçeption in Marseille, France described significant response rates in pleural mesothelioma after intrapleural instillation of IFN-γ protein, including several complete pathologic responses in patients who had stage IA disease (tumor limited to the parietal and diaphragmatic pleura).

Investigators at Queen Elizabeth II Hospital in Perth, Australia conducted the first clinical trial of direct intratumoral delivery of cytokine genes in patients who had MPM using a recombinant VV that expressed the human IL-2 gene (see Table 1). A vaccinia vector was chosen because of its large genome, proven safety in human vaccines, and availability of anti-VV antibodies for evaluation of vector-induced immune responses. Insertion of the IL-2 gene into the thymidine kinase region of the VV also rendered the vector partially replication-restricted, which allowed for semiselective tumor cell expression. The Perth team serially injected the VV–IL-2 vector (at a dose of 1×10^7 pfu) into palpable chest wall lesions of six patients with advanced malignant mesothelioma. Toxicities were minimal, and there was no clinical or serologic evidence of spread of vaccinia vector to patient contacts. Modest intratumoral T-cell infiltration was detected on postvector delivery tumor biopsies, but no significant tumor regression was seen in any of the patients. VV–IL-2 mRNA was detected by reverse transcriptase polymerase chain reaction in serial tumor biopsies for up to 6 days after injection but declined to low levels by day 8. The prolonged nature of IL-2 gene expression in this trial was remarkable considering that all patients generated significant serum titers of anti-VV–neutralizing antibodies [71].

The use of cellular vectors to deliver the IL-2 gene in patients who have pleural mesothelioma also has been studied in a phase II European clinical trial sponsored by Transgene, Inc (Strasburg, France). Mertelsmann and colleagues in Freiburg, Germany conducted a phase II randomized study of nonspecific immunotherapy of malignant mesothelioma by repeated intratumoral injection of Vero cells engineered to produce human IL-2. The results of this trial have not yet been published. Vero cells are immortalized monkey fibroblasts capable of constitutive expression of therapeutic human proteins, such as inflammatory cytokines. Vero cells can be grown in culture, packaged in vials, tested for quality, stored, and administered to a patient like a standard medicinal product. Transgene scientists engineered Vero cells to secrete high levels of human IL-2 or other cytokines, including IFN-γ. The first two patients who had mesothelioma in this study were enrolled in March 1999 with a total planned enrollment of 20 patients. This phase II trial was based on earlier animal studies that demonstrated efficacy of Vero IL-2 therapy in the treatment of spontaneously occurring tumors and two phase I clinical trials completed in France and Switzerland that documented safety of this product in human subjects and preliminary evidence of antitumoral activity [72].

The Future of Genetic Immunotherapy for Mesothelioma
Several other candidate cytokine genes are being evaluated for therapeutic effectiveness in animal models of mesothelioma. Caminschi and colleagues

[73] at Queen Elizabeth II Medical Center in Perth studied murine meso-thelioma transduction with the gene encoding for IL-12, one of the most active immunomodulatory cytokines. This same group previously demonstrated that systemic administration of exogenous IL-12 induced strong antitumoral immune responses in an immunocompetent murine mesothelioma model. The Perth investigators demonstrated that injection of murine mesothelioma cells trans-fected ex vivo with the IL-12 gene (AB1-IL-12) prevented tumor growth in immunocompetent mice but produced typical tumors in athymic nude mice, implicating a T-cell–dependent mechanism of IL-12 activity. Immune competent mice injected with AB1-IL-12 were protected from subsequent challenge with parental, non–IL-12 expressing tumor, which confirmed induction of long-term immunity. AB1-IL-12 injection reduced the incidence of tumor develop-ment from parental cell challenge at a distant site [74].

Because IFN-γ protein seems from the medical literature to be among the most active cytokines in inducing antitumoral immune responses (and clinically meaningful tumor regressions) in clinical trials in patients who have mesothe-lioma, it is not surprising that the efficacy IFN-γ gene delivery has been studied in animal models of the disease. Investigators at the Institut Gustave Roussy in France studied the effect of local IFN-γ gene transfer in a murine mesothelioma cell line, AK7, which had strong similarities similar to human mesothelioma, particularly the sarcomatoid variant [75]. AK7 cells expressed low levels of major histocompatibility class I and class II antigens and secreted high levels of latent transforming growth factor-beta (TGF-β). Human sarcomatoid mesotheliomas express low levels of major histocompatibility complex class I antigens that can be induced by exposure to cytokines such as IFN-γ. The TGF-β pathway in AK7 cells is operative but inefficient because endogenous TGF-β is predominantly inactive. Typically, mesothelioma serves as a good example of a nonimmunogenic tumor given its dense fibrous stroma and paucity of infiltrating T lymphocytes. Immune tolerance toward mesothelioma has been attributed, in part, to high levels of TGF-β produced by the tumor cells.

One mechanism of cytokine gene transfer efficacy in immunocompetent murine models of mesothelioma may be reversal of this intratumoral immune tolerance induced by tumor/stroma–derived compounds, such as TGF-β. The Institut Gustave Roussy group characterized and treated pre-established AK7 tumors by direct intratumoral injection of an adenovirus vector that expressed murine IFN-γ, Ad.mIFN-γ, which resulted in significant tumor regression. Peripheral tumor infiltration by CD4 + and CD8 + T lymphocytes in the treated tumors confirmed the induction of an immune response. Tumor relapse in several mice was observed, possibly because of local TGF-β secretion by residual mesothelioma cells [75].

Another mechanism of genetic immunotherapy in animal models of meso-thelioma involves intratumoral delivery of genes that encode for costimulatory molecules, which, when expressed at high levels, may reverse the tolerant state of tumor-infiltrating lymphocytes. For example, Friedlander and colleagues [76] at Louisiana State Health Sciences Center in New Orleans delivered the gene for the costimulatory molecule CD40 ligand (CD40L) in an immunocompetent murine model of malignant mesothelioma. They hypothesized that CD40L gene therapy would be effective in local and distant tumor suppression. Using an rAd encoding murine CD40L (AdCD40L), they demonstrated no suppression of in vitro cell growth for the AC29 (mesothelioma) cell line. Inoculation of immunocompetent CBA/J mice with AC29 cells transduced ex vivo with AdCD40L resulted in significant suppression of tumor formation in vivo when compared with controls ($P<0.001$). Injection of AdCD40L into previously established AC29 tumors in CBA/J mice yielded evidence of tumor regression associated with increased recruitment of CD8 + tumor-infiltrating lymphocytes. Adoptive transfer of CD8 + T cells from AdCD40L-treated tumor-bearing mice conferred protection to naive mice challenged with AC29 tumor cells. Finally, in mice implanted with two synchronous tumors at distant sites, treatment of one of the tumors with AdCD40L resulted in bilateral regression. Overall, this report by Friedlander and colleagues [76] confirmed the induction of tumor-specific CD8 + T cells by AdCD40L gene transfer and supported the further development of AdCD40L for the treatment of malignant mesothelioma, perhaps in combination with delivery of suicide or cytokine genes.

Nonspecific Immune Stimulation

Innate and adaptive antitumoral immune responses also can be elicited by targeted expression of nonspecific immunostimulatory genes. As an example of this paradigm, Lukacs and colleagues [77] delivered a mycobacterial heat shock protein gene-65 via cationic liposomes into the abdominal cavities of mice bearing intraperitoneal sarcomas, which resulted in significant antitumoral responses. The rationale for the in vivo antitumoral efficacy of heat shock protein-65 gene transfer was that heat shock proteins expressed in tumor cells would serve as molecular chaperones and facilitate more efficient tumor antigen presentation via endogenous major histocompatibility complex molecules. Lanuti and colleagues [78] found that the antitumoral effects of heat shock protein-65 gene transfer via cationic liposomes could be reproduced in an immunocompetent murine mesothelioma model but appeared secondary to nonspecific effects of lipid pDNA complexes. Plasmid delivery of heat shock protein-65, the *E coli* β-galactosidase marker gene *lacZ*, or a null vector all conferred significant survival advantages compared with saline control. Significantly, there was no survival benefit for heat shock gene transfer compared with instillation of the null vector alone. Lanuti and colleagues [78] postulated that the unmethylated cytosine-guanine (CpG) motifs of the prokaryotic DNA in the null vector were sufficient to activate danger signals and induce innate and adaptive antitumoral immune responses.

These findings were similar to those of Lukacs and colleagues [79] in their study of intraperitoneal β-galactosidase gene delivery in immunocompetent mice bearing intra-abdominal mesotheliomas. Transfection of tumor cells with plasmid-liposome complexes or replication-incompetent retroviruses encoding for β- galactosidase produced marked decreases in intra-abdominal mesothelioma burden in immunocompetent—but not immunodeficient—mice. Although the retrovirus-liposome constructs provided the greatest β- galactosidase expression, this did not correlate with superior antitumoral response. Lukacs and colleagues [79] also demonstrated generation of tumor-specific CTLs in mesothelioma-bearing mice treated with intraperitoneal β-galactosidase–plasmid/liposome complexes. The antitumoral effect induced by intratumoral expression of bacterial antigens was likely T cell mediated.

Rudginsky and colleagues [80] investigated the effects of prokaryotic DNA delivery in in vivo mesothelioma models. They conducted a series of experiments that demonstrated antitumoral responses and increased survival with liposomal delivery of fragments of bacterial plasmid DNA, genomic *E coli* DNA, and synthetic CpG oligonucleotides. Liposomal delivery of eukaryotic DNA or methylated bacterial DNA was not associated with increased survival or tumor reduction. Intraperitoneal lavage after liposomal delivery revealed elevations in the proinflammatory cytokines TNF-α and IL-12 only with those complexes that induced antitumoral immunity [80]. The work of Rudginsky's group suggests that the unmethylated CpG motifs of prokaryotic DNA play a crucial role in the development of innate and adaptive antitumoral immune responses.

Interferon-β Gene Therapy

Type I (α, β) and type II (γ) IFN proteins have demonstrable antitumoral activity when administered systemically or locally to patients who have pleural mesothelioma. IFN-β, for example, has potent antiproliferative effects on mesothelioma cells in vitro and strong immunostimulatory actions in animal models but is limited in clinical use by toxicity of systemic administration [81]. Odaka and colleagues [82] in the Thoracic Oncology Research Laboratory at the University of Pennsylvania Medical Center investigated the effects of IFN-β gene therapy in murine models of mesothelioma. The Penn Thoracic Oncology Research Laboratory investigators showed that a single intraperitoneal injection of an rAd expressing the murine IFN-β gene (Ad.muIFN-β) eradicated established mesothelioma tumors and significantly prolonged survival in an immunocompetent mouse model of the disease. Intraperitoneal Ad. muIFN-β gene therapy (in mice bearing intra-abdominal tumors) also resulted in marked responses in distant subcutaneous tumors. A subsequent series of experiments by Odaka and colleagues [82] confirmed that the antitumoral effects of Ad.muIFN-β were mediated by induction and recruitment of CD8 + T lymphocytes.

Based on these results, in 2003, investigators at the University of Pennsylvania Medical Center, in conjunction with the Biogen-IDEC Corporation, initiated a phase 1 trial of Ad.IFN-β (BG00001) in patients who had MPM (or metastatic pleural tumors) (see Table 1). We have completed enrollment in this phase I clinical trial but continue active follow-up of surviving patients and evaluation of patients' peripheral blood and pleural fluid samples for evidence of IFN-β gene transfer and for induced antivector or antitumoral immune responses.

In this phase I trial, ten patients underwent intrapleural (IPl) infusion of a single dose of Ad.IFN-β (at two dose levels) after pretreatment leukopheresis. The purpose of the single blood volume leukopheresis was to obtain enough peripheral blood mononuclear cells for sophisticated immunologic testing, including tetramer analysis. Seven of the patients enrolled had mesothelioma, two patients had metastatic non–small cell lung cancer, and the other patient had metastatic ovarian cancer to the pleural space.

The first three patients received (9×10^{11} viral particles) of Ad.IFN-β. They all tolerated dosing with mild to moderate (grade 1–2) toxicities. None of the patients experienced a dose-limiting toxicity or a serious adverse event. Transitory lymphopenia was the most common toxicity seen; other side effects included chest pain, coryza, fever, anemia, and elevated liver enzymes. Two of three patients in the first cohort are still alive 24 and 19 months, respectively, after receiving vector.

Four patients with mesothelioma were enrolled at dose level 2 (3×10^{12} viral particles). One patient experienced an episode of transient hypoxia (grade 3) approximately 11 hours after dosing and rapidly recovered to baseline. This patient has completed more than 1 year of evaluations without any further complications. The next two patients at dose level 2 tolerated dosing well with no immediate or delayed complications. The fourth patient treated at dose level 2 developed grade 3 elevations in liver function tests without clinical evidence of hepatic dysfunction. These liver function test elevations gradually decreased to baseline levels over a period of several months. Although these side effects caused no real clinical problems, they were by definition classed as dose-limiting toxicities. Subsequently, as per protocol, three additional patients were treated at dose level 1 (9×10^{11} viral particles) without evidence of serious adverse events. In this phase I trial, 9×10^{11} viral particles was determined to be the maximally tolerated dose.

All of the ten patients who were dosed with IPl Ad.IFN-β underwent repeat imaging studies 60 days after discharge. In our first cohort of patients, two are still alive at 24 months and 19 months after therapy. One patient who had mesothelioma had slight progression of disease at his 60-day follow-up and was subsequently started on palliative chemotherapy with stabilization of his disease. Another patient in this cohort who had ovarian cancer had a dramatic response of her abdominal and pleural disease by PET scan that lasted 4 months after IPl Ad.IFN-β instillation. Progression of her abdominal disease regressed after initiation of therapy with an antivascular endothelial growth factor monoclonal antibody (bevacizumab) . The third patient who had metastatic lung cancer had disease progression at day 60 and died with progressive disease 8 months after therapy.

In our second cohort of patients (all with mesothelioma), three patients had stable disease at 60 days. The first patient is currently at 14 months after treatment, with stable disease on CT and PET scan without additional therapies. The second and third patients had stable disease (per modified Response Evaluation Criteria in Solid Tumors [RECIST]) at 60 days. Both patients had subsequent evidence of disease progression and were recommended for salvage chemotherapy, however. The final patient in this cohort had rapidly progressive disease and died approximately 4 months after treatment.

In our last cohort of patients (three additional patients at dose level 1), all patients have been evaluated at 60 days. Both patients who had mesothelioma had stable disease by modified RECIST criteria at the 2-month follow-up; one patient with stage IV non–small cell lung cancer showed disease progression but has since had a dramatic response to the addition of erlotinib.

Although only a phase 1 trial, we have seen five patients who demonstrated stabilization of their disease, several at the 6-month follow-up. This delayed type of response may reflect induction of immune response to the tumor by local injection of the Ad.IFN-β vector [83].

Although we have completed successfully an initial phase 1 trial that tested the safety and efficacy of single dose of Ad.IFN-β in patients who had mesothelioma and malignant pleural effusions, our preclinical data posit that multiple doses of Ad.IFN-β will result in increased efficacy with more advanced tumors (data not shown). We are scheduled to begin a second phase 1 trial in which two doses of Ad.IFN-β vector will be administered 7 days apart in patients who have malignant mesothelioma and malignant pleural effusion (MPE). Patient evaluation in this repeated dose trial will include (1) assessment of the overall toxicity via clinical observation and standard laboratory tests, (2) assessment of the immune response to the tumor and the adenoviral vector, and (3) measurement of gene transfer by ELISA analysis of pre- and postvector delivery pleural fluid specimens obtained from the indwelling pleural catheter. We will assess tumor response via chest CT and ^{18}FDG PET scanning.

Recent efforts in the Thoracic Oncology Research Laboratory of the University of Pennsylvania Medical Center have focused on augmenting the response to immuno-gene therapy. Marked augmentation of efficacy has been obtained with combinations, including Ad.IFN-β plus cyclo-oxygenase-2 inhibition, surgical debulking, vascular disruptive agents, and neoadjuvant chemotherapy with cisplatin and gemcitabine [84,85]. We plan to incorporate several of these innovative approaches in future phase II clinical trials.

INDUCTION OF APOPTOSIS

The most common cancer gene therapy modality used in human clinical trials to date has been mutation compensation, which is intracellular insertion of normal copies of absent or mutated tumor suppressor genes responsible for the malignant phenotype of the cancer cell. Intratumoral delivery of the wild-type p53 gene has been the standard bearer in human cancer gene therapy trials, because mutations in the p53 tumor suppressor gene account for a significant proportion of genetic abnormalities in solid tumors. Most mesotheliomas, however, contain wild-type p53 and a normal copy of the cell cycle regulator pRB. The most common molecular abnormality found in pleural mesotheliomas is loss of expression of the cyclin-dependent kinase inhibitor, p16^{INK4a}. Mutations in p16^{INK4a} result in unchecked cell cycle progression, despite the presence of normal pRB expression and wild-type p53, which engenders a neoplastic phenotype [86].

Frizelle and colleagues [86] at the University of Minnesota School of Medicine showed that re-expression of p16^{INK4a} in mesothelioma cells in vitro and in vivo results in cell cycle arrest, cell growth inhibition, apoptosis, and tumor reduction [87]. They also demonstrated prolonged survival in athymic nude mice with established human mesothelioma xenografts repeated administration of an Ad vector expressing wild-type p16^{INK4a} [86]. Successful translation of p16 mutation compensation to human clinical trials depends on the development of more efficient means of tumor cell transduction, perhaps via tumor-selective, replication-restricted viral vectors.

Yang and colleagues [88] at the University of California, San Francisco Thoracic Oncology Laboratory have targeted another common genetic abnormality in mesothelioma for mutation compensation gene therapy: homozygous deletion of the INK4a/ARF locus. The p14(ARF) protein encoded by the INK4a/ARF locus promotes degradation of the p53 inhibitor MDM2. Deletion of the INK4a/ARF locus abrogates p14(ARF) protein expression, which decreases MDM2 degradation and accelerates p53 inactivation. The University of California, San Francisco group transfected human mesothelioma cell lines in vitro with an Ad vector that encoded for human p14(ARF) complementary DNA (Ad.p14). Overexpression of p14(ARF) within mesothelioma cells enhanced intracellular levels of p53 and p21 and dephosphorylation of pRb. Adp14 also inhibited mesothelioma cell growth via induction of G(1)-phase cell cycle arrest and apoptotic cell death. This novel gene therapy approach using p14 gene transfer has not yet been tested in human clinical trials [88].

The UCSF investigators [88a] also investigated the efficacy of the ONYX-015 adenovirus in mesothelioma cells and found that the cytolytic effect of this agent in mesothelioma depends on the absence of p14(ARF) expression. ONYX-015 is a conditionally replication-competent adenovirus that lacks the E1b55 kDa gene. The protein product of the E1b55 kDa gene can bind and inactivate wild-type p53. ONYX-015 is replication restricted to tumor cells that lack functional p53. Clinical trials of ONYX-015 in patients with head and neck and lung cancers revealed preliminary evidence of tumor responses with minimal toxicity. In mesothelioma, unlike most other solid tumors, genetic alterations in p53 are uncommon, but functional inhibition of p53 can be achieved via deletions in the INK4a/ARF locus. Yang and colleagues reported the cytotoxic effects of ONYX-015 in vitro on mesothelioma cell lines lacking p14(ARF) and increased resistance of these same cell lines to ONYX-015 after transduction of the tumor cells with Adp14 [88a].

Despite the fact that most mesotheliomas contain wild-type p53, this tumor suppressor gene is often functionally impaired in mesothelioma cells secondary to binding by inhibitor proteins, such as MDM-2 and simian virus (SV) 40 large T antigen (Tag). There may be a rationale for gene therapy of mesothelioma via overexpression of wild-type p53 within the tumor cell to overwhelm this blockade. Giuliano and colleagues [89] performed a series of experiments that involved transduction of human mesothelioma cells with a replication-deficient Ad wild-type p53 vector. They demonstrated significant inhibition of in vitro tumor cell growth with documentation of apoptotic processes in the dying tumor cells. Giuliano and colleagues also showed that ex vivo wild-type p53 gene transfer to mesothelioma cells inhibited growth of tumor implants in nude mice. In immunodeficient mice with established human mesothelioma xenografts, intratumoral wild-type p53 gene injection inhibited tumor growth and prolonged survival [89]. Despite the relative absence of p53 mutations or deletions in mesothelioma, it may be reasonable to initiate human clinical trials of Ad wild-type p53 gene therapy in mesothelioma similar to those completed in lung cancer, head and neck cancer, and metastatic colon cancer (see Table 1).

Other investigators have proposed alternate methods of inhibiting mesothelioma cells, such as the introduction of downstream promoters of apoptosis (eg, the pro-apoptotic Bcl-2 family member, Bak). Pataer and colleagues [90] at M.D. Anderson Cancer Center in Houston codelivered binary adenoviral-Bak/GV-16 vectors into p53 wild-type and p53 mutated mesothelioma cell lines in vitro along with binary Ad.*lacZ*/GV-16 control vectors. The M.D. Anderson group demonstrated marked induction of apoptosis and decreased cellular viability with Bak gene transfer in p53 sensitive and resistant cell lines. Apoptosis was not noted, however, with *lacZ* delivery. If hurdles surrounding transduction efficiency could be surmounted, in vivo gene transfer with pro-apoptotic Bcl-2 family members would be a reasonable strategy for future mesothelioma gene therapy clinical trials.

SIMIAN VIRUS 40: IS THERE A ROLE IN THERAPY FOR MESOTHELIOMA?

One of the most remarkable and controversial developments in mesothelioma research in recent years has been the identification of simian virus 40 (SV40) sequences in mesothelioma tumor specimens from the United States and several European countries. SV40, a nonhuman polyomavirus that was a contaminant of some polio vaccines in the 1950s and 1960s, has the capacity to transform normal cells via the oncogenic properties of its Tag. SV-40 has been shown to induce mesothelioma formation in hamsters after intrapleural or intraperitoneal injection [91]. Laboratory analysis of human mesothelioma specimens demonstrated co-immunoprecipitation of SV40 Tag with tumor suppressor gene products, such as p53 and pRB [92]. The presence and multifunctionality of SV40 Tag within mesothelioma cells may explain the persistence of wild-type p53 and pRb in MPM, unlike most other solid tumors.

The evolving role pf SV40 as a co-carcinogen in mesothelioma has spawned several novel gene therapy approaches. For example, Schrump and Waheed [93] at the Surgical Brach of the National Cancer Institute demonstrated that antisense oligonucleotides directed against SV40 Tag mRNA induce apoptosis and enhance sensitivity to chemotherapeutic agents in SV40 (+) mesothelioma cells in vitro. Imperiale and colleagues [94] at the University of Michigan and Wayne

State University Medical Centers proffered an alternative strategy that involved a genetically engineered vaccine to SV40 Tag. SV40 is an ideal candidate for antigen-specific immunotherapy because Tag is a viral antigen, which, unlike most other human tumor-associated antigens, does not readily induce immune tolerance. The Michigan collaborators devised a recombinant, truncated version of Tag (mTag) modified to exclude the J domain and the p53/pRB binding domains: regions with oncogenic function. They cloned the mTag gene into a vaccinia vector (vac-mTag) and demonstrated significant antitumoral immune responses in Balb/c mice that bore Tag(+) tumors.

SUMMARY

Gene therapy for mesothelioma is currently in its adolescence. Multiple novel preclinical investigations and ongoing phase I trials offer significant hope for the future. Several early-stage clinical studies that involve intrapleural and intra-tumoral delivery of viral and cellular vectors carrying various therapeutic genes have proved safe in humans, with evidence of intratumoral gene transfer and anecdotal tumor responses. The expansion of knowledge regarding molecular aspects of mesothelioma carcinogenesis has facilitated the development of prom-ising gene therapy modalities that target specific oncoproteins and mutant tumor suppressor genes. Although implementation of any of these gene therapy approaches as part of standard medical care for patients who have mesothelioma remains years in the future, the field is finally progressing toward more definitive phase II/III efficacy studies. Unfortunately, the marginal benefits garnered from standard anticancer treatments in mesothelioma argue strongly for continued participation in clinical studies of various experimental approaches, particularly gene therapy [95]. These trials serve multiple purposes: to establish safety, determine proper dosing, evaluate for efficacy, and, in an iterative fashion, guide future avenues of laboratory investigation.

References

[1] Sterman D, Kaiser L, Albelda S. Advances in the treatment of malignant pleural meso-thelioma. Chest 1999;116:504–20.
[2] Carmen IH. A death in the laboratory: the politics of the Gelsinger aftermath. Mol Ther: J Am Soc Gen Ther 2001;3(4):425–8.
[3] Lambright ES, Force SD, Lanuti ME, et al. Efficacy of repeated adenoviral suicide gene therapy in a localized murine tumor model. Ann Thorac Surg 2000;70(6):1865–70 [discussion 1870–1].
[4] Al-Hendry A, Magliocco AM, Al-Tweigeri T, et al. Ovarian cancer gene therapy: repeated treatment with thymidine kinase in an adenovirus vector and ganciclovir improves survival in a novel immunocompetent murine model. Am J Obstet Gynecol 2000;182:553–9.
[5] Black ME, Newcomb TG, Wilson HMP, et al. Creation of drug-specific herpes simplex virus type 1 thymidine kinase mutants for gene therapy. Proc Natl Acad Sci U S A 1996; 93:3525–9.
[6] Qiao HJ, Black ME, Caruso M. Enhanced ganciclovir killing and bystander effect of human tumor cells transduced with retroviral vector carrying a herpes simplex thymidine kinase gene mutant. Hum Gene Ther 2000;11:1569–76.
[7] Robinson BW, Mukherjee SA, Davidson A, et al. Cytokine gene therapy or infusion as treatment for solid human cancer. J Immunother 1998;21:211–7.

[8] Tiberghien P. Use of suicide genes in gene therapy. J Leukoc Biol 1994;56:203–9.
[9] Huber BE, Austin EA, Richards CA, et al. Metabolism of 5-fluorocytosine to 5-fluorouacil in human colorectal tumor cells transduced with the cytosine deaminase gene: significant antitumor effects when only a small percentage of tumor cells express cytosine deaminase. Proc Natl Acad Sci U S A 1994;91:8302–6.
[10] Hoganson DK, Batra RK, Olsen JC, et al. Comparison of the effects of three different toxin genes and their levels of expression on cell growth and bystander effect in lung adenocarcinoma. Cancer Res 1996;56:1315–23.
[11] Matthews T, Boehme R. Antiviral activity and mechanism of action of ganciclovir. Rev Infect Dis 1988;10:S490–4.
[12] Rubsam LZ, Davidson BL, Shewach DS. Superior cytotoxicity with ganciclovir compared with acyclovir and 1-β-D-arabinofuranosylthymine in herpes simplex virus-thymidine kinase expressing cells: a novel paradigm for cell killing. Cancer Res 1998;58:3873–82.
[13] Pope IM, Poston GJ, Kinsella AR. The role of the bystander effect in suicide gene therapy. Eur J Cancer 1997;33:1005–16.
[14] Moolten FL, Wells JM, Mroz PJ. Multiple transduction as a means of preserving ganciclovir chemosensitivity in sarcoma cells carrying retrovirally transduced herpes thymidine kinase genes. Cancer Lett 1992;64:257–63.
[15] Treat J, Kaiser LR, Sterman DH, et al. Treatment of advanced mesothelioma with the recombinant adenovirus H5.010RSVTK: a phase 1 trial (BB-IND 6274). Hum Gene Ther 1996;7:2047–57.
[16] Schwarzenberger P, Harrison L, Weinacker A, et al. Gene therapy for malignant mesothelioma: a novel approach for an incurable cancer with increased incidence in Louisiana. J La State Med Soc 1998;150:168–74.
[17] Ram Z, Culver KW, Walbridge B, et al. In situ retroviral-mediated gene transfer for the treatment of brain tumors in rats. Cancer Res 1993;53:83–8.
[18] Freeman SM, Abboud CN, Whartenby KA, et al. The "bystander effect": tumor regression when a fraction of the tumor mass is genetically modified. Cancer Res 1993;53:5274–83.
[19] Hasegawa Y, Emi N, Shimokata K, et al. Gene transfer of herpes simplex virus type I thymidine kinase gene as a drug sensitivity gene into human lung cancer lines using retroviral vectors. Am J Respir Cell Mol Biol 1993;8:655–61.
[20] Caruso M, Panis Y, Gagandeep S, et al. Regression of established macroscopic liver metastases after in situ transduction of a suicide gene. Proc Natl Acad Sci U S A 1993;90:7024–8.
[21] Elshami AA, Saavedra A, Zhang HB, et al. Gap junctions play a role in the bystander effect of the herpes simplex virus thymidine kinase/ganciclovir system in vitro. Gene Ther 1996;3:85–92.
[22] Mesnil M, Yamasaki H. Bystander effect in herpes simplex virus-thymidine kinase/ganciclovir cancer gene therapy: role of gap-junctional intercellular communication. Cancer Res 2000;60:3989–99.
[23] Smythe WR, Hwang HC, Amin KM, et al. Use of recombinant adenovirus to transfer the herpes simplex virus thymidine kinase (HSVtk) gene to thoracic neoplasms: an effective in vitro drug sensitization system. Cancer Res 1994;54:2055–9.
[24] Smythe WR, Kaiser LR, Amin KM, et al. Successful adenovirus-mediated gene transfer in an in vivo model of human malignant mesothelioma. Ann Thorac Surg 1994;57:1395–401.
[25] Smythe WR, Hwang HC, Elshami AA, et al. Successful treatment of experimental human mesothelioma using adenovirus transfer of the herpes simplex-thymidine kinase gene. Ann Surg 1995;222:78–86.
[26] Hwang HC, Smythe WR, Elshami AA, et al. Gene therapy using adenovirus carrying the herpes simplex thymidine kinase gene to treat in vitro models of human malignant mesothelioma and lung cancer. Am J Respir Cell Mol Biol 1995;13:7–16.
[27] Elshami A, Kucharczuk J, Zhang H, et al. Treatment of pleural mesothelioma in an immunocompetent rat model utilizing adenoviral transfer of the HSV-thymidine kinase gene. Hum Gene Ther 1996;7:141–8.
[28] Esandi MC, van Someren GD, Vincent AJ, et al. Gene therapy of experimental malignant

mesothelioma using adenovirus vectors encoding the HSV*tk* gene. Gene Ther 1997;4: 280–7.

[29] Kucharczuk JC, Raper S, Elshami AA, et al. Safety of adenoviral-mediated transfer of the herpes simplex thymidine kinase cDNA to the pleural cavity of rats and non-human primates. Hum Gene Ther 1996;7:2225–33.

[30] Treat J, Kaiser LR, Sterman DH, et al. Treatment of advanced mesothelioma with the recombinant adenovirus H5.010RSV*TK*: a phase 1 trial (BB-IND 6274). Hum Gene Ther 1996;7:2047–57.

[31] Sterman DH, Treat J, Litzky LA, et al. Adenovirus-mediated herpes simplex virus thymidine kinase gene delivery in patients with localized malignancy: results of a phase 1 clinical trial in malignant mesothelioma. Hum Gene Ther 1998;9:1083–92.

[32] Molnar-Kimber KL, Sterman DH, Chang M, et al. Humoral and cellular immune responses induced by adenoviral-based gene therapy for localized malignancy: results of a phase 1 clinical trial for malignant mesothelioma. Hum Gene Ther 1998;9:2121–33.

[33] Sterman DH, Molnar-Kimber K, Iyengar T, et al. A pilot study of systemic corticosteroid administration in conjunction with intrapleural adenoviral vector administration in patients with malignant pleural mesothelioma. Cancer Gene Ther 2000;7(12):1511–8.

[34] Gao GP, Yang Y, Wilson JM. Biology of adenovirus vectors with E1 and E4 deletions for liver-directed gene therapy. J Virol 1996;70:8934–43.

[35] Sterman DH, Recio A, Molnar-Kimber K, et al. Herpes simplex virus thymidine kinase (HSV*tk*) gene therapy utilizing an E1/E4-deleted adenoviral vector: preliminary results of a phase I clinical trial for pleural mesothelioma. Am J Respir Crit Care Med 1999; 159:A237.

[36] Alavi JB, Eck SL. Gene therapy for malignant gliomas. Hematol Oncol Clin North Am 1998;12:617–29.

[37] Perez-Cruet MJ, Trask TW, Chen SH, et al. Adenovirus-mediated gene therapy of experimental gliomas. J Neurosci Res 1994;39:506–11.

[38] Morris JC, Ramsey WJ, Wildner O, et al. Phase I study of intralesional administration of an adenovirus vector expressing the HSV-1 thymidine kinase gene (AdV.RSV-*TK*) in combination with escalating doses of ganciclovir in patients with cutaneous metastatic melanoma. Hum Gene Ther 2000;11:487–503.

[39] Black ME, Kokoris MS, Sabo P. Herpes simplex virus-1 thymidine kinase mutants created by semi-random sequence mutagenesis improve prodrug-mediated tumor cell killing. Cancer Res 2001;61(7):3022–6.

[40] Wiewrodt R, Amin K, Kiefer M, et al. Adenovirus-mediated gene transfer of enhanced herpes simplex virus thymidine kinase mutants improves prodrug-mediated tumor cell killing. Cancer Gene Ther 2003;10(5):353–64.

[41] Alemany R, Balague Curiel C. Replicative adenoviruses for cancer therapy. Nat Biotechnol 2000;18:723–7.

[42] Tsukuda K, Wiewrodt R, Molnar-Kimber K, et al. An E2F-responsive replication-selective adenovirus targeted to the defective cell cycle in cancer cells: potent antitumoral efficacy but no toxicity to normal cells. Cancer Res 2002;62(12):3438–47.

[43] Kahlos K, Anttila S, Asikainen T, et al. Manganese superoxide dismutase in healthy human pleural mesothelium and in malignant pleural mesothelioma. Am J Respir Cell Mol Biol 1998;18:579–80.

[44] Doglioni C, Dei Tos AP, Laurino L, et al. Calretinin: a novel immunocytochemical marker for mesothelioma. Am J Surg Pathol 1996;20:1037–46.

[45] Gotzos V, Vogt P, Celio M. The calcium binding protein calretinin is a selective marker for malignant pleural mesotheliomas of the epithelial type. Path Res Pract 1996;192:137–47.

[46] Chang K, Pastan I. Molecular cloning of mesothelin, a differentiation antigen present on mesothelium, mesotheliomas, and ovarian cancers. Proc Natl Acad Sci U S A 1996;93: 136–40.

[47] Ambrosini G, Adid C, Altieri DC. A novel anti-apoptosis gene, surviving, expressed in cancer and lymphoma. Nat Med 1997;3:917–21.

[48] Ishiwata N, Inase N, Fujie T, et al. Suicide gene therapy using keratin 19 enhancer and promoter in malignant mesothelioma cells. Anticancer Res 2003;23(2B):1405–9.

[49] Berlinghoff S, Veldwijk MR, Laufs S, et al. Susceptibility of mesothelioma cell lines to adeno-associated virus 2 vector-based suicide gene therapy. Lung Cancer 2004;46(2):179–86.

[50] Hall SJ, Sanford MA, Atkinson G, et al. Induction of potent antitumor natural killer cell activity by herpes simplex virus-thymidine kinase and ganciclovir therapy in an orthotopic mouse model of prostate cancer. Cancer Res 1998;58:3221–5.

[51] Freeman SM, Ramesh R, Marogi AJ. Immune system in suicide gene therapy. Lancet 1997;349:2–3.

[52] Vile RG, Castleden S, Marshall J, et al. Generation of an anti-tumor immune response in a non-immunogenic tumour: HSV*tk* killing *in vivo* stimulates a mononuclear cell infiltrate and a Th1-like profile of intratumoural cytokine expression. Int J Cancer 1997;71:267–74.

[53] Melcher A, Todryk S, Hardwick N, et al. Tumor immunogenicity is determined by the mechanism of cell death via induction of heat shock protein expression. Nat Med 1998;4:581–7.

[54] Chen SH, Li Chen XH, Wang Y, et al. Combination gene therapy for liver metastasis of colon carcinoma in vivo. Proc Natl Acad Sci U S A 1995;92:2577 81.

[55] O'Malley Jr B, Cope KA, Chen SH, et al. Combination gene therapy for oral cancer in a murine model. Cancer Res 1996;56:1737–41.

[56] Castleden SA, Chong H, Garcia-Ribas I, et al. A family of bicistronic vectors to enhance both local and systemic antitumor effects of HSV*tk* or cytokine expression in a murine melanoma model. Hum Gene Ther 1997;8:2087–102.

[57] Coll J, Mesnil M, Lefebvre M, et al. Long-term survival of immunocompetent rats with intraperitoneal colon carcinoma tumors using herpes simplex thymidine kinase/ganciclovir and IL-2 treatments. Gene Ther 1997;4:1160–6.

[58] Kolls J, Freeman S, Ramesh R, et al. The treatment of malignant pleural mesothelioma with gene modified cancer cells: a phase I study. Am J Respir Crit Care Med 1998;157:A563.

[59] Schwarzenberger P, Lei D, Freeman SM, et al. Antitumor activity with the HSV-tk-gene cell line PA-1-STK in malignant mesothelioma. Am J Respir Cell Mol Biol 1998;19(2):333–7.

[60] Harrison Jr LH, Schwarzenberger PO, Byrne PS, et al. Gene-modified PA1-STK cells home to tumor sites in patients with malignant pleural mesothelioma. Ann Thorac Surg 2000;70(2):407–11.

[61] Byrne PS, Schwarzenberger PO, Harrison L, et al. Cytokine profile assessment of mesothelioma patients treated with escalating doses of intrapleurally administered, genetically modified PA1STK cells and a twice daily regimen of ganciclovir: a phase I clinical trial [American Society of Gene Therapy 2004 abstract]. Mol Ther 2004;605.

[62] Leong CC, Marley JV, Loh S, et al. The induction of immune responses to murine mesothelioma by IL-2 gene transfer. Immunol Cell Biol 1997;75:356–9.

[63] Fakharai H, Shawler D, Gjerset R, et al. Cytokine gene therapy with interleukin-2-transduced fibroblasts: effects of IL-2 dose on anti-tumor immunity. Hum Gen Ther 1995;6:591–601.

[64] Christmas T, Manning LS, Garlepp MJ, et al. Effect of interferon-alpha 2a on malignant mesothelioma. Interferon Res 1993;13:9–12.

[65] Astoul P, Viallat JR, Laurent JC, et al. Intrapleural IL-2 in passive immunotherapy for malignant pleural effusion. Chest 1993;103(1):209–13.

[66] Astoul P, Picat-Joossen D, Viallat J, et al. Intrapleural administration of interleukin-2 for the treatment of patients with malignant pleural mesothelioma: a phase II study. Cancer 1998;83:2099–104.

[67] Boutin C, Viallat J, VanZandwijk N, et al. Activity of intrapleural recombinant gamma-interferon in malignant mesothelioma. Cancer 1991;67:2033–7.

[68] Boutin C, Nussbaum E, Monnet I, et al. Intrapleural treatment with recombinant gamma-interferon in early stage malignant pleural mesothelioma. Cancer 1994;74:2460–7.

[69] Robinson B, Bowman R, Manning L, et al. Interleukin-2 and lymphokine-activated killer cells in malignant mesothelioma. Eur Respir Rev 1993;3:220–2.

[70] Goey SH, Eggermont AM, Punt CJ, et al. Intrapleural administration of interleukin-2 in pleural mesothelioma: a phase I–II study. Br J Cancer 1995;72:1283–8.

[71] Mukherjee S, Haenel T, Himbeck R, et al. Replication-restricted vaccinia as a cytokine gene therapy vector in cancer: persistent transgene expression despite antibody generation. Cancer Gen Ther 2000;7(5):663–70.

[72] Rochlitz C, Jantscheff P, Bongartz G, et al. Gene therapy study of cytokine-transfected xenogeneic cells (Vero-interleukin-2) in patients with metastatic solid tumors. Cancer Gene Ther 1999;6(3):271–8.

[73] Caminschi I, Venetsanakos E, Leong CC, et al. Interleukin-12 induces an effective antitumor response in malignant mesothelioma. Am J Respir Cell Mol Biol 1998;19: 738–46.

[74] Caminschi I, Venetsanakos E, Leong CC, et al. Cytokine gene therapy of mesothelioma: immune and antitumor effects of transfected interleukin-12. Am J Respir Cell Mol Biol 1999;21:347–56.

[75] Cordier Kellerman L, Valeyrie L, Fernandez N, et al. Regression of AK7 malignant mesothelioma established in immunocompetent mice following intratumoral gene transfer of interferon gamma. Cancer Gene Ther 2003;10(6):481–90.

[76] Friedlander PL, Delaune CL, Abadie JM, et al. Efficacy of CD40 ligand gene therapy in malignant mesothelioma. Am J Respir Cell Mol Biol 2003;29(3 Pt 1):321–30.

[77] Lukacs KV, Nakakes A, Atkins CJ, et al. In vivo gene therapy of malignant tumors with heat shock protein-65 gene. Gen Ther 1997;4:345–50.

[78] Lanuti M, Rudginsky S, Force S, et al. Cationic lipid:bacterial DNA complexes elicit antitumor effects and adaptive immunity in murine intraperitoneal tumor models. Cancer Res 2000;60:2955–63.

[79] Lukacs KV, Porter CD, Pardo OE, et al. In vivo transfer of bacterial marker genes results in differing levels of gene expression and tumor progression in immunocompetent and immunodeficient mice. Hum Gene Ther 1999;10(14):2373–9.

[80] Rudginsky S, Siders W, Ingram L, et al. Antitumor activity of cationic lipid complexed with immunostimulatory DNA. Mol Med 2001;4(4):347–55.

[81] Rosso R, Rimoldi R, Salvati F, et al. Intrapleural natural beta interferon in the treatment of malignant pleural effusions. Oncol 1988;45:253–6.

[82] Odaka M, Sterman DH, Wiewrodt R, et al. Eradication of intraperitoneal and distant tumor by adenovirus-mediated interferon-β gene therapy is attributable to induction of systemic immunity. Cancer Res 2001;61:6201–12.

[83] Sterman DH, Albelda SM. Advances in the diagnosis, evaluation, and management of malignant pleural mesothelioma. Respirology 2005;10(3):266–83.

[84] DeLong P, Tanaka T, Kruklitis R, et al. Use of cyclooxygenase-2 inhibition to enhance the efficacy of immunotherapy. Cancer Res 2003;63(22):7845–52.

[85] Kruklitis RJ, Singhal S, Delong P, et al. Immuno-gene therapy with interferon-beta before surgical debulking delays recurrence and improves survival in a murine model of malignant mesothelioma. J Thorac Cardiovasc Surg 2004;127(1):123–30.

[86] Frizelle SP, Rubins JB, Zhou JX, et al. Gene therapy of established mesothelioma xenografts with recombinant p16^{INK4a} adenovirus. Cancer Gene Ther 2000;7:1421–5.

[87] Frizelle SP, Grim J, Zhou JX, et al. Re-expression of p16^{INK4a} in mesothelioma cells results in cell cycle arrest, cell death, tumor suppression, and tumor regression. Oncogene 1998;16:3087–95.

[88] Yang C, You L, Yeh C, et al. Cell cycle arrest and induction of apoptotic death in mesothelioma cells by the adenovirus-mediated p14^{ARF} expression. J Natl Cancer Inst 2000; 19;92(8):636–41.

[88a] Yang C, You L, Yeh C, et al. p14^{ARF} modulates the cytolytic effect of ONYX-015 in mesothelioma cells with wild-type p53. Cancer Res 2001;61:5959–63.

[89] Giuliano M, Catalano A, Strizzi L, et al. Adenovirus-mediated wild-type p53 overexpression reverts tumourigenicity of human mesothelioma cells. Int J Mol Med 2000; 5(6):591–6.

[90] Pataer A, Smythe WR, Yu R, et al. Adenovirus-mediated Bak gene transfer induces apoptosis in mesothelioma cell lines. J Thorac Cardiovasc Surg 2001;121(1):61–7.
[91] Cicala C, Pompetti F, Carbone M. SV40 induces mesothelioma in hamsters. Am J Pathol 1993;142(5):1524–33.
[92] Carbone M, Rizzo P, Grimley PM, et al. Simian virus-40 large-T antigen binds p53 in human mesotheliomas. Nat Med 1997;3(8):908–12.
[93] Schrump DS, Waheed I. Strategies to circumvent SV40 oncoprotein expression in malignant pleural mesothelioma. Semin Cancer Biol 2001;11:73.
[94] Imperiale MJ, Pass HI, Sanda MG. Prospects for an SV40 vaccine. Semin Cancer Biol 2001;11:81–5.
[95] Vogelzang NJ, Rusthoven JJ, Symanowski J, et al. Phase III study of pemetrexed in combination with cisplatin versus cisplatin alone in patients with malignant pleural mesothelioma. J Clin Oncol 2003;21(14):2636–44.

Further Readings

Chen SH, Shine HD, Goodman JC, et al. Gene therapy for brain tumors: regression of experimental gliomas by adenovirus-mediated gene transfer in vivo. Proc Natl Acad Sci U S A 1994;91:3054–7.

Culver KW, Ram Z, Wallbridge S, et al. In vivo gene transfer with retroviral vector-producer cells for treatment of experimental brain tumors. Science 1992;256:1550–2.

Kozarsky K, Wilson JM. Gene therapy: adenovirus vectors. Curr Opin Genet Dev 1993;3:499–503.

Martini N, McCormack PM, Bains MS, et al. Pleural mesothelioma. Ann Thorac Surg 1987;43:113–20.

Moolten FL. Drug sensitivity ("suicide") genes for selective cancer therapy. Cancer Gene Ther 1994;1:279–87.

Rusch V. Pleurectomy/decortication and adjuvant therapy for malignant mesothelioma. Chest 1993;103:382S–4S.

Rusch V. Trials in malignant mesothelioma: LCSG 851 and 882. Chest 1994;106:359S–62S.

Rusch VW, Figlin R, Godwin D, et al. Intrapleural cisplatin and cytarabine in the management of malignant pleural effusions: a Lung Cancer Study Group trial. J Clin Oncol 1991;9:313–9.

Vile RG, Hart IR. Use of tissue-specific expression of the herpes simplex virus thymidine kinase gene to inhibit growth of established murine melanomas following direct intratumoral injection of DNA. Cancer Res 1993;53:3860–4.

Vile RG, Nelson JA, Castleden S, et al. Systemic gene therapy of murine melanoma using tissue specific expression of the HSVtk gene involves an immune component. Cancer Res 1994;54:6228–34.

Hematol Oncol Clin N Am 19 (2005) 1175–1190

HEMATOLOGY/ONCOLOGY CLINICS
OF NORTH AMERICA

Mesothelioma from the Patient's Perspective

Helen Clayson, MBBS, FRCP, FRCGP[a,b,*],
Jane Seymour, RGN, BA (hons), MA, PhD[c],
Bill Noble, MB ChB, MRCGP, MD[d]

[a]Hospice of St. Mary of Furness, Ford Park, Ulverston, Cumbria LA12 7JP, UK
[b]University of Sheffield, Sheffield, UK
[c]Palliative and End-of-Life Studies, School of Nursing, University of Nottingham, Nottingham, UK
[d]Academic Unit of Supportive Care, University of Sheffield, Sheffield, UK

The UK incidence of mesothelioma continues to rise. In 2002, there were 1862 reported deaths caused by mesothelioma, and this number is expected to peak at 1950 to 2450 cases per annum between 2011 and 2015 [1,2]. Treatments thus far have failed to make significant improvements in survival in most cases [3,4]. In view of the acknowledged symptom burden and lack of effective disease-modifying or curative treatments, physicians recommend that patients who have mesothelioma have access to palliative care from the point of diagnosis [5]. An understanding of the illness from a patient's perspective is necessary to shape effective palliative care services [6,7], but little is known about the patient's experience of mesothelioma. In the past three decades there has been a shift in focus from the biomedical approach in health care to a patient-centered perspective. Various national policies reflect this change in emphasis, which requires individual patients to be considered as experiencing individuals rather than the objects of some disease entity [6–8].

This article reports findings from interviews with 15 patients who had malignant pleural mesothelioma. The qualitative research interview is a specific conversational technique in which an understanding of the lived experience of the patient and the meanings that they ascribe to their situation are elicited by the interviewer [9]. Qualitative interviews do not provide statistically representative data; rather they illuminate social phenomena [10]. Interview transcripts may not represent literal truth but may be a rehearsed negotiated report that represents an agreed public account of their situation.

This article was supported by Scientific Foundation Board of the Royal College of General Practitioners grant SFB 2001/07.

* Corresponding author. Hospice of St. Mary of Furness, Ford Park, Ulverston, Cumbria LA12 7JP, UK. E-mail address: h.clayson@sheffield.ac.uk (H. Clayson).

The interviews were one aspect of a doctoral study undertaken by the author (H.C.) at the University of Sheffield entitled "Palliative care in mesothelioma: What are the needs of patients and their families?" The wider study is a four-part, community-based, multimethod case study conducted in three areas in northern England, all with a high incidence of mesothelioma: Barrow-in-Furness, Leeds, and Doncaster. The full study includes (1) interviews with 15 patients who suffered from mesothelioma, (2) six focus groups with bereaved relatives of patients who had died as a result of mesothelioma, (3) interviews with relevant health care professionals, and (4) a review of general practice, hospital, and hospice (where applicable) medical records of 80 patients who died because of mesothelioma. Ethical approval was obtained from the Local Research Ethics Committees in the three locations. The aim of the interviews with patients was to determine the experience of mesothelioma and its meaning for them.

METHODS
Participants
The interview sample consisted of 13 men and 2 women, mean age 69 years, all of whom knew that they had malignant pleural mesothelioma (Table 1). Participants were recruited by clinical nurse specialists who worked with multidisciplinary lung cancer teams. Patients had to be well enough to participate in an interview, know their diagnosis, and give informed consent. An information leaflet was provided, and full written consent was obtained. Thirteen patients were married; in 12 cases their spouses were present during the interviews. Fourteen patients were interviewed at home, and 1 patient was interviewed at the hospice where he was an inpatient. Two patients were interviewed the week before they died.

Interview Process
The interviews took place between December 2000 and June 2003. Participants were invited to give a brief account of their family and occupational history and tell the story of their illness. An interview guide was used where necessary to ensure coverage of key areas (Box 1). Specific questions about dying were not included, but the area was addressed if the patient indicated willingness via verbal or nonverbal clues. Interviews varied in length from 27 to 75 minutes, with the exception of a terminally ill man whose contribution was just one word ("devastated") but whose wife talked for more than 1 hour. This couple was insistent that they wanted the interview to occur despite his rapidly deteriorating condition. The wife's contribution was not treated as an interview but provided useful background information regarding her husband's situation. Patients' stories of their experiences may be understood as reflecting a process of narrative reconstruction in which ill people redefine their self-identity in the face of loss and attempt to make sense of the chaos and disruption caused by illness [11,12].

Data analysis followed the principles of the grounded theory approach, with key themes distilled from the data through a process of constant comparison [13,14]. Analysis was conducted by a single researcher, and reliability was not

Table 1
Sample characteristics and asbestos exposure

Patient ID	Age (y)	Sex	Occupation(s) when exposed	Industry	Asbestos exposure
Mrs. N	72	F	Market stallholder	Retail	From asbestos in market roof
			Housewife (husband and son worked in the shipyard)	—	From husband's and son's overalls
Mr. D	62	M	Cabin lad	Railway	Occupational
			Shunter	Railway	Occupational
Mr. M	Missing data	M	Labourer	Shipbuilding	Occupational
Mr. J	66	M	Apprentice millwright	Shipbuilding	Occupational
Mr. U	68	M	Sheet metal worker	Shipbuilding	Occupational
Mr. I	61	M	Engineering apprentice (9 mo)	Shipbuilding	Occupational
			Foreman (28 y)	Paper mill	Occupational
Mr. K	72	M	Shipyard labourer	Shipbuilding	Occupational
Mr. Y	75	M	Marine engineer (4 y)	Shipbuilding	Occupational
			Maintenance engineer (>10 y)	Railway and gasworks maintenance	Occupational
Mr. S	58	M	Store manager	Retail	Asbestos ceiling was replaced in the store
Mr. C	66	M	Maintenance engineer	Power station	Occupational
Mr. A	79	M	Labourer	Railways maintenance	Occupational
Mr. Q	81	M	Floor layer	Construction	Occupational
Mr. V	68	M	Welder	Construction	Occupational
Mr. H	81	M	Lagger	Railways maintenance	Occupational
Mrs. T	55	F	Housewife	—	Lived next to an asbestos shed while it was demolished

checked by comparison with multiple coders [9]. However, critical discussion regarding the themes identified and their development was undertaken between the first author (H.C.) and the coauthors, who provided doctoral supervision for the wider study.

The main themes from the interviews are discussed later and are illustrated by quotations. The quotations have been "tidied up," with hesitations, repetitions, and pauses removed unless these are essential to convey the sense of the extract. Validity was checked by reference to data from bereaved relatives' focus groups (H. Clayson, MBBS, FRCP, FRCGP, thesis in preparation, 2005) and presentations to health care professionals with knowledge of mesothelioma: Northern Mesothelioma Nurses Network, Association for Palliative Medicine Congress,

BOX 1: INTERVIEW GUIDE

Personal history
    Can you tell me about your family background and then your work history?
Medical history
    Can you tell me about the start of this illness?

    How was the diagnosis made?

    What symptoms are you experiencing?
Asbestos exposure
    What do you believe about the cause of this illness?

    Were you aware of the risks of asbestos at any time?

    How did you learn about asbestos risks?
Impact of the disease and coping strategies
    Can you describe how you learned of the diagnosis?

    Can you describe your reaction?

    How have you dealt with those feelings?

    Who or what has been helpful?

    What effects has this illness had on your family?
Financial matters
    Can you tell me how you are getting on with state benefits and compensa-
        tion claims?
Plans
    Can you tell me about any future plans?
Screening question
    Are there any other matters that you would like to raise?
The questions regarding financial matters and future plans were added after the
first three interviews.

European Association for Palliative Care, British Thoracic Oncology Group, and International Mesothelioma Interest Group.

Ethical Considerations

Interviews with terminally ill patients may cause additional distress; alternatively there may be benefits for patients who contribute to research that pays attention to their concerns. Although patients may have physical and emotional problems at the time of the interview, they have the right to be offered opportunities to contribute to research and make informed choices about doing so. Various authors have emphasized that patients can benefit from participation in terms of empowerment, altruism, and giving voice to the voiceless, provided that care is taken to avoid actual or potential harm [15–18]. It must be acknowledged, however, that direct benefit to patients is not always obtained and distress inadvertently may be caused. The interviewer (H.C.) is a hospice doctor and experienced general practitioner. To address any potential distress the interviewers ascertained that all participants were in touch with their clinical nurse specialist. At the end of each interview, researchers again verified that patients had access to their clinical nurse specialists for support if needed.

FINDINGS

Four main themes arose from the data: coping with symptoms, the burden of medical interventions, finding out about mesothelioma, and psychosocial issues.

Coping with Symptoms

The symptoms experienced by patients at onset and the mode of disease progression agreed with previous accounts of mesothelioma [5,19,20] (Box 2).

Symptoms were reported by patients in terms of their impact on normal activities, which echoed theories of cognitive representations of illness that emphasize the need for patients to understand their illness identity in terms of its effects on their daily lives [21] (Box 3). Patients redefined the meaning of their symptoms as the disease developed, with initial interpretations of symptoms changing as they developed a greater understanding of their illness. In some cases this redefinition led to a sense of empowerment. Some patients felt able to tell their doctors when pleural effusions had recurred and expected appropriate intervention. It also gave rise to anxieties, however, as knowledge of the disease made it harder for patients to ignore or deny the symptoms that indicated disease progression. Not knowing what might happen in the future was a common experience, and most patients and their families reported that they struggled with the lack of any definite information about the significance of their symptoms. Many patients seemed reluctant to seek help for what were clearly severe symptom issues. Researchers recognize that this is a common characteristic in traditionally configured communities, such as those in this study.

Dyspnea, which was the main symptom that affected most of the patients, was associated with profound anxiety associated with the terms "fighting for breath" and "gasping for air" used by many patients. Patients reported continuing to be breathless after treatment, but none described learning any self-help techniques, such as breathing control. Fear was exacerbated in some patients who had heard of people with mesothelioma "suffocating to death" or "drowning in fluid." It was clear that patients' families found it deeply distressing to

---

BOX 2: PRESENTATION OF MESOTHELIOMA AND NUMBER OF PATIENTS AFFECTED

Shortness of breath: 7
Chest pain: 2
Fatigue: 2
Chest infection and/or weight loss: 2
Incidental (abnormal chest radiograph after rib injury): 1
Screening (annual chest radiograph advised by general practitioner in view of past asbestos exposure): 1

BOX 3: COPING WITH SYMPTOMS

(1) Mrs. T (55-year-old patient and her husband, environmental exposure): "Well, I get to the point where I cough and cough, get wind or want to burp, then I'm sick, and the last twice I've been sick I've nearly choked. It's a good job (husband) was there, I seem to lose my airways or whatever…"

Mr. T: "…at midnight last night we were both laid on the bathroom floor with Ann going (gasping) and absolutely panic stricken that that was her last breath, and I am trying to console her, trying to rescue her… We are coping."

Later in the interview:

Mr. T: "But within 6 weeks you can't walk round town… I mean, do we have 12 weeks where you can still walk around the house and then 12 weeks in bed? We just don't know."

Mrs. T: "And nobody knows, no one can answer that can they? It depends how I react to treatment, if I get any."

(2) Mr. Y (75-year-old retired engineer): "Oh dear, I started with violent pains. I was jumping about on that settee like no-one's business, and Jenny said 'Get the doctor.' I said 'It'll go away, it went away last week, it'll be all right, it'll go away.' She says 'Get the doctor, we're not having that noise all day!' So we rang for the doctor. They asked if it was urgent, I said 'No,' and anyway the doctor arrived after he'd finished his surgery in about an hour. He arrived, examined me, gave me a severe chastising for not getting him here earlier. I said I didn't think it was urgent. 'I'll be the judge of that' he said, and rang for an ambulance."

(3) Mr. A (79-year-old retired railway laborer): "…and the pain's always there but I can control it with the medication I'm on to a point… it varies day by day, sometimes it'll pull in my back, other times it'll pull in my front, other times it'll pull where I had my biopsy and it's really nasty when it gets to that area."

(4) Mr. S (58-year-old store manager): "If you could call it stable, it's stable. Or if it's creeping on I don't know about it. I suppose it will creep on eventually won't it?"

witness patients struggling to breathe. This factor, together with the obvious loss of weight of most patients, was a major contributor to the difficulties and emotional burden experienced (Box 3).

Pain was only a major problem for one of the patients interviewed, and the pain had responded to treatment by the time of the interview. Another patient seemed to accept constant low-grade pain while admitting that it was severe at times.

Deteriorating bodily appearance because of loss of weight also caused great distress. Two male patients showed photographs that portrayed them in previous good health, which was in marked contrast to their appearance at interview. One of the women flapped her oversized blouse to demonstrate how much weight she had lost, obviously distressed about her altered appearance.

The Burden of Medical Interventions

Patients' experiences of medical treatment and interventions varied considerably. For some patients, the investigations or interventions were unpleasant and distressing; other patients seemed to tolerate the procedures well (Box 4).

Twelve patients required several pleural aspirations to relieve pleural effusions. The unpredictability and often the speed of onset of pleural effusions caused great distress, compromised patients' abilities to manage their illness, and

BOX 4: THE BURDEN OF MEDICAL INTERVENTIONS

(1) Mr. I (61-year-old paper mill foreman describing problems during pleural aspiration): "It was a terrible ordeal. No pain, no. Not painful at all, but it's the weirdest experience. He said this will happen to one say, one in a hundred... I was practically in shock. Only took about 500 mL... and I was going 'Oh God, I feel as though I'm dying.' He (consultant) walked in and said 'You'd better stop now... can't you see that he's close to going into shock.' Soon as the needle came out I was alright."

(2) Mr. T: "The gentleman, we don't know his name, who came to do the talcum powder..."

Mrs. T (55-year-old patient and her husband describing medical pleurodesis on the ward): "I was sat there and he came in an all green gown and he came into the nurse station and said he'd got to do this talcum powder thing, and the matron said 'Yes, have you done it before?' 'He said I've never done this before'."

(3) Mr. Y (75-year-old clinical trial participant describing chemotherapy side effects and continuing pain): "Oh yes, I've had 3 days at radiotherapy and I've had 12 sessions of chemotherapy. I've seen the doctor, is it 3 or 4 times? I saw the consultant first... then they transferred me from Dr. (A) to Dr. (B) and he got me to go on to this trial thing they're running... And so far so good... Shortness of breath, tingling in my arms... Yes. Pins and needles and burning, burning sensations... The pain is manageable, but it seems to be getting bigger."

(4) Mrs. V (nurse and wife of 68-year-old retired welder explaining her concerns about his treatment): "Mr. C the surgeon referred him to the oncologist with a view to multimodular treatment. Well he didn't have the multimodular treatment, he just had the radiotherapy and it wasn't the correct amount because of the liver, and he didn't have the chemo. The oncologist wasn't in favor of that, so we've had to go along with that. I did question him and you don't like questioning the specialist, do you? But I did say 'Is there any more?' in the nicest possible way of course. You don't want to tread on peoples' toes."

(5) Mr. I (56-year-old maintenance engineer who suffered a steroid-induced psychosis on holiday abroad): "Well, I thought I was Jesus, that was the crunch... I thought I could cure anything and do anything... Wasn't sleeping, an hour's sleep was enough and I was wide awake and so as a consequence I was up all night and so was she. She was frightened what the hell I was going to do next... I was terrible, you know, just totally, uncontrollable, as far as mood swings."

disrupted their treatment calendars [22]. Patients seemed to understand the concept of draining fluid on the lung as a practical solution that gave rapid results, but they did not always find pleural aspiration to be a straightforward procedure.

Nine patients underwent successful pleurodesis; for two patients in one location this meant traveling to a cardiothoracic center 72 miles from home. Patients recalled unpleasant side effects of the medication, and subsequently one patient described tumor that extended along the thoracoscopy wound track and resulted in painful lumps on her chest wall. Three patients reported concerns that inexperienced junior doctors had performed practical procedures.

Patients who received active treatments often had to attend several hospitals. Some patients reported being bewildered by the various doctors, feeling uncertain as to who was in charge of their treatment—chest physicians, oncologists, thoracic surgeons, and, occasionally, palliative medicine specialists—and seeing their family doctor for day-to-day management.

Two patients were offered enrollment in chemotherapy trials, only one of whom was well enough to proceed, and two others had radical surgery. Although after surgery the patients reported that they had been informed that surgery was unlikely to be curative, at the same time they reported disappointment and unfulfilled expectations in relation to the management of their disease. One patient who had radical surgery 3 months before his interview was doing well and hoped at least for an extended survival. He and his wife, a nurse, were concerned that adjuvant chemotherapy was not being given, however, contrary to their expectations shaped by information they obtained from a North American website. This incident revealed some of the complexities surrounding patient involvement in the treatment decision-making process [23,24].

FINDING OUT ABOUT MESOTHELIOMA

Most patients described how they were referred for a chest radiograph at their first or second consultation with a general practitioner. After the chest radiograph indicated that results were abnormal, patients were seen quickly by a hospital consultant—within 2 weeks at the most. Some patients had prior knowledge of workmates or family members with mesothelioma, and this knowledge gave rise to anticipatory anxiety, the so-called "Damocles syndrome" [25]. For most patients this anxiety prompted their search for help and influenced their expectations of the diagnostic process, although their prior knowledge often was incomplete. All the patients acknowledged asbestos as the cause of their disease, although some expressed a degree of disbelief about causation, perhaps because they felt a degree of loyalty to an industry in which they had worked for many years.

Most patients were informed of the diagnosis by the chest medicine physician, although one was informed by his general practitioner. Patients recalled that doctors communicated that the disease was incurable and associated with a limited lifespan. The status of mesothelioma in the United Kingdom as a prescribed disease meant that disclosure of diagnosis was quickly followed by an explanation of the procedures necessary to pursue claims for state benefits and civil compensation. (Prescribed disease is defined in UK regulations as being caused by particular recognized occupations. People who satisfy the criteria are entitled to state industrial disease benefits.) Only one of the 15 patients reported questioning the doctor about the diagnosis or asking for further information. Patients' immediate reactions to the diagnosis appeared to occur in two forms: either as shock or stoic acceptance. Patients spoke of feeling numb and overwhelmed by the sheer quantity and shocking nature of the news, despite what were, for most, accurate suspicions. Although in some cases patients remembered that doctors had expressed sympathy, the predominant recollection was of a hopeless message: incurable disease with no treatments offered in most cases. Accompanying spouses often recalled more of the consultation than did the patient (Box 5).

BOX 5: FINDING OUT ABOUT MESOTHELIOMA

(1) Mr. J (66-year-old worker exposed to asbestos as an apprentice millwright in a shipyard): "Oh yeah, I realize how bad my father got, so I'm expecting the same. How I'll handle it when it does arrive, I don't know."

(2) Mr. U (68-year-old retired sheet metal worker): "I'd always been aware that I might have it because me friends around me were going one by one... 'cos the lad I worked with, he only went in January, he went up at the hospice as well actually... they were from the sheet metal shop... whole family wiped out, father and two sons."

Later, when his wife had been told the diagnosis before him:

Mr. U: "I looked at her face and I said 'You know something I don't, they've found cancer, haven't they?' She just broke down. So then back to the doctor and he said 'Well I'm sorry you've got cancer of the lung. It wasn't a good way of doing it but, on the other score, she got to know, or I wouldn't have told her. And that's the thing that annoyed me really, I could have told her but I didn't have the chance, she had to tell me."

H.C.: "What do you feel would have been the best way of dealing with it?"

Mr. and Mrs. U in unison: "Both together."

(3) Mr. S (58-year-old store manager, describing his worries after being told the diagnosis by a nurse on the telephone): "I didn't know what the hell mesothelioma was, I'd no idea. I'd heard about it, there'd been a lot of cases locally and I'd read about these people in the factories... I'd got an idea, I was getting worried. Well, you've never been told this in your life, probably, but you think the worst, you think 'Are they going to be taking my lung out? Cut a tumour out?'"

(4) Mr. Y: "...I just turned to wood. The doctor said 'You've got mesothelioma' and I can't remember anything after that."

Mrs. Y: "She said 'It's mesothelioma, it's malignant, it's terminal and there's no treatment.' They wouldn't take the lung out because it was too big an operation that would only give him another 6 months."

(5) Mrs. T: "...and I just says to him 'Can you give me a time?' ...and he just says 'No, I don't want to give you any false hope, and I can't give you much hope.'"

Mr. T: "He said 'It's very, very serious and it's in a position where we don't think we can help you.'" (Mrs. T and her husband talking to the consultant after protracted investigations eventually confirmed mesothelioma.)

(6) Mr. D (62-year-old ex-railway worker recalling the impact of the diagnosis and fear generated by mention of Macmillan nurses): "...doctor told me what I'd got... we didn't know what to do... he mentioned Macmillan nurses and my first thought was... I was going to die."

(7) Mr. V (68-year-old retired welder explaining that it was important for him to see the specialist more often): "I have never been one for going to the doctors but it's just, and I'm not belittling the nurses at all, I just feel that I'd like to see the skilled man a little bit more, the tradesman, in my mind, I'd like to see a little bit more often, to tell me how things are going."

Despite the problems perceived to surround the breaking of bad news, good relationships with doctors were often reported and much appreciated. In general terms, however, communication issues throughout the illness experience were a continuing cause of distress. For example, one patient was telephoned by a clinical nurse specialist who incorrectly assumed that he already had been told his diagnosis. He was left with many unanswered questions and unresolved fears after the nurse told him he had mesothelioma. In two additional cases, patients' wives were told the diagnosis before them, which caused much tension and distress. Reference to the possibility of a referral to a Macmillan nurse (clinical nurse specialists who support cancer patients and their families as funded by the UK charity Macmillan Cancer Relief) at the time of disclosing the diagnosis was perceived as distressing for one person who associated them only with dying.

Psychosocial Issues

Despite the initial shock of the diagnosis, at the time of their interview all the patients seemed to display an unquestioning acceptance of the diagnosis of mesothelioma, although they sometimes questioned the way in which they had been exposed to asbestos. Most patients expressed their determination to cope as well as possible with support from their close family. Couples often seemed to have agreed on an approach to the situation characterized by quiet stoicism.

Patients often balanced their accounts of knowing that the disease was incurable with descriptions of how they would attempt to stay healthy for as long as possible . This approach may represent a way of regaining control over chaos and trying to influence the outcome (Box 6).

Patients who have mesothelioma differed from many cancer patients because it was explained at diagnosis that the disease is essentially incurable. Even radical surgery was explained as possibly extending survival but not curative. Despite this particularly dire prognosis, most patients still managed to reframe their expectations of life, often exhibited hope and humor, and were at pains to emphasize that they were coping, albeit with some admission that emotions surfaced at times. The need to convince the researcher that they were coping may have been an additional strategy to reduce emotional tension in the interview and in their lives. It also may have been a device to avoid further questioning in a sensitive area.

Stoic reactions to the diagnosis were described by patients in positive terms. This group is so overwhelmed by the physical and emotional burden of the disease and the additional demands of benefits and compensation processes that they may have no energy left to support a more active reaction, however.

Most patients exhibited a fatalistic outlook typical of older patients who had grown up in the economic recession of post-war Britain [26,27]. One patient, 72-year-old Mrs. N, clearly displayed a fatalistic outlook and seemed particularly accepting of the terminal nature of her illness, balancing relative risks of other causes of death at her age. Only one patient openly expressed anger. This patient's father had died because of asbestos-related disease, and they both worked in the same shipyard. He wanted to apportion blame but had difficulty attributing it to the company that had employed him and his father.

Several male patients disclosed emotional distress, but in each case it was minimized in the interviews, and the emphasis was on making the best use of the time left. Some patients expressed hope of living much longer than anticipated but at the same time acknowledged they were dying. Mr. I said he was looking

BOX 6: PSYCHOSOCIAL ISSUES

(1) Mr. M (retired shipyard laborer): "It took me by surprise like, but I couldn't do owt about it so you've just got to accept it."

(2) Mr. J (68-year-old worker exposed as a shipyard apprentice): "I'm not just going to carry on, I'm going to crack on. Well what we're going to do is to enjoy each day."

Mrs. J: "It's a waste of time getting upset."

Mr. J: "Aye, a waste of time... I've had my upsets, I've had my tears... and after that I just said 'Sod it, I'll just take each day as it comes.'"

Later in the interview, talking about causation:

Mr. J: "It makes you feel angry 'cos I don't know if it's them that's caused it or what, but somebody should be responsible for it, because I don't know what's caused it."

(3) Mrs. N (72-year-old patient with paraoccupational and environmental exposure): "How've I dealt with it? Well, I'm 72 years old and I've got to die sometime and I've got to die with something. I mean I could go outside and get knocked down and die, I could get the flu and die, so I've got this and I'm going to die, so what can I do? Especially living to 72... I think that it would upset me if I'd only been 30 or 40 but not now."

(4) Mrs. T (55-year-old woman exposed to asbestos when a building was demolished adjacent to her home): "... it's just continually on your mind when you're sat thinking, you think 'Why me?' and then you think 'Well why not me?' As you say, 1 in 3 people have got it so why not me? I've been perfectly healthy up to 55 so I've had 55, a lot of people don't get that long."

(5) Mr. R: "... it could be 12 months, it could be 2 years. They just don't know. And they said I'd be upset, and I was a bit weepy every time..."

H.C.: "You did mention keeping fit, doing what you can."

Mr. R: "Yep, I try and occupy myself, make sure I go out every day if I can... I try, doing what I can, I've got to keep my heart going if nothing else. And deep breathing, away from the traffic" [laughing].

Later in the interview talking about benefits and claims procedures:

Mr. R (58-year-old store manager describing how he tries to keep well and the demands of financial claims): "...filling in form after form for the government and solicitors... I've been told to make a claim, so whether that comes off or not I don't know, but I'm constantly getting letters from them. I've got a file about that big from solicitors, Social Security keep writing to me..."

(6) Mr. D: "Well I believe there's two pensions I can pick up. One is er..."

Mrs. D: "Disability living allowance. The other one is industrial injury."

Mr. D (68-year-old ex-railway worker worrying about state benefits and doubting that he would be eligible): "We filled all the forms in... and we haven't received anything yet. Luckily I have been paid [by his employer]. The second one I'm still waiting for some crazy doctor to come to disprove what the hospital proved. And that's my worry, that's my biggest worry."

forward to his fiftieth wedding anniversary in 8 years' time but admitted that he joked and "put on a false front" while actually thinking about his situation all the time. Others expressed ways in which they tried to make sense of the devastating diagnosis by making plans to deal with death and ensure that their possessions were distributed in accordance with their wishes. For some patients, making practical arrangements for the future seemed to be a means of positive action and an important way in which to reduce the burden for their spouses and wider family.

LIMITATIONS

Recruitment problems in terminally ill patients are well documented [15,16]. The sample of patients interviewed in this study was recruited by clinical nurse specialists. These practitioners may have acted as gatekeepers and not approached patients who they felt were too ill or distressed for interview, who were in the middle of demanding treatment regimens, or who were inpatients in hospital or hospice. Patients who were experiencing severe symptoms or psychological distress may have declined to be interviewed. Other patients were deteriorating so rapidly that they became too ill for interview in the 1 or 2 weeks between recruitment and interview. One patient's wife cancelled his interview because she did not want him to be upset when he was doing well at that time. The interviewer (H.C.) was known to be a doctor by all the participants, which may have influenced their responses. The 11 patients whose spouses were present at the interviews may have moderated their accounts to avoid upsetting them. Although the initial proposal was to interview some patients twice, this did not happen, partly because of lack of time and partly because there was a sense that the patients had said as much as they wished by the end of each interview. It would have been intrusive and unnecessary to ask for a second interview of people who had such a limited time to live.

DISCUSSION

A patient who receives a diagnosis of mesothelioma is in a uniquely difficult position because the cause of the illness is known to be exposure to asbestos, the disease is incurable, and it is known to cause breathlessness, pain, and imminent death. Symptoms are similar to those in lung cancer, but intractable pain and recurrent pleural effusions are more common in mesothelioma [5,19,28]. Hawley and colleagues [29], who reported an interview study with Australian patients who had mesothelioma, their informal carers, and health professionals, suggested that severe pain, breathlessness, and anxiety occur more frequently in cases of mesothelioma than in cancers of other organs, such as breast and colon. Psychosocial distress has been shown to be related to the symptom burden in patients who had lung cancer [30,31].

After the disclosure of diagnosis, patients who had mesothelioma had to revise their hopes and expectations in the new and devastating knowledge that they were dying [11,32]. Symptoms acquired different meanings along the disease trajectory as knowledge was acquired and as physical functions altered. In addition to the usual difficulties of living with a terminal disease, the unpredictable nature of recurrent pleural effusions and the associated severe symptom and treatment burdens caused existential and physical suffering. As illustrated by the interview data, dyspnea is a particularly distressing symptom. It may represent a life-threatening acute event, it may confirm disease progression, it is physically and emotionally exhausting, and it may be truly terrifying. A popular current definition of dyspnea as the subjective experience of difficulty in breathing concentrates on the feeling of being breathless and tends to ignore the sheer physicality of the work that goes into the breathing process, particularly in the presence of effusion, lung fixation, or chest wall involvement [33,34].

Dyspnea directly reduces physical competence and opportunities for social interaction and generates existential and practical anxieties [35]. Krishnasamy and Wilkie [31] illustrated that a practical or pharmacologic medical response to symptoms may ignore the meaning of symptoms for the patient and may exclude opportunities for the patient to explore nonpharmacologic and complementary therapies that can make a significant contribution to symptom control [34].

Refractory pain is reported as a particular problem in mesothelioma; one study reported it as the only cancer in which morphine requirements continue to increase even in the final stage of the illness [36]. Pain control was not reported as a frequent problem in this sample, which was surprising, but stoic attitudes to pain and perhaps an acceptance that cancer pain is inevitable were evident. This finding may represent a cohort effect of expectations coupled with stoicism of the older generation [37].

In most cases, the patient and family become engaged in complex time-consuming procedures to claim state benefits and civil compensation. These processes are an additional cause of distress that interferes with patients' and families' coping strategies [38]. The diagnosis may be received against background knowledge of workmates or relatives who have died because of the disease or previous asbestos hazard warnings.

Interventions in mesothelioma caused distress and patients reported a great need to feel confident in their doctors, particularly physicians who performed invasive procedures. Sometimes this confidence was lacking. Communication issues arose and centered around the breaking bad news consultation but also extended beyond this. Previous studies have indicated that the way in which bad news is broken to this vulnerable group can have a devastating effect if done badly [39,40]. The problems that doctors have in breaking bad news are well documented, however, and this topic is included in communication skills training for medical students [41,42]. It is possible that mesothelioma is a particularly difficult diagnosis to impart because of the lack of effective treatments to offer, the short prognosis, and the benefits/claims issues related to asbestos. Telling a spouse—especially a wife—the diagnosis instead of the patient may have occurred more frequently in the past, before it became usual practice to inform cancer patients of their diagnosis. In the past it may have been a facet of the benign paternalism that once characterized doctor-patient relationships. It is currently accepted, however, that this approach ignored patient autonomy, relied on often incorrect assumptions by doctors, and contributed to tensions and anxieties for patients and families [39].

Earlier studies that examined psychological reactions to a diagnosis of mesothelioma reported depression, anxiety, helplessness, and fatalistic attitudes [43–45]. The current interview study did not include a clinical evaluation of psychological reactions; transient emotional difficulties were reported by the participants in the context of coping with the illness. One patient in this interview study reported feeling angry and was reluctant to blame his employer, which reflected similar findings in the earlier study that examined a group of employees who had been furnished previously with information concerning asbestos risk. This type of reaction may indicate an unexpressed or subconscious acceptance of risk of asbestos-related disease. Another interpretation is that these patients were facing overwhelming stresses—mental and physical—and, with one exception, did not have the mental energy left for an angry reaction. Some of the participants demonstrated a fatalistic outlook, which has been described as a characteristic of the heavy engineering industry. It may be relevant that some of the male patients had lived longer than many of their workmates or peers, they had been in reserved occupations in World War II, and they had lived with significant risks to their health during their working lives [26,46,47].

Although several of the patients mentioned overt emotional crises and breakdowns at the time of diagnosis, they tended to be minimized in the interviews. In all cases the emphasis was on coping as well as possible in the circumstances. In some ways this finding echoes reports of the quiet and uncomplaining way in which men tend to cope with prostate cancer [48]. Unfortunately, denial is not an option for patients who have mesothelioma. There is no escape from the diagnosis because of constant reminders caused by the high symptom burden, unpredictable disease trajectory, and frequent contacts with benefits advisors and lawyers to obtain financial entitlements.

Many authors have described the impact of terminal disease and the ways in which patients and their families construct new meanings and new roles and responsibilities to manage the illness [11,21,32]. The adaptive responses of the patients interviewed did not differ substantially from previous reports concerning patients with terminal illnesses and confirmed the oscillations that patients may make, even in the same sentence, between belief and disbelief, acceptance and denial, hope and despair, which echo the uncertainties of the illness and illustrate the quest for meaning. This occurrence has been described as ambiguous or fluctuating awareness [11,32].

SUMMARY

Patients who have mesothelioma experience a chaotic illness with a high symptom burden and traumatic distressing medical interventions that are palliative rather than curative in virtually all cases. Patients interviewed for this study tended to deal with the illness and its consequences with stoicism and relied heavily on their spouses for support and encouragement in the privacy of their homes. Benefit and compensation processes aggravated the situation and persist for relatives to deal with after patients die. Patients who have mesothelioma are in a particularly disadvantaged situation. These interviews reveal considerable unmet need for relief of symptoms and distress. These issues are being widely reported in the interests of informing service development.

References

[1] Peto J, Decarli A, La Vecchia C, et al. The European mesothelioma epidemic. Br J Cancer 1999;79:666–72.

[2] Hodgson JT, McElvenny DM, Darnton AJ, et al. The expected burden of mesothelioma mortality in Great Britain from 2002–2050. Br J Cancer 2005;92(3):587–93.

[3] Muers MF, Rudd RM, O'Brien ME, et al. British Thoracic Society randomised feasibility study of active symptom control with or without chemotherapy in malignant pleural mesothelioma. Thorax 2004;59(2):144–8.

[4] Treasure T, Sedrakyan A. Pleural mesothelioma: little evidence, still time to do trials. Lancet 2004;364:1183–5.

[5] British Thoracic Society Standards of Care Committee. Statement on malignant mesothelioma in the United Kingdom. Thorax 2001;56:250–65.

[6] Mead N, Bower P. Patient-centredness: a conceptual framework and review of the empirical literature. Soc Sci Med 2000;51:1087–110.

[7] Small N, Rhodes P. Too ill to talk? User involvement and palliative care. London: Routledge; 2000.

[8] Improving supportive and palliative care for adults with cancer. London: National Institute for Clinical Excellence; 2004.

[9] Kvale S. InterViews. Thousand Oaks (CA): Sage Publications; 1996.

[10] Bowling A. Research methods in health: investigating health and health services. Buckingham (UK): Open University Press; 1999.

[11] Seale C. Constructing death: the sociology of dying and bereavement. Cambridge (UK): Cambridge University Press; 1998.

[12] Mathieson CM, Stam HJ. Renegotiating identity: cancer narratives. Sociol Health Illn 1995; 17(3):283–306.

[13] Glaser B, Strauss A. The discovery of grounded theory. Chicago: Aldine; 1967.

[14] Grbich C. Qualitative research in health: an introduction. London: Sage; 1999.

[15] Dean RA, McClement SE. Palliative care research: methodological and ethical challenges. Int J Palliat Nurs 2002;8(8):376–80.

[16] Karim K. Conducting research involving palliative patients. Nurs Stand 2000;15(2):34–6.

[17] Renzetti CM, Lee RM. Researching sensitive topics. Newbury Park (CA): Sage Publications; 1993.

[18] Seymour J, Ingelton C, Payne S, et al. Specialist palliative care: patients' experiences. J Adv Nurs 2003;44(1):24–33.

[19] Edwards JG, Abrams KR, Leverment JN, et al. Prognostic factors for malignant mesothelioma in 142 patients: validation of CALGB and EORTC scoring systems. Thorax 2000;55(9):731–5.

[20] Yates DH, Corrin B, Stidolph PN, et al. Malignant mesothelioma in south east England: clinicopathological experience of 272 cases. Thorax 1997;52(6):507–12.

[21] McNamara B. Fragile lives: death, dying and care. Buckingham (UK): Open University Press; 2001.

[22] Costain Schou K, Hewison J. Being treated: navigating the treatment calendar. In: Experiencing cancer. Buckingham (UK): Open University Press; 1999. p. 110–52.

[23] Barnard D. Unsung questions of medical ethics. Soc Sci Med 1985;21(3):243–9.

[24] Bowling A, Ebrahim S. Measuring patients' preferences for treatment and perceptions of risk. Qual Health Care 2001;10(Suppl 1):i2–8.

[25] de Villiers C, Weskamp K, Bryer A. The sword of Damocles: the psychosocial impact of familial spinocerebellar ataxia in South Africa. Am J Med Genet 1997;74(3):270–4.

[26] Field D. Older people's attitudes towards death in England. Mortal 2000;5(3):277–97.

[27] Williams R. A protestant legacy: attitudes to death and illness among older Aberdonians. Oxford (UK): Clarendon Press; 1990.

[28] Cooley ME. Symptoms in adults with lung cancer: a systematic literature review. J Pain Symptom Manage 2000;19:137–53.

[29] Hawley R, Monk A, Wiltshire J. The mesothelioma journey: developing strategies to meet the needs of people with mesothelioma, their family carers and health professionals involved in their care. Sydney (Australia): Research Centre for Adaptation in Health and Illness; 2004.

[30] Zabora J, Brintzenhofeszoc K, Curbow B, et al. The prevalence of psychological distress by cancer site. Psychooncology 2001;10:19–28.

[31] Krishnasamy M, Wilkie E. Lung cancer: patients', families' and professionals' perceptions of health care need: a national needs assessment study. London: Macmillan Practice Development Unit; 1999.

[32] Hinton J. The progress of awareness and acceptance of dying assessed in cancer patients and their caring relatives. Palliat Med 1999;13:19–35.

[33] Bredin M, Corner J, Krishnasamy M, et al. Multi-centre randomised controlled trial of nursing intervention for breathlessness in patients with lung cancer. BMJ 1999;318: 901–4.

[34] Corner J, Dunlop R. New approaches to care. In: Clark D, Hockley, Ahmedzai S, editors. New themes in palliative care. Buckingham (UK): Open University Press; 1997. p. 288–302.

[35] O'Driscoll M, Corner J, Bailey C. The experience of breathlessness in lung cancer. Eur J Cancer Care (Engl) 1999;8:37–43.

[36] Mercadante S. Problems with opioid dose escalation in cancer pain: differential diagnosis and management strategies. In: Bruera E, Portenoy K, editors. Topics in palliative care. Oxford (UK): Oxford University Press; 2001. p. 213–44.

[37] Vig EK, Pearlman RA. Quality of life while dying: a qualitative study of terminally ill older men. J Am Ger Soc 2003;51(11):1595–601.

[38] Downs FM, Giles GM, Johnson MJ. Palliative physicians persuade procurators fiscal. Palliat Med 2002;16:532–9.

[39] Brennan J. Cancer in context: a practical guide to supportive care. Oxford (UK): Oxford University Press; 2004.

[40] Macdonald E, Murphy K. The patient's perspective. In: Macdonald E, editor. Difficult conversations in medicine. Oxford (UK): Oxford University Press; 2004. p. 36–44.

[41] Macdonald E. The doctor's perspective. In: Difficult conversations in medicine. Oxford (UK): Oxford University Press; 2004. p. 46–75.

[42] Schofield T. A curriculum for communication in medical education. In: Macdonald E, editor. Difficult conversations in medicine. Oxford (UK): Oxford University Press; 2004. p. 208–21.

[43] Lebovits AH, Chahinian AP, Gorzynski JG, et al. Psychological aspects of asbestos-related mesothelioma and knowledge of high risk for cancer. Cancer Detect Prev 1981;4:181–4.

[44] Lebovits AH, Chahinian AP, Holland JC. Exposure to asbestos: psychological responses of mesothelioma patients. Am J Ind Med 1983;4:459–66.

[45] Lebovits AH. Industrially acquired pulmonary disease. Adv Psychosom Med 1985;14: 78–92.

[46] Johnston R, McIvor A. Lethal work: a history of the asbestos tragedy in Scotland. East Lothian (Scotland): Tuckwell Press; 2000.

[47] Connell RW. Masculinities. Oxford (UK): Polity Press in association with Blackwell Publishers Ltd; 1995.

[48] Brennan J. Cancer in context: a practical guide to supportive care. Oxford (UK): Oxford University Press; 2004.

HEMATOLOGY/ONCOLOGY CLINICS
OF NORTH AMERICA

CUMULATIVE INDEX 2005

A

Abciximab, as an antiplatelet agent, 93–94

Acceleration, of radiotherapy, for non-small cell lung cancer, stages I and II, 243–245

Acquired immunodeficiency syndrome (AIDS), primary central nervous system lymphoma related to, **665–687**
  diagnostic considerations, 671–674
    baseline evaluations, 671–672
    biopsy for, 698–699
    early biopsy *versus* empiric toxoplasmosis therapy, 673–674
    evaluation of cerebrospinal fluid, 672–673
  epidemiology and link with Epstein-Barr virus, 666–667
  histopathology, 667
  radiographic features, 667–671, 693–694
    CT and MRI assessment, 667–670
    metabolic imaging, 670–671
  treatment options, 674–681
    antiretroviral therapy, 674–675
    chemotherapy and combined modality therapy, 675–678
    Epstein-Barr virus-targeted therapies, 679–681
    radiation therapy, 674

Acute chest syndrome, in sickle cell disease, **857–879**
  clinical presentation, 860–861
  diagnosis, 865–868
  epidemiology, 858–860
  future directions, 872–873
  laboratory features, 863–865
  management, 868–872
    recurrent, chronic transfusions for, 813–814
    transfusion for, 807–808
  pathophysiology, 861–863

Acute coronary syndromes, use of antiplatelet drugs in, 96–100
  ximelagatran for prevention of cardio-vascular events after, 79

Acute ischemic stroke, thrombolytic therapy for, current clinical practice, 158–162

Acute sickle cell pain, 786–797
  clinical picture, 788
  pain management for, 789–797
    assessment, 790–791
    pharmacologic management, 791–797
  pathogenesis, 786–788
  phases and objective signs, 788–789

Acute transfusions, in sickle cell disease, indications for, 806–811

Adenotonsillectomy, in patients with sickle cell disease, 897

Adenoviral-mediated gene therapy, in mesothelioma, 1148

Adjuvant therapy, chemotherapy, for lung cancer, **263–281**
  compared with breast cancer, 272–273
  in stage IIIA non-small cell lung cancer, 305–307
  Japanese trials with oral uracil-tegafur, 273–274
  large simple randomized trials of, 270–272
  methodologic considerations in trials of, 268–270
  older randomized trials of, 266–268
  postoperative, for resected non-small cell lung cancer, 292–294
  recent North American trials, 274–275
  for extremity soft tissue sarcomas, **489–500**
  for sarcoma in adolescents and young adults, 540–541
  radiation, for resected non-small cell lung cancer, **283–302**
    central nervous system relapse, 294–296

Note: Page numbers of article titles are in **boldface** type.

0889-8588/05/$ – see front matter
doi:10.1016/S0889-8588(05)00133-4

general considerations, 283–284
patterns of failure following
  surgery, 284–286
postoperative chemotherapy and,
  292–294
reported results of, 286–291
toxicity and technical
  considerations, 291–292

Adjuvants, for acute sickle cell pain, 795–797

Adolescents, sarcomas in young adults and,
  527–546
  demographics of, 527–530
  etiology of, 533–534
  late effects of therapy, 542–544
  management outside clinical trials,
    539–542
  presentation of, 534
  psychosocial aspects, 535–536
  treatment issues, 536–539
  tumor biology, 530–533

Age, as prognostic factor in primary central
  nervous system lymphoma, 630–631
  at diagnosis of primary central nervous
    system lymphoma, 689

AIDS. *See* Acquired immunodeficiency syndrome.

Akt, in lung cancer therapy, 353
  Rb-p53-Akt axis in sarcomagenesis, 434

Algorithm, for treatment of primary
  intraocular lymphoma, 744–746

Alkylating agents, for malignant
  mesothelioma, 1120–1121

Allogeneic stem cell transplantation, for
  Ewing's sarcoma family of tumors,
  514–515

Alloimmunization, as complication of
  transfusion in sickle cell disease patients,
  816–818

Alopecia, as complication of heparin
  therapy, 44

Alteplase, structure, function, and
  procoagulant effect of, 148–152

Altered fractionation radiotherapy, for
  non-small cell lung cancer, stages I
  and II, 243–245

Alveolar rhabdomyosarcoma, molecular
  mechanisms of, 439

Anaphylaxis, in acute reaction to heparin, 40

Anatomic distribution, of lesions in primary
  central nervous system lymphoma,
  690–91

Anemia, maternal, during pregnancy in
  women with sickle cell disease, 904
  treatment-related, in lung cancer
    patients, supportive care for,
    380–381

Anesthesia, general, for major surgery in
  sickle cell disease patients, preparation
  for transfusions in, 809–811

Angina, chronic, use of antiplatelet drugs in,
  100–101

Angiogenesis, as target in lung cancer therapy,
  353–354

Angiogenesis inhibitors, for malignant
  mesothelioma, 1129–1130

Angiography, fluorescein, in diagnosis of
  primary intraocular lymphoma, 741

Angiosarcoma, paclitaxel for advanced or
  metastatic, 582–583
  and STA-4783, 583

Anthracyclines, for malignant mesothelioma,
  1120–1121

Anti-adhesion therapy, for sickle cell disease
  with, prospects for, 978–978

Antiangiogenic therapies, for mesothelioma,
  1137–1145
  bevacizumab, 1140–1141
  imatinib mesylate, 1142
  other agents in early studies,
    1142–1143
  PTK787, 1141–1142
  SU5416, 1139–1140
  tetrathiomolybdate, 1142
  thalidomide, 1140

Antibiotics, in management of acute chest
  syndrome in sickle cell disease,
  868–869

Anticoagulant therapy, with unfractionated
  heparin, 1–4
  with vitamin K antagonists, **69–85**

Anticoagulation, in sickle cell patients with
  pulmonary hypertension, 892
  of central venous catheters in clinical
    practice, 195–197

Anticonvulsants, as adjuvants for acute sickle
  cell pain, 795–796

Antidepressants, tricyclic, as adjuvants for
  acute sickle cell pain, 795–796

Antiepileptic medications, for seizures in
  primary central nervous system
  lymphoma, 623

Antihistamines, as adjuvants for acute sickle
  cell pain, 795–796

Antimetabolites, for malignant mesothelioma,
  1122–1124

Antimicrobial agents, for leg ulcers in sickle
  cell disease patients, 950

Antimicrotubule agents, for malignant
  mesothelioma, 1121

Antiplatelet agents, **87–117**
    adverse effects of, 107–108
        bleeding complications, 107–108
        with aspirin, 107
    clinical use of, 96–107
        in acute coronary syndrome,
            96–100
        in cerebrovascular disease, 106
        in chronic angina, 100–101
        in percutaneous coronary
            intervention, 101–106
        in peripheral occlusive arterial
            disease, 106–107
    drugs currently in use, 91–96
        aspirin, 91–93
        indirect-acting drugs, 95–96
        phosphodiesterase inhibitors,
            94–95
        platelet glycoprotein IIb/IIIa
            complex inhibitors, 93–94
        thienopyridines, 93
    future agents for, 109–110
    research on pathogenesis of thrombosis
        and, 90–91
    research on physiology and, 89–90
    resistance to, 108

Antiretroviral therapy, for AIDS-related
    primary central nervous system
    lymphoma, 674–675

Antisense therapy, B-cell leukemia and, in
    lung cancer, 356

Antithrombotic therapy, 1–202
    antiplatelet agents, **87–117**
        adverse effects of, 107–108
        clinical use of, 96–107
        drugs currently in use, 91–96
        future agents for, 109–110
        research on pathogenesis of
            thrombosis and, 90–91
        research on physiology and,
            89–90
        resistance to, 108
    central venous catheter-related
        thrombosis in cancer patients,
        183–202
        anticoagulation of, in clinical
            practice, 195–197
        costs of, 193
        diagnosis of, 191–192
        prevention of, with heparin,
            194–195
            with low-dose warfarin,
                193–194
        risk factors for, 189–191
        sequelae of, 188–189
        treatment of, 192–193
        types of, 184–188
    development of generic low molecular
        weight heparins, **53–68**

direct thrombin inhibitors, **77–80,
    119–145**
    as alternative to vitamin K
        antagonist therapy, 76–80
        ximelagatran, 77–80
    current status and clinical use of,
        argatroban, 132–134
        bivalirudin, 131
        melagatran and ximelagatran,
            134–139
        recombinant hirudine
            (lepirudin), 128–131
    role and use for rational
        anticoagulation, **119–145**
        current status and clinical use
            of, 128–139
        indirect agents, current status
            and clinical use,
            124–126
        indirect *versus* direct
            inhibitors, 124
        rationale and function of, 126
        role of thrombin in thrombo-
            genesis, 119–124
thrombolytic therapy, current clinical
    practice, **147–181**
    agents for, structure, function, and
        procoagulant effects,
        148–152
    cerebrovascular thrombosis,
        158–162
    complications of, 170–171
    miscellaneous disorders, 170
    myocardial infarction, 152–158
    overview of, 148
    peripheral arterial thrombosis,
        166–169
    venous thromboembolism,
        162–166
unfractionated heparin, low molecular
    weight heparins, and pentasaccha-
    ride, **1–51**
    mechanism of action,
        pharmacology, and clinical
        use, pentasaccharides
        (fondaparinux), **24–30**
        unfractionated heparin,
            1–4
    side effects and adverse reactions
        to, **31–46**
        acute heparin reaction
            (anaphylaxis?), 40
        alopecia, 44
        altered liver function tests, 44
        bleeding, 38–40
        heparin and eosinophilia, 44
        heparin-associated
            osteoporosis, 40–43
        heparin-induced thrombo-
            cytopenia, 31–38

heparin-related dermal
reactions, 43–44
hyperkalemia, hypoaldo-
steronism, and meta-
bolic disorders, 44
in patients with prosthetic
heart valves, 45
in pregnancy, 45–46
priapism, 44
vitamin K antagonists, **69–85**
adverse effects of, 74–76
alternatives to, for long-term
treatment, 76–80
pharmacology of, 70–74

Aplasia, transient red cell, acute transfusion
for, in sickle cell disease, 806

Apoptosis, induction of, in gene therapy for
mesothelioma, 1165–1167

Ardeparin, 5–8, 10
See also Low molecular weight heparins.

Argatroban, as a direct thrombin inhibitor,
132–134
as an antiplatelet agent, 95–96

Arixtra. *See* Fondaparinux

Arterial blood pressure, in sickle cell disease,
827–837
elevated, 831
hyperviscosity syndrome,
832–834
hypotheses on, 830–831
regulation of, 827–830
treatment of hypertension,
831–832
whole blood viscosity, 832

Arterial disease. *See* Peripheral
arterial thrombosis.

Aspiration and irrigation, for priapism in
sickle cell disease, 922–923

Aspirin, as an antiplatelet agent, 91–93
adverse effects of, 107

Assessment, of acute sickle cell pain, 790–791

Atrial fibrillation, antiplatelet therapy in, 106
ximelagatran for stroke prevention in
patients with, 79

Autoinfarction, ocular, in sickle cell
disease, 966

Autologous stem cell transplantation, for
central nervous system involvement in
non-Hodgkin's lymphoma, 605–606
with intensive chemotherapy for
primary central nervous system
lymphoma, 722–725

Autonomic vascular control, role in leg
ulceration in sickle cell disease patients,
945–946

Avascular necrosis, of femoral head, in sickle
cell disease, 929–934
clinical identification, 930
femoral infarcts, 929–934
growth disturbances, 930–931
non-surgical disease, 931–932
pathophysiology and risk factors,
929–930
prevalence and incidence, 930
radiography, 931
staging, 931
surgical treatment, 932–934
core decompression, 933
osteotomies, 933
total hip arthroplasty,
933–934

AZD2171, antiangiogenic therapy for
mesothelioma with, 1142–1143

B

B-cell leukemia, and antisense therapy in lung
cancer, 356

B-cell primary central nervous system
lymphoma, indolent, 661–662

BAY43-9006, antiangiogenic therapy for
mesothelioma with, 1142–1143

Benzodiazepines, as adjuvants for acute sickle
cell pain, 795–796

Bevacizumab, antiangiogenic therapy for
mesothelioma with, 1140–1141

Biomarker studies, screening for malignant
mesothelioma with, 1027–1029

Biopsy, in diagnosis of primary central
nervous system lymphoma, 698–699
in AIDS patients, 673–674,
698–699
in immunocompetent patients, 698
of suspected sarcoma, 453–457
prior excisional, surgical
management after, 460–461
vitreous, in diagnosis of primary
intraocular lymphoma, 742

Birth weight. low, in neonates of women with
sickle cell disease, 908–909

Bivalirudin, as a direct thrombin
inhibitor, 131
as an antiplatelet agent, 95–96

Black sunburst lesion, ocular, due to sickle cell
disease, 960–961

Bleeding complications, of antiplatelet
therapy, 107–108
of heparin therapy, 38–40
of pentasaccharide therapy, 38–40
of vitamin K antagonist therapy,
74–75

Blood pressure, arterial, in sickle cell disease, **827–837**
    elevated, 831
    hyperviscosity syndrome, 832–834
    hypotheses on, 830–831
    regulation of, 827–830
    treatment of hypertension, 831–832
    whole blood viscosity, 832

Blood products, selection of, for transfusion in sickle cell disease patients, 819–821

Blood transfusion. *See* Transfusion management.

Blood-brain barrier disruption, enhancement of chemotherapy by, in primary central nervous system lymphoma, 725

Bone and joint disease, in sickle cell disease, **929–941**
    bone marrow disturbances, 937–938
    femoral infarcts, 929–934
        clinical identification, 930
        growth disturbances, 930–931
        non-surgical disease, 931–932
        pathophysiology and risk factors, 929–930
        prevalence and incidence, 930
        radiography, 931
        staging, 931
        surgical treatment, 932–933
    humeral infarcts, 934–935
    osteomyelitis, 936–937
    other bony effects, 938
    surgical treatment, 932–934
        core decompression, 933
        osteotomies, 933
        total hip arthroplasty, 933–934
    vertebral infarcts, 935–936

Bone marrow disturbances, in sickle cell disease, 937–938

Bone marrow transplantation, for primary central nervous system lymphoma, 622–623

Bony metastases, in lung cancer patients, supportive care for, 375

Bortezomib, novel therapy with, for metastatic sarcomas, 583–585

Brain delivery, of chemotherapy, enhancement of by blood-brain barrier disruption in primary central nervous system lymphoma, 725

Breast cancer, adjuvant chemotherapy for, compared with lung cancer, 272–273

Bronchial obstruction, in lung cancer patients, dyspnea and, 371–372

Bystander effect, in gene therapy for mesothelioma, 1150

C

c-Kit, in lung cancer therapy, 351–352
    in malignant mesothelioma, 1005

c-Met, in lung cancer therapy, 352
    in malignant mesothelioma, 1003–1005

Cachexia, in lung cancer patients, supportive care for, 377–378

Cancer and Leukemia Group B system, for malignant mesothelioma prognosis, 1042
    validation of, 1043–1047

Cancer patients, catheter-related thrombosis in, **183–202**
    anticoagulation of, in clinical practice, 195–197
    costs of, 193
    diagnosis of, 191–192
    prevention of, with heparin, 194–195
        with low-dose warfarin, 193–194
    risk factors for, 189–191
    sequelae of, 188–189
    treatment of, 192–193
    types of, 184–188

Cardiovascular events, ximelagatran for prevention of, after acute coronary syndromes, 79

Catheter-related thrombosis, in cancer patients, **183–202**
    anticoagulation of, in clinical practice, 195–197
    costs of, 193
    diagnosis of, 191–192
    prevention of, with heparin, 194–195
        with low-dose warfarin, 193–194
    risk factors for, 189–191
    sequelae of, 188–189
    treatment of, 192–193
    types of, 184–188

CD56. *See* Neural cell adhesion molecule.

Cell cycle, and cyclin-dependent kinases in lung cancer therapy, 356
    in malignant mesothelioma, 1000–1001

Cell cycle regulatory proteins, sarcomas and, 431–434
    p53 tumor suppressor protein pathway, 433–434
    Rb-p53-Akt axis, 434

retinoblastoma tumor suppressor
protein pathway, 433
signal transduction, 431–433

Cellular adhesion molecules, in malignant
mesothelioma, 1010

Central nervous system, involvement of, in
non-Hodgkin's lymphoma, **597–609**
diagnosis, 600–602
cerebrospinal fluid analysis,
601–602
neuroimaging, 600–601
prophylaxis, 602
risk factors, 599
treatment, 602–606
transplantation, 605–606
metastases of lung cancer to, relapse and
prevention, 294–296
relapse to, in lymphoma patients,
751–763

Central nervous system lymphoma, primary,
611–749
AIDS-related, **665–687**
diagnostic considerations,
671–674
epidemiology and link with
Epstein-Barr virus,
666–667
histopathology, 667
radiographic features,
667–671
treatment options, 674–681
clinical features, **689–692**
age and gender, 689
anatomic distribution of
lesions, 690–691
predisposing conditions, 690
symptoms and signs,
691–692
time from symptom onset to
diagnosis, 692
diagnosis, **692–700**
biopsy, 698–699
cerebrospinal fluid analysis,
694–697
differentials, 692–693
neuroimaging, 693–694
ocular evaluation, 697–698
staging, 699–700
indolent B-cell, 661–662
new treatment approaches,
719–728
blood-brain barrier
disruption and intra-
arterial chemo-
therapy, 725
intensive chemotherapy and
autologous stem cell
transplantation,
722–725

Phase II trials of single-
agent chemotherapy
regimens, 719–721
rituximab, 721–722
pathology and genetics, **705–717**
gross pathology, 706
incidence, 705–706
microscopic pathology
and immunopheno-
type, 706–707
molecular pathology,
712–714
pathogenesis, 711–712
prognostic factors, 612, **629–649**
age and performance status,
630–631
new variables with potential
value as, 636–643
predictors of treatment-
related toxicity,
643–645
scoring systems for, 631–636
T-cell, 658–661
treatment, **611–627**
bone marrow transplanta-
tion, 622–623
chemotherapy, 614–622
for recurrent, 623
radiotherapy alone, 613–614
steroids, 612–613
symptomatic treatment, 623
treatment-related neurotoxicity,
729–738
mechanisms of, 729–730
neuroimaging findings,
730–731
neurologic and neurocognitive sequelae, 732–735
white matter changes and
cognitive outcome,
731–732
unusual variants of, **651–664**
neurolymphomatosis,
652–653
primary leptomeningeal
lymphoma, 653–657
rare pathologic variants,
657–662
secondary, **751–763**
clinical features and diagnosis,
754–755
incidence, 751–754
outcome after relapse, 758–760
prophylaxis for, 760–761
risk factors for relapse, 755–758

Central venous catheters, thrombosis of, in
cancer patients, **183–202**
anticoagulation of, in clinical
practice, 195–197
costs of, 193

diagnosis of, 191–192
prevention of, with heparin,
194–195
with low-dose warfarin,
193–194
risk factors for, 189–191
sequelae of, 188–189
treatment of, 192–193
types of, 184–188
Cerebral infarction, overt and incomplete
(silent), in children with sickle cell
anemia, **839–855**
acute management, 848
clinical diagnosis, 843–844
hydroxyurea, 850–851
management algorithm for, 842
neuroimaging, 844–847
neurorehabilitation, 851–852
prevention, 848
risk factors, 840–843
transfusion therapy, 848–850
See also Stroke.
Cerebrospinal fluid analysis, in primary
central nervous system lymphoma,
694–697
AIDS-related, 672–673, 697
in immunocompetent patients,
695–697
in suspected central nervous system
involvement in non-Hodgkin's
lymphoma, 601–602
Cerebrovascular disease, current clinical
practice for antithrombotic therapy for,
antiplatelet drugs for, 106
current clinical practice in
antithrombotic therapy for,
158–162
in acute ischemic stroke,
160–162
Certoparin, 5–6, 11, 14
See also Low molecular weight heparins.
Chemotherapy, adjuvant and neoadjuvant,
for extremity soft tissue sarcomas,
489–500
adjuvant, for sarcoma in adolescents and
young adults, 540–541
adjuvant, of lung cancer, **263–281**
compared with breast cancer,
272–273
in stage IIIA non-small cell lung
cancer, 305–307
Japanese trials with oral
uracil-tegafur, 273–274
large simple randomized trials of,
270–272
methodologic considerations in
trials of, 268–270
older randomized trials of,
266–268

postoperative, for resected
non-small cell lung cancer,
292–294
recent North American trials,
274–275
combined with radiotherapy, for small
cell lung cancer, **321–342**
chemotherapy dosing, 335
chemotherapy schedules,
334–335
choice of chemotherapy
agents, 330–334
novel approaches to,
335–337
radiotherapy dosing,
328–329
radiotherapy volume, 330
rationale, 322
sequential *versus* concurrent,
322–324
standard *versus* hyper-
fractionated radiation,
325–328
for stage IIIA non-small cell lung
cancer, induction, followed
by surgery, 310–312
other randomized trials of,
312–314
without surgery, 308–310
for central nervous system involvement
in non-Hodgkin's lymphoma,
602–604
for mesothelioma, **1117–1135**
agents for, anthracyclines and
alkylating agents, 1120–1121
antimetabolites, 1122–1124
antimicrotubule agents, 1121
platinums, 1121
topoisomerase inhibi-
tors, 1121
goals of, 1125–1128
advanced disease, 1125–1126
perioperative therapy, 1127
second-line, 1126–1127
novels agents, 1128–1130
angiogenesis inhibitors,
1129–1130
histone deacetylase
inhibitors, 1130
ranpirnase, 1128–1129
tyrosine kinase inhibi-
tors, 1129
for primary central nervous system
lymphoma, 614–622
AIDS-related, 675–678
enhancement of, by blood-brain
barrier disruption, 725
high-dose methotrexate, 616–622
intensive, with autologous stem
cell transplantation, 722–725

intra-arterial, 725
phase II trials of single-agent
regimens, 719–721
systemic lymphoma regimens,
615–616
for primary intraocular lymphoma,
744–746
induction, followed by surgery in
stage IIIA non-small cell lung
cancer, 307–308
metastatic sarcomas, novel therapies for,
573–590
9-nitrocamptothecin, 585–586
bortezomib, 585
ecteinascidin, 583–585
everolimus, 580
gemcitabine and combinations,
573–578
imatinib, in dermatofibrosarcoma
protuberans, 580–581
in desmoid tumors and other
sarcomas, 581–582
safety and tolerability of,
578–579
oblimersen, 587
paclitaxel, and STA-4783, 583
in angiosarcoma, 582–583
pegylated liposomal doxorubicin,
586–587
SU11248, 579–580
with radiotherapy for non-small cell
lung cancer, stages I and II,
253–254

Chest radiographs, findings in initial
evaluation of suspected lung cancer,
220–221
screening for lung cancer with, history
of, 211

Chest syndrome, acute. *See* Acute
chest syndrome.

Children, with sickle cell anemia, overt and
incomplete (silent) cerebral infaction in,
839–855
acute management, 848
clinical diagnosis, 843–844
hydroxyurea, 850–851
management algorithm for, 842
neuroimaging, 844–847
neurorehabilitation, 851–852
prevention, 848
risk factors, 840–843
transfusion therapy, 848–850
with sickle cell disease, prevalence of
pulmonary hypertension in,
885–886

Cholecystectomy, in patients with sickle cell
disease, 897–898

Choroidal occlusions, due to sickle cell
disease, 963

Chromosomal aberrations, in malignant
mesothelioma, 999–1000

Chronic sickle cell pain, 797–799
due to avascular necrosis, 798
due to leg ulcers, 797–798
intractable, without obvious pathology,
798–799

Chronic transfusions, in sickle cell disease,
indications for, 811–814

Cilostazol, as an antiplatelet agent, 95

Classification, of sarcomas, histologic,
428–430
systems for, in adolescents and young
adults, 530

Clexane. *See* Enoxaparin.

Clinical evaluation, of lung cancer, **219–235**
clinical presentation, 220
diagnosing the primary tumor,
221–225
radiographic findings based on cell
type, 220–221

Clinical presentation, initial, of patients with
sarcoma, 451–452

Clivarin. *See* Reviparin.

Clopidogrel, as antiplatelet agent, 93

Coagulation factors, plasma, potential role of
thrombogenesis in sickle cell disease,
778–779

Cognitive outcome, with treatment-related
neurotoxicity in primary central nervous
system lymphoma, neurocognitive
sequelae, 732–735
white matter abnormalities and,
731–732

Collagen, inhibitors of interaction with
platelets, future applications of, 110

Computed tomography (CT), conventional,
in evaluation of response to therapy in
soft tissue sarcomas, 472–475
in diagnosis of overt and incomplete
(silent) cerebral infarction in
children with sickle cell anemia,
844–847
low-dose scans, lung cancer screening
with, **209–217**

Congestive heart failure, antiplatelet therapy
in, 107

Conjunctival vasculature, effects of sickle cell
disease on, 957–958

Contrast media, transfusion before infusion
of, in sickle cell disease patients,
815–816

Core decompression, for avascular necrosis of
femoral head in sickle cell disease
patients, 933

Coronary syndromes, acute, use of
    antiplatelet drugs in, 96–100
    ximelagatran for prevention of
        cardiovascular events after, 79

Corticosteroids, for primary central
    nervous system lymphoma,
    612–613, 623

Cough, in lung cancer patients, supportive
    care for, 375–376

Coumarins. *See* Warfarin *and*
    Vitamin K antagonists.

COX-2 inhibitors. *See*
    Cyclo-oxygenase inhibitors.

Crises. *See* Acute sickle cell pain.

Cryotherapy, for treatment of sickle cell
    disease affecting the eyes, 968

Cyclin-dependent kinases, in lung cancer
    therapy, 356

Cyclo-oxygenase (COX) inhibitors, for acute
    sickle cell pain, 791–793
        non-selective, 791–792
        selective (COX-2), 791–793

Cytokine analysis, in diagnosis of primary
    intraocular lymphoma, 743

Cytokine gene therapy, for mesothelioma,
    1159–1165

Cytology, of cerebrospinal fluid, in primary
    central nervous system lymphoma,
    695–696

D

Dactylitis, in sickle cell disease, 936–937

Dalteparin, 5–12, 14, 16
    development of generic low molecular
        weight heparins, **53–68**
    versus ximelagatran for treatment
        of acute venous thrombo-
        embolism, 78
    See also Low molecular weight heparins.

Debridement, of leg ulcers in sickle cell
    disease patients, 949–950

Deep fibromatoses. *See* Desmoid tumors.

Deep vein thrombosis, central venous
    catheter-related, 186–188
    thrombolytic therapy in, 163–164
        current clinical practice, 165–166

Dental effects, of sickle cell disease, 938

Depression, in lung cancer patients,
    supportive care for, 382

Dermal reactions, heparin-related, 43–44

Dermatofibrosarcoma protuberans, imatinib
    mesylate in, 580–581

Desmoid tumors, and deep fibromatoses,
    565–571
    clinical presentation, 566
    diagnosis, 567
    etiology, 565–566
    genetics, 567
    histology, 566–567
    treatment, 567–569
    imatinib mesylate in, 581–582

Dexamethasone, in management of acute
    chest syndrome in sickle cell
    disease, 872

Diagnosis, of primary central nervous system
    lymphoma, **692–700**
    biopsy, 698–699
    cerebrospinal fluid analysis,
        694–697
    differentials, 692–693
    neuroimaging, 693–694
    ocular evaluation, 697–698
    staging, 699–700
    of primary tumor in lung cancer,
        221–225

Diagnostic evaluation, of suspected sarcoma,
    452–453

Differential diagnosis, of primary
    central nervous system lymphoma,
    692–693

Dipyridamole, as an antiplatelet agent,
    94–95

Direct thrombin inhibitors, as alternative to
    vitamin K antagonist therapy, 76–80
    ximelagatran, 77–80
    role and use for rational anticoagulation,
        119–145
        current status and clinical use of,
            128–139
            argatroban, 132–134
            bivalirudin, 131
            melagatran and ximelagatran,
                134–139
            recombinant hirudine
                (lepirudin), 128–131
        indirect agents, current status and
            clinical use, 124–126
        indirect *versus* direct inhibi-
            tors, 124
        rationale and function of, 126
        role of thrombin in
            thrombogenesis, 119–124

Doppler ultrasonography, transcranial, in
    diagnosis of overt and incomplete
    (silent) cerebral infarction in children
    with sickle cell anemia, 844–847

Doxorubicin, pegylated liposomal, novel
    therapy with, for metastatic sarcomas,
    586–587

Dyspnea, in lung cancer patients, supportive
      care for, 369–374
            bronchial obstruction and,
                  371–372
            hemoptysis and, 372
            pharmacologic treatment, 370–371
            pleural effusion and, 372–375

E

Ecteinascidin, novel therapy with, for
      metastatic sarcomas, 583–585

Educational effects, of leg ulcers in sickle cell
      disease patients, 951–952

Embolism. *See* Pulmonary embolism.

Enoxaparin, 5–11, 13–14, 20–21, 22–23
            adverse effects in pregnant women with
                  prosthetic heart valves, 45–46
            development of generic low molecular
                  weight heparins, **53–68**
            teratogenic effects of, 45–46
            See also Low molecular weight heparins.

Eosinophilia, related to heparin therapy, 44

Epidermal growth factor receptors, in lung
      cancer therapy, 345–350

Epstein-Barr virus, AIDS-related primary
      central nervous system lymphoma and,
      role in epidemiology, 666–667
            therapies targeting, 679–681
                  disruption of viral
                        functions, 680
                  selective drug activation,
                        680–681
                  targeting viral antigens,
                        679–680

Eptifibatide, as an antiplatelet agent, 94

Erection, of penis. *See* Priapism.

Erythrocytes, in sickle cell anemia, adhesion
      mechanisms, 772–773
            contributions of sickling of, 772

Etilephrine, for prevention of priapism in
      sickle cell disease, 925

Etoposide, role in therapy of Ewing's sarcoma
      family of tumors, 507–508

European Organization for the Research and
      Treatment of Cancer, scoring system for
      malignant mesothelioma prognosis,
      1042–1043
            validation of, 1043–1047

Everolimus, for imatinib-resistant
      gastrointestinal stromal tumors, 580

Ewing's sarcoma, and primitive neuroecto-
      dermal family of tumors, **501–525**
            current clinical trials, 516–517
            epidemiology and clinical
                  features, 502

            genetic and molecular
                  characteristics, 502–503
            localized, treatment of, 503–509
            metastatic, treatment of, 509–511
            progressive and relapsed, 511
            risk for secondary malignancy
                  after curative therapy,
                  515–516
            stem cell transplantation for,
                  511–515
      molecular mechanisms of, 439–440
      outcomes after surgery for, 465–467
            functional, 466
            oncologic, 465

Exanta. *See* Ximelagatran

Exchange transfusion, method for, in sickle
      cell disease, 804–805

Extremities, soft tissue sarcomas of, **489–500**
            adjuvant chemotherapy, 492–495
            neoadjuvant chemotherapy,
                  495–497
            prognostic variables, 490–492

Eye. *See* Intraocular lymphoma.

Eyes, effects of sickle cell disease on,
      957–972
            clinical features, 957–966
                  autoinfarction, 966
                  black sunburst, 960–961
                  choroidal occlusions, 963
                  conjunctival vasculature,
                        957–958
                  hyphema, 958–959
                  iridescent spots, 959–960
                  macula, 962
                  optic nerve head, vascular
                        changes at, 963
                  proliferative sickle
                        retinopathy, 963–966
                  retinal vasculature, 961
                  salmon patch
                        hemorrhage, 959
            treatment, 967–970
                  cryotherapy, 968
                  feeder vessel
                        photocoagulation, 967
                  pars plana vitrectomy,
                        968–969
                  scatter photocoagulation,
                        967–968
                  scleral buckling surgery,
                        969–970

F

Fatigue, treatment-related, in lung cancer
      patients, supportive care for, 380–381

Fatty acids, omega-3, new therapy for sickle
      cell disease with, 976–977

Femoral infarcts, in sickle cell disease, 929–934
  clinical identification, 930
  femoral infarcts, 929–934
  growth disturbances, 930–931
  non-surgical disease, 931–932
  pathophysiology and risk factors, 929–930
  prevalence and incidence, 930
  radiography, 931
  staging, 931
  surgical treatment, 932–934
    core decompression, 933
    osteotomies, 933
    total hip arthroplasty, 933–934

Fever, neutropenic, treatment-related, in lung cancer patients, supportive care for, 379–380

Fibrin sheath formation, catheter-related thrombosis due to, 184–185

Fibromatoses, deep. *See* Desmoid tumors.

Fluid administration, in management of acute chest syndrome in sickle cell disease, 869–870

Fluorescein angiography, in diagnosis of primary intraocular lymphoma, 741

Fluxum. *See* Panaparin.

Fondaparinux, as an antiplatelet drug, 95–96
  mechanism of action, pharmacology, and clinical use, **24–30**

Fragmin. *See* Dalteparin.

Fraxiparin. *See* Nadroparin.

Functional Assessment of Cancer Therapy–Lung Scale, as measure of quality of life, **389–420**
  Lung Cancer Subscale, 404–411
  published evidence on reliability and validity of, 390–399
  validated translations and cultural adaptations, 399–404

Functional outcomes, after surgical management of sarcoma, 466–467
  osteosarcoma and Ewing's sarcoma, 466
  soft tissue sarcoma, 466–467

Fusion gene products, as target of sarcoma therapy, 441–442

Fusion product down-regulation, in targeted sarcoma therapy, 442

G

Gardos channel blockers, new therapy for sickle cell disease with, 977–978

Gastrin-releasing peptide, in lung cancer therapy, 357–358

Gastrointestinal stromal tumors (GISTs), **547–564**
  imaging of response to therapy in, 482–483
  medical management, 552–560
    before targeted molecular therapies, 552–553
    targeted therapy with imatinib mesylate, 553–560
      clinical management of resistance to, 558–560
      determinants of response to, 556–557
      progression of tumor while on, 557
  molecular mechanisms of, 440
  novel therapies for metastatic,
    everolimus, 580
    imatinib mesylate, 575–579
    SU11248, 579–580
  surgical management, 548–552
    emerging approaches combining imatinib and, 552
    outcomes, 549–550
    preoperative assessment, 548
    primary disease, 548–549
    recurrent or metastatic, 550–552

Gemcitabine, novel therapy with, for metastatic sarcomas, 573–575

Gender, and diagnosis of primary central nervous system lymphoma, 689

Gene therapy, for malignant pleural mesothelioma, **1147–1173**
  cytokine gene therapy, 1159–1165
  induction of apoptosis, 1165–1167
  principles and vectors, 1147–1158
  simian virus 40, 1167
  suicide gene vaccines, 1158–1159

Generic drugs, low molecular weight heparins, development of, **53–68**

Genetic variables, potential for primary central nervous system lymphoma prognosis, 639

Genetics, and pathology of primary central nervous system and intraocular lymphoma, **705–717**

Glycoprotein Ib inhibitors, as future antiplatelet agents, 109–110

Glycoprotein IIb/IIIa complex inhibitors, as antiplatelet agents, 93–94

Granulocyte-macrophage colony-stimulating factor, for leg ulcers in sickle cell disease patients, 950

Growth disturbances, and bone and joint disease in sickle cell disease, 930–931

Growth retardation, intrauterine, in fetuses of women with sickle cell disease, 908–909

H

HAART. *See* Antiretroviral therapy.

Heart valves, prosthetic, adverse reactions to heparins in pregnant women with, 45–46

Heat shock protein, in lung cancer therapy, 355–356

Hematopoietic stem cell transplantation, for central nervous system involvement in non-Hodgkin's lymphoma, 605–606

Hemoglobin, polymerization of, in sickle cell anemia, 772

Hemolytic reactions, as complication of transfusion in sickle cell disease patients, 816–818

Hemoptysis, in lung cancer patients, dyspnea and, 372

Heparin, as an antiplatelet agent, 95–96
  clinical use as an indirect thrombin inhibitor, 124–126
  development of generic low molecular weight, **53–68**
  for long-term treatment of venous thromboembolism, 76–77
  in prevention of central venous catheter-related deep venous thrombosis, 193–194
  mechanism of action, pharmacology, and clinical use, low molecular weight, **4–23**
    pentasaccharides (fondaparinux), **24–30**
    unfractionated, **1–4**
  side effects and adverse reactions to unfractionated heparin, low molecular wieght heparin, and pentasaccharide, **31–46**
    acute heparin reaction (anaphylaxis?), 40
    alopecia, 44
    altered liver function tests, 44
    bleeding, 38–40
    dermal reactions related to, 43–44
    eosinophilia, 44
    heparin-induced thrombo-cytopenia, 31–38
    hyperkalemia, hypoaldosteronism, and metabolic disorders, 44
    in patients with prosthetic heart valves, 45
    in pregnancy, 45–46
    osteoporosis associated with, 40–43
    priapism, 44

Heparin-induced thrombocytopenia, 31–38
  treatment of, 38

Hepatic sequestration, acute, transfusion for, in sickle cell disease, 806–807

Herpes simplex virus-1 thymidine kinase suicide gene therapy, for mesothelioma, 1150–1158

Hip arthroplasty, total, for avascular necrosis of femoral head in sickle cell disease patients, 933–934
  preparation for, in patients with sickle cell disease, 898

Hirudin, as an antiplatelet agent, 95–96
  recombinant (lepirudin), as a direct thrombin inhibitor, 128–131

Hirulog. *See* Bivalirudin.

Histine deacetylase inhibitors, for malignant mesothelioma, 1130

Histologic classification, of sarcomas, 428–430

Histology, of desmoid tumors and deep fibromatoses, 566–567
  of sarcomas in adolescents and young adults, 530–533

Histopathologic variables, potential for primary central nervous system lymphoma prognosis, 636–639

Histopathology, of AIDS-related primary central nervous system lymphoma, 667

Human epidermal growth factor 2/neu, in lung cancer therapy, 350–351

Humeral infarcts, in sickle cell disease, 934–935

Hydration, of patients with sickle cell disease undergoing surgical procedures, 900–901

Hydroxyurea therapy, 974–976
  for leg ulcers in sickle cell disease patients, 951
  for overt and incomplete (silent) cerebral infarction in children with sickle cell anemia, 850–851
  in sickle cell patients with pulmonary hypertension, 890–891

Hyperkalemia, related to heparin therapy, 44

Hypertension, in sickle cell disease, arterial, and hyperviscosity, 831–835
  pulmonary, **881–896**
    diagnosis, 887–889
    hemodynamics and risk factors, 883–884
    incidence and prevalence, 884–887
    management, 813–814, 890–893
    prognosis, 889–890

Hyperviscosity, arterial blood pressure and, in sickle cell disease, **827–837**

Hyphema, due to sickle cell disease, 958–959

Hypoaldosteronism, related to heparin therapy, 44

Hypofractionation, of radiotherapy, for non-small cell lung cancer, stages I and II, 244–245

I

Ifosfamide, role in therapy of Ewing's sarcoma family of tumors, 506–507

Imaging, of response to therapy in soft tissue sarcomas, **471–487**
  conventional CT and MRI, 472–475
  dynamic contrast-enhanced MRI, 478–481
  gastrointestinal stromal tumors, 482–483
  magnetic resonance spectroscopy, 481
  positron emission tomography, 475–478
  thallium-201 scintigraphy, 482
  screening for malignant mesothelioma with, 1027

Imaging. *See* Neuroimaging.

Imatinib mesylate, antiangiogenic therapy for mesothelioma with, 1142
  for gastrointestinal stromal tumors, 553–560
    clinical management of resistance to, 558–560
      combination therapies, 560
      other tyrosine kinase inhibitors, 559–560
      SU11248, 558–559
    determinants of response to, 556–557
    novel therapies with, 575–578
      safety and tolerability of, 578–579
    progression of tumor while on, 557
  for sarcomas, 443–444
  in dermatofibrosarcoma protuberans, 580–581
  in desmoid tumors and other sarcomas, 581–582

Immunophenotype, in diagnosis of primary intraocular lymphoma, 743
  in primary central nervous system lymphoma, 706-707

Immunotherapy, genetic, future of for mesothelioma, 1160–1162
  in targeted sarcoma therapy, 441–442

Incentive spirometry, in management of acute chest syndrome in sickle cell disease, 870

Incomplete cerebral infarction. *See* Cerebral infarction.

Indeparin. *See* Ardeparin.

Indirect thrombin inhibitors, clinical use of heparin and warfarin as, 124–126
  versus direct thrombin inhibitors, 124

Indolent B-cell primary central nervous system lymphoma, 661–662

Infection, due to central venous catheter thrombosis, 188

Infection control, in patients with sickle cell disease undergoing surgical procedures, 901

Infections, as complication of transfusion in sickle cell disease patients, 818
  of leg ulcers in sickle cell disease patients, 949, 950

Inflammation, chronic vascular, sickle cell disease as syndrome of, 773–775

INK4 family, in malignant mesothelioma, 1001–1002

Innohep. *See* Tinzaparin.

Intensity-modulated radiotherapy, for malignant mesothelioma, 1111–1112

Interferon-beta gene therapy, for mesothelioma, 1163–1165

International Extranodal Lymphoma Study Group Prognostic Score, for primary central nervous system lymphoma, 632–636

International Prognostic Index, for primary central nervous system lymphoma, 631–632

Intra-arterial chemotherapy, in primary central nervous system lymphoma, 725

Intraluminal thrombosis, of central venous catheters, 186

Intraocular lymphoma
  diagnosis and management, **739–749**
    clinical features, 709, 739–741
      fluorescein angiography, 741
      ophthalmic examination, 740
    diagnosis, 710, 741–744
      cytokine analysis, 743
      differentials for, 708
      immunophenotyping, 743
      molecular analysis, 743–744
      pathology, 742–743
      vitreous biopsy and specimen analysis, 742
    treatment, 744–746
      algorithm for, 744–746
      current options for, 746
      future therapies for, 746
  pathology and genetics, **707–711**

Intrauterine growth retardation, in fetuses of women with sickle cell disease, 908–909

Iridescent spots, due to sickle cell disease, 959–960

Iron chelation therapy, in sickle cell patients with pulmonary hypertension, 892

Iron overload, in sickle cell disease patients as complication of transfusion, 818–819
new oral therapy for, 981

Irrigation, aspiration and, for priapism in sickle cell disease, 922–923

Ischemic stroke, acute, thrombolytic therapy for, current clinical practice, 158–162

J

Joint disease. *See* Bone and joint disease.

K

Karyotype abnormalities, in sarcomagenesis, 434–437
complex karyotypes, 436–437
general concepts, 434
simple karyotypes, 434–436

Kinases. *See* Tyrosine kinases.

L

Late effects, of sarcoma therapy in adolescents and young adults, 542–543

Leg ulceration, in sickle cell disease, **943–956**
characteristics of, 947–949
complications of, 951–952
history, 943
incidence and prevalence, 943–944
risk factors, 944–947
autonomic vascular control, 945
gender, 944
hematology, 944–945
role of venous incompetence, 946–947
treatment of, 949–951
antimicrobial agents, 950
controversial indication for transfusions, 815–816
debridement and dressings, 949–950
other interventions, 950–951

Lepirudin, as a direct thrombin inhibitor, 128–131

Leptomeningeal lymphoma, primary, 653–657

Leukemia, B-cell, and antisense therapy in lung cancer, 356

Leukocyte adhesion, as prerequisite to vaso-occlusion in sickle cell disease, 775–778

Leuprolide, for prevention of priapism in sickle cell disease, 925–926

Limb salvage surgery, in sarcoma, 457–460

Liposarcomas, molecular mechanisms of, 437–438
targeted therapy of, 443

Liposomal doxorubicin, pegylated, novel therapy with, for metastatic sarcomas, 586–587

Liver function tests, altered, with long-term heparin administration, 44

Logiparin. *See* Tinzaparin.

Lovenox. *See* Enoxaparin.

Low birth weight, in neonates of women with sickle cell disease, 908–909

Low molecular weight heparin, as an antiplatelet agent, 95–96

Low molecular weight heparins, development of generic, **53–68**
for long-term treatment of venous thromboembolism, 76–77
mechanism of action, pharmacology, and clinical use, **4–23**

Lung cancer, multidisciplinary approach to, 209–420
adjuvant chemotherapy of, **263–281**
compared with breast cancer, 272–273
Japanese trials with oral uracil-tegafur, 273–274
large simple randomized trials of, 270–272
methodologic considerations in trials of, 268–270
older randomized trials of, 266–268
recent North American trials, 274–275
clinical evaluation and staging of, **219–235**
clinical presentation, 220
diagnosing the primary tumor, 221–225
radiographic findings based on cell type, 220–221
staging
non-small cell lung cancer, 225–229
small cell lung cancer, 230–231
non-small cell, postoperative radiation therapy for resected, **283–302**
central nervous system relapse, 294–296

general considerations,
    283–284
patterns of failure following
    surgery, 284–286
postoperative chemotherapy
    and, 292–294
reported results of, 286–291
toxicity and technical consid-
    erations, 291–292
stage IIIA, **303–319**
    chemoradiotherapy without
        surgery in, 308–310
    competing risks of patients
        with, 315–316
    heterogeneity of, 304
    induction chemoradio-
        therapy followed by
        surgery in, 310–312
    induction chemotherapy
        followed by surgery in,
        307–308
    other randomized trials
        including surgery,
        312–314
    results of surgery alone in,
        304–305
    toxicity considerations of
        surgery in, 314–315
    trials of adjuvant chemo-
        therapy in, 305–307
    trimodality including surgery
        versus bimodality, 312
stages I and II, nonsurgical therapy
    for, **237–261**
    altered fractionation,
        243–245
    combined modality therapy,
        253–254
    ongoing trials, 255
    other radiotherapy
        techniques, 253
    radiation dose escalation,
        240–243
    radiofrequency ablation,
        254–255
    standard fractionation
        radiotherapy, 239–240
    stereotactic radiotherapy,
        245–252
novel therapies in, **343–367**
    B-cell leukemia 2 and antisense
        therapy, 356–357
    cell cycle and cyclin-dependent
        kinases, 356
    heat shock proteins, 355–356
    nonreceptor tyrosine kinases,
        353–354
        Akt, 353
        angiogenesis and VEGF,
            353–354

mammalian target of
    rapamycin, 353
phosphatidylinositol-
    3'-kinase, 353
proteasome inhibitors,
    354–355
receptor tyrosine kinases,
    344–352
    c-Kit, 351–352
    c-Met, 352
    epidermal growth factor
        receptors, 345–350
    human epidermal growth
        factor 2/neu,
        350–351
retinoid signaling pathways, 354
tumor-associated antigens,
    357–360
    gastrin-releasing peptide,
        357–358
    neural cell adhesion molecule
        (CD56), 357
    tumor vaccines, 358–360
quality of life in, using Functional
    Assessment of Cancer Therapy–
    Lung Scale, **389–420**
screening, **209–217**
    associated studies, 215–216
    biases associated with, 210
    consensus recommendations, 214
    CT-detected nodules, guidelines
        for treating, 212–214
    current trials of, 212–
    reasons for, 209–210
    with chest radiographs, history
        of, 211
small cell, combined chemoradiotherapy
    in, **321–342**
    chemotherapy dosing, 335
    chemotherapy schedules,
        334–335
    choice of chemotherapy
        agents, 330–334
    novel approaches to,
        335–337
    radiotherapy dosing,
        328–329
    radiotherapy volume, 330
    rationale, 322
    sequential *versus* concurrent,
        322–324
    standard *versus* hyper-
        fractionated radiation,
        325–328
supportive care in, **369–387**
    for disease-related symptoms,
        369–378
    for treatment-related symptoms,
        378–382
    psychosocial issues, 382

Lymphoma, intraocular, primary
  diagnosis and management,
    739–749
  pathology and genetics, **707–711**
  leptomeningeal, primary, 653–657
  non-Hodgkin's, central nervous system
    involvement in, **597–609**
    diagnosis, 600–602
      cerebrospinal fluid analysis,
        601–602
      neuroimaging, 600–601
    prophylaxis, 602
    risk factors, 599
    treatment, 602–606
      transplantation, 605–606
  primary central nervous system,
    611–749
    AIDS-related, **665–687**
      diagnostic considerations,
        671–674
      epidemiology and link with
        Epstein-Barr virus,
        666–667
      histopathology, 667
      radiographic features,
        667–671
      treatment options, 674–681
    clinical features, **689–692**
      age and gender, 689
      anatomic distribution of
        lesions, 690–691
      predisposing conditions, 690
      symptoms and signs,
        691–692
      time from symptom onset to
        diagnosis, 692
    diagnosis, **692–700**
      biopsy, 698–699
      cerebrospinal fluid analysis,
        694–697
      differentials, 692–693
      neuroimaging, 693–694
      ocular evaluation, 697–698
      staging, 699–700
    indolent B-cell, 661–662
    new treatment approaches,
      719–728
      blood-brain barrier disrup-
        tion and intra-arterial
        chemotherapy, 725
      intensive chemotherapy and
        autologous stem
        cell transplantation,
        722–725
      Phase II trials of single-agent
        chemotherapy regi-
        mens, 719–721
      rituximab, 721–722
    pathology and genetics, **705–717**
      gross pathology, 706
      incidence, 705–706

      microscopic pathology
        and immunopheno-
        type, 706–707
      molecular pathology,
        712–714
      pathogenesis, 711–712
    prognostic factors, 612, **629–649**
      age and performance status,
        630–631
      new variables with potential
        value as, 636–643
      predictors of treatment-
        related toxicity, 643–645
      scoring systems for, 631–636
    T-cell, 658–661
    treatment, **611–627**
      bone marrow transplanta-
        tion, 622–623
      chemotherapy, 614–622
      for recurrent, 623
      radiotherapy alone, 613–614
      steroids, 612–613
      symptomatic treatment, 623
    treatment-related neurotoxicity,
      729–738
      mechanisms of, 729–730
      neuroimaging findings,
        730–731
      neurologic and neuro-
        cognitive sequelae,
        732–735
      white matter changes and
        cognitive outcome,
        731–732
    unusual variants of, **651–664**
      neurolymphomatosis,
        652–653
      primary leptomeningeal
        lymphoma, 653–657
      rare pathologic variants,
        657–662
  secondary central nervous system,
    751–763
    clinical features and diagnosis,
      754–755
    incidence, 751–754
    outcome after relapse, 758–760
    prophylaxis for, 760–761
    risk factors for relapse, 755–758

M

Macula, effects of sickle cell disease on, 962

Magnetic resonance imaging (MRI), in
  diagnosis of overt and incomplete
  (silent) cerebral infarction in children
  with sickle cell anemia, 844–847
  in evaluation of response to therapy in
    soft tissue sarcomas, conventional,
    472–475
    dynamic contrast-enhanced,
      478–481

Magnetic resonance spectroscopy imaging, in evaluation of response to therapy in soft tissue sarcomas, 481

Malignant mesothelioma. *See* Mesothelioma.

Mammalian target of rapamycin (mTOR), in lung cancer therapy, 353

Margins, surgical, of suspected sarcoma, 461–

Melagatran, as a direct thrombin inhibitor, 134–139

Mesothelin, in detection of malignant mesothelioma, 1029–1035

Mesothelin-related protein, soluble, in detection of malignant mesothelioma, 1029–1035

Mesothelioma, malignant, 997–1190
 antiangiogenic therapies for, **1137–1145**
 chemotherapy for, **1117–1135**
 detection of, **1025–1040**
  lessons learned from CA125 in early ovarian cancer detection, 1035–1036
  mesothelin and soluble mesothelin-related protein, 1029–1035
  screening, 1026–1029
  uses of multiple serum markers for, 1037
 gene therapy for, **1147–1173**
 molecular biology of, **997–1023**
 multimodality treatment of, **1089–1097**
 nonpleural, **1067–1087**
  of the tunica vaginalis, 1080–1081
  pericardial, 1081–1082
  peritoneal, 1067–1080
 patient's perspective on, **1175–1190**
  burden of medical interventions, 1180–1182
  coping with symptoms, 1179–1180
  finding out about, 1182–1186
 prognostic factors for, **1041–1052**
  clinical scoring systems, 1041–1043
   validation, 1043–1047
  molecular prognostic markers, 1047–1048
  other predictors, 1050–1051
  predictors of survival in patients treated surgically, 1048–1049
 radiologic measurement of, **1053–1066**
  clinical trials of, 1055–1056
  computer-assisted, 1062–1064
  measuring lesions, 1054–1055
  response evaluation criteria in solid tumors and mesothelioma, 1056–1058
  variability in, 1058–1062
  volumetric measurements, 1064
 radiotherapy for, **1099–1115**

Metabolic disorders, related to heparin therapy, 44

Metabolic imaging, of AIDS-related primary nervous system lymphoma, 670–671

Metastases, after surgical management of gastrointestinal stromal tumors, 550–553
 bony, in lung cancer patients, supportive care for, 375
 of Ewing's sarcoma family of tumors, treatment of, 509–510
 of sarcomas, novel therapies for, **573–590**
  9-nitrocamptothecin, 585–586
  bortezomib, 585
  ecteinascidin, 583–585
  everolimus, 580
  gemcitabine and combinations, 573–578
  imatinib, in dermatofibrosarcoma protuberans, 580–581
   in desmoid tumors and other sarcomas, 581–582
   safety and tolerability of, 578–579
  oblimersen, 587
  paclitaxel, and STA-4783, 583
   in angiosarcoma, 582–583
  pegylated liposomal doxorubicin, 586–587
  SU11248, 579–580

Methotrexate, high-dose, for primary central nervous system lymphoma, 616–622

Miscarriage, in women with sickle cell disease, 907

Mitogen-activated protein kinase pathway, in malignant mesothelioma, 1009

Molecular analysis, in diagnosis of primary intraocular lymphoma, 743–744

Molecular biology, of malignant mesothelioma, **997–1023**
 cellular adhesion molecules, 1010
 chromosomal aberrations, 999–1000
 etiology, 997–999
 INK4 family, 1001–1002
 normal cell cycle, 1000–1001
 $p16^{INK4a}/p14^{ARF}$ alterations, 1002–1003
 reactive oxygen species, 1009–1010
 receptor tyrosine kinases, 1003
  c-Kit, 1005
  c-Met, 1003–1005
  vascular endothelial growth factor receptor, 1005–1006

signal pathways, 1006–1007
  mitogen-activated protein
    kinase pathway, 1009
  mTOR pathway, 1007–1009
  SV40, 1010–1012

Molecular markers, for prognosis in
  malignant mesothelioma, 1047–1048

Molecular pathology, of primary central
  nervous system lymphoma, 712–714

Molecular variables, potential for primary
  central nervous system lymphoma
  prognosis, 639

Monoclonal antibodies, for primary
  intraocular lymphoma, 746
  rituximab, for central nervous system
    involvement in non-Hodgkin's
    lymphoma, 604–605
    for primary central nervous system
      lymphoma, phase II trials of,
      721–722

Mortality, during pregnancy in women
  with sickle cell disease, maternal,
  905–907
    perinatal, 908

mTOR pathway, in malignant mesothelioma,
  1007–1009

Mucositis, oral, treatment-related, in lung
  cancer patients, supportive care for,
  381–382

Multiple organ failure, in sickle cell disease,
  acute transfusion for, 809

Myocardial infarction, thrombolytic therapy
  in, current clinical practice, 152–158
    delivery of reperfusion therapy,
      156–157
    faciliatated percutaneous coronary
      intervention, 156
    primary percutaneous coronary
      intervention, 157–158
    thrombolysis *versus* primary
      percutaneous coronary
      intervention, 153–156

N

Nadroparin, 5–6
  See also Low molecular weight heparins.

Nausea, treatment-related, in lung cancer
  patients, supportive care for, 378–379

Neoadjuvant therapy, for extremity soft tissue
  sarcomas, **489–500**

Neural cell adhesion molecule (CD56), in
  lung cancer therapy, 357

Neurocognitive sequelae, to treatment-related
  neurotoxicity in primary central nervous
  system lymphoma, 732–735

Neuroimaging, in diagnosis of overt and
  incomplete (silent) cerebral infarction in
  children with sickle cell anemia,
  844–847
  of primary nervous system lymphoma,
    693–694
    AIDS-related, 667–671
      CT and MRI assessment,
        667–670
      metabolic imaging, 670–671
    in treatment-related neurotoxicity,
      730–731
  of suspected central nervous system
    involvement in non-Hodgkin's
    lymphoma, 600–601

Neurologic sequelae, to treatment-related
  neurotoxicity in primary central nervous
  system lymphoma, 732

Neurologic syndromes, acute, in sickle cell
  disease, transfusion for, 808–809

Neurolymphomatosis, 652–653

Neuropathic pain, in sickle cell disease, 799

Neurorehabilitation, for overt and incomplete
  (silent) cerebral infarction in children
  with sickle cell anemia, 851–852

Neurotoxicity, treatment-related, in primary
  central nervous system lymphoma,
  729–738
    mechanisms of, 729–730
    neuroimaging findings, 730–731
    neurologic and neurocognitive
      sequelae, 732–735
    white matter changes and cognitive
      outcome, 731–732

Neutropenia, treatment-related, in lung cancer
  patients, supportive care for, 379–380

Neutropenic fever, treatment-related, in lung
  cancer patients, supportive care for,
  379–380

Nitric oxide, in management of acute chest
  syndromein sickle cell disease, 872–873

Nitrocamptothecin, 9-, novel therapy with, for
  metastatic sarcomas, 585–586

Nodules, lung, CT-detected, guidelines for
  treatment of, 212–213

Non-Hodgkin's lymphoma, central nervous
  system involvement in, **597–609**
    diagnosis, 600–602
      cerebrospinal fluid analysis,
        601–602
      neuroimaging, 600–601
    prophylaxis, 602
    risk factors, 599
    treatment, 602–606
      transplantation, 605–606

Non-small cell lung cancer, postoperative
  radiation therapy for resected,
  283–302
    central nervous system relapse,
      294–296
    general considerations, 283–284
    patterns of failure following
      surgery, 284–286
    postoperative chemotherapy and,
      292–294
    reported results of, 286–291
    toxicity and technical
      considerations, 291–292
  stage IIIA, **303–319**
    chemoradiotherapy without
      surgery in, 308–310
    competing risks of patients with,
      315–316
    heterogeneity of, 304
    induction chemoradiotherapy
      followed by surgery in,
      310–312
    induction chemotherapy followed
      by surgery in, 307–308
    other randomized trials including
      surgery, 312–314
    results of surgery alone in,
      304–305
    toxicity considerations of surgery
      in, 314–315
    trials of adjuvant chemotherapy in,
      305–307
    trimodality including surgery *versus*
      bimodality, 312
  stages I and II, nonsurgical therapy for,
    237–261
    altered fractionation, 243–245
      accelerated, 243–244
      hypofractionation, 244–245
    combined modality therapy,
      253–254
    ongoing trials, 255
    other radiotherapy techniques, 253
    radiation dose escalation,
      240–243
    radiofrequency ablation, 254–255
    standard fractionation
      radiotherapy, 239–240
    stereotactic radiotherapy,
      245–252
  staging of, 225–229
    extrathoracic, 226–227
    intrathoracic, 227–229
Nonreceptor tyrosine kinases, in lung cancer
  therapy, 353–354
    Akt, 353
    angiogenesis and VEGF, 353–354
    mammalian target of
      rapamycin, 353
    phosphatidylinositol-3'-kinase, 353

Nonsteroidal anti-inflammatory drugs
  (NSAIDs), aspirin, as an antiplatelet
  agent, 91–93
  for acute sickle cell pain, 791, 792
Normiflo. *See* Ardeparin.
NSAIDs. *See* Nonsteroidal anti-
  inflammatory drugs.
Nuclear factor-kB pathway, in malignant
  mesothelioma, 1009

O

Oblimersen, novel therapy with, for
  metastatic sarcomas, 587
Obstetrics. *See* Pregnancy.
Ocular evaluation, in primary central nervous
  system lymphoma, 697–698
  See also Intraocular lymphoma.
Omega-3 fatty acids, new therapy for sickle
  cell disease with, 976–977
Oncologic outcomes, after surgical
  management of sarcoma, 465–466
    osteosarcoma and Ewing's
      sarcoma, 465
    soft tissue sarcoma, 465–466
Ophthalmic examination, in diagnosis of
  primary intraocular lymphoma, 740
Opioids, for acute sickle cell pain, 793–795
  classification of, 794
Optic nerve head, vascular changes at, due to
  sickle cell disease, 963
Oral mucositis, treatment-related, in lung
  cancer patients, supportive care for,
  381–382
Organ failure, multiple, in sickle cell disease,
  acute transfusion for, 809
Osteomyelitis, in sickle cell disease, 936–937
Osteonecrosis. *See* Bone and joint disease.
Osteopenia, in sickle cell disease, 938
Osteoporosis, heparin-associated, 40–43
Osteosarcoma, outcome after surgery for,
  functional, 466
    oncologic, 465
Osteotomies, for avascular necrosis of femoral
  head in sickle cell disease patients, 933
Outcome, after central nervous system relapse
  in lymphoma patients, 758–760
  of treatment-related neurotoxicity in
    primary central nervous system
    lymphoma, 731–735
Outcomes, after surgical management of
  sarcoma, 465–467
    functional, 466–467
    oncologic, 465–466
  of surgical management of gastro-
    intestinal stromal tumors, 549–550

Ovarian cancer, early detection with CA 125, lessons learned from, 1035–1036

Overanticoagulation, due to vitamin K antagonist therapy, 74–75
See also Bleeding complications.

Overt cerebral infarction. *See* Cerebral infarction.

Oxygenation, of patients with sickle cell disease undergoing surgical procedures, 901

P

P-selectin blockade, in management of acute chest syndrome in sickle cell disease, 873

p16^{INK4a}/p14^{ARF} alterations, in malignant mesothelioma, 1002–1003

p53 tumor suppressor protein pathway, in sarcomagenesis, 433–434
Rb-p53-Akt axis, 434

Paclitaxel, in advanced or metastatic angiosarcoma, 582–583
and STA-4783, 583

Pain, in lung cancer patients, supportive care for, 374
in sickle cell disease, classification of painful episodes, 785–787
See also Pain management.

Pain management, in sickle cell disease, **785–802**
acute pain syndromes, 786–797, 869
chronic pain syndromes, 797–799
neuropathic pain, 799
specific recommendations for, 799–800

Palliative radiotherapy, for malignant mesothelioma, 1100–1102

Panaparin, 5–6
See also Low molecular weight heparins.

Patent foramen ovale, antiplatelet therapy in, 107

Pathogenesis, of primary central nervous system lymphoma, 711–712

Pathology, of intraocular lymphoma, **707–711**
of primary central nervous system lymphoma, **705–717**
gross pathology, 706
incidence, 705–706
microscopic pathology and immunophenotype, 706–707
molecular pathology, 712–714
pathogenesis, 711–712

Patients, viewpoints on mesothelioma, **1175–1190**

Pegylated liposomal doxorubicin, novel therapy with, for metastatic sarcomas, 586–587

Pentasaccharides (fondaparinux), bleeding as complication of therapy with, 39–40
mechanism of action, pharmacology, and clinical use, **24–30**
thrombocytopenia induced by, 37–38

Percutaneous coronary intervention, antiplatelet therapy in, 101–106
ADP receptor antagonists, 101–103
aspirin, 101
platelet glycoprotein IIb/IIIa inhibitors in, 103–106
in myocardial infarction, delivery of reperfusion therapy, 156–157
facilitated, 156
primary, 157–158
versus thrombolysis, 153–156

Performance status, as prognostic factor in primary central nervous system lymphoma, 630–631

Pericardial mesothelioma, 1081–1082

Peripheral arterial thrombosis, current clinical practice, 166–169
antiplatelet agents for, 106

Peritoneal mesothelioma, **1067–1087**
clinical presentation, 1071
epidemiology, 1067–1068
intraperitoneal and systemic chemotherapy for, 1077–1078
pathology, 1068–1069
adenomatoid (benign), 1070–1071
deciduoid, 1070
diffuse, 1069–1070
multicystic, 1070
well-differentiated papillary, 1070
prognosis, 1079–1080
radiation and biologic agents for, 1078–1079
surgical treatment protocols of cytoreduction and hyperthermic chemotherapy, 1071–1077

Pharmacogenetics, potential for primary central nervous system lymphoma prognosis, 639–642

Pharmacokinetics, potential for primary central nervous system lymphoma prognosis, 642–643

Phenothiazines, as adjuvants for acute sickle cell pain, 795–796

Phosphatidylinositol-3'-kinase (PI3K), in lung cancer therapy, 353

Phosphodiesterase inhibitors, as antiplatelet agents, 94–95

Photocoagulation, for treatment of sickle cell disease affecting the eyes, 967–968
  feeder vessel, 967
  scatter, 967–968

Physical examination, initial, of patients with sarcoma, 451–452

Physicians, effect of, on adolescents and young adults with sarcoma, 538–539

Physiology, in research on antiplatelet drugs, 89–90

Plars plana vitrectomy, for nonclearing vitreous hemorrhage due to sickle cell disease, 968–969

Plasma coagulative factors, potential role of thrombogenesis in sickle cell disease, 778–779

Plasminogen activator, recombinant (r-PA), structure, function, and procoagulant effect of, 148–152

Platelets, potential role of thrombogenesis in sickle cell disease, 778–779

Platinums, for malignant mesothelioma, 1121

Pleural effusion, in lung cancer patients, dyspnea and, 372–374

Pleural mesothelioma, malignant, multi-modality treatment of, **1089–1097**
  See also Mesothelioma, malignant.

Pleurectomy, and decortication, radiation after, for mesothelioma, 1103–1105

Pneumonectomy, extrapleural, radiation after, for mesothelioma, 1105–1107

Polymerase chain reaction, for cerebrospinal fluid analysis in primary central nervous system lymphoma, 696–697

Positron emission tomography (PET), in diagnosis and staging of lung cancer, 219–235
  in evaluation of response to therapy in soft tissue sarcomas, 475–478

Postoperative therapies. *See* Adjuvant therapy.

Postphlebitic syndrome, due to central venous catheter thrombosis, 188–189

Predisposing conditions, in diagnosis of primary central nervous system lymphoma, 690

Pregnancy, adverse reactions to enoxaparin in pregnant women with prosthetic heart valves, 45–46
  sickle cell disease and, **903–916**
    controversial indication for transfusions in, 814–815
    fetal implications of maternal disease, 908–909
      fetal monitoring during painful events, 909

      intrauterine growth retardation/low birth-weight, 908–909
      perinatal mortality, 908
    in women with sickle cell trait, 914
    maternal issues, 905–908
      intrapartum complications, 907–908
      miscarriage, 907
      mortality, 905–907
      postpartum complications, 908
    obstetric management
      recommendations, 909–910
      labor and delivery, 910
      monitoring, 909–910
    other issues related to, 910–914
      other sickle cell disease comorbidities, 913–914
      transfusion therapy in, 911–913
      treatment of sickle cell pain episodes, 910–911
      urinary tract infections, 910
    potential pathophysiologic interactions, 903–904
      maternal anemia, 904
      red cell sickling, 903–904
      vascular occlusion, 904
    studies of, 904–905

Preoperative blood transfusions, in patients with sickle cell disease, 898–900

Presentation, clinical, initial, of patients with sarcoma, 451–452

Priapism, as complication of heparin therapy, 44
  in sickle cell disease, **917–928**
    epidemiology and natural history, 918–920
    management of acute episodes, 920–924
      aspiration and irrigation, 922–923
      surgical shunts, 924
      transfusion, 814, 924
      vasoactive agents, 921–922
    physiology, 917–918
    strategies for secondary prevention of, 924–926

Primary central nervous system lymphoma. *See* Lymphoma, primary central nervous system.

Primary intraocular lymphoma. *See* Intraocular lymphoma.

Primitive neuroectodermal tumor of bone, and Ewing's sarcoma family of tumors, **501–525**
  current clinical trials, 516–517
  epidemiology and clinical features, 502

genetic and molecular
    characteristics, 502–503
localized, treatment of, 503–509
metastatic, treatment of, 509–511
progressive and relapsed, 511
risk for secondary malignancy
    after curative therapy,
    515–516
stem cell transplantation for,
    511–515
Prognostic factors, for malignant
    mesothelioma, malignant, **1041–1052**
    clinical scoring systems,
        1041–1043
        validation, 1043–1047
    molecular prognostic markers,
        1047–1048
    other predictors, 1050–1051
    predictors of survival in patients
        treated surgically, 1048–1049
in primary central nervous system
    lymphoma, 612, **629–649**
    age and performance status,
        630–631
    new variables with potential value
        as, 636–643
        histopathologic, 636–639
        molecular and genetic, 639
        pharmacogenetics, 639–642
        pharmacokinetics, 642–643
    predictors of treatment-related
        toxicity, 643–645
    scoring systems for, 631–636
        International Extranodal
            Lymphoma Study
            Group Prognostic
            Score, 632–636
        International Prognostic
            Index, 631–632
        others, 636
Prognostic variables, in extremity soft tissue
    sarcomas, 490–492
Prophylaxis, against central nervous system
    relapse in lymphoma patients, 760–761
    in suspected central nervous system
        involvement in non-Hodgkin's
        lymphoma, 602
Prosthetic heart valves, adverse reactions to
    heparins in pregnant women with,
    45–46
Proteasome inhibitors, in lung cancer therapy,
    354–355
Pseudoephedrine, for prevention of priapism
    in sickle cell disease, 925
Psychosocial issues, depression in lung cancer
    patients, supportive care for, 382
    in adolescents and young adults with
        sarcoma, 535–536

PTK787, antiangiogenic therapy for
    mesothelioma with, 1141–1142
Pulmonary embolism, due to central venous
    catheter thrombosis, 189
    thrombolytic therapy in, 164–165
        current clinical practice, 165–166
Pulmonary hypertension, in sickle cell disease,
    881–896
    chronic transfusions for, 813–814
    diagnosis, 887–889
        Doppler echocardiography,
            887–888
        exercise measurements of pul-
            monary pressure, 889
        right heart catheterization,
            888–889
    hemodynamics and risk factors,
        883–884
    incidence and prevalence, 884–887
        in adult patients, 884–885
        in non- U.S. population,
            886–887
        in pediatric patients, 885–886
    management, 890–893
        anticoagulation, 892
        intensifying sickle cell disease
            treatment, 890–892
        new treatments for, 979–980
        pulmonary vasodilating and
            remodeling medica-
            tions, 892–893
    prognosis, 889–890
Pulmonary vasodilator and remodeling
    agents, in sickle cell patients with
    pulmonary hypertension, 892–893

Q

Quality of life, in lung cancer, validity of the
    Functional Assessment of Cancer
    Therapy-Lung Scale, **389–420**

R

Radiation therapy, combined with
    chemotherapy, for small cell lung
    cancer, **321–342**
        chemotherapy dosing, 335
        chemotherapy schedules,
            334–335
        choice of chemotherapy
            agents, 330–334
        novel approaches to,
            335–337
        radiotherapy dosing,
            328–329
        radiotherapy vol-
            ume, 330
        rationale, 322

sequential *versus* concurrent, 322–324
standard *versus* hyperfractionated radiation, 325–328
for stage IIIA non-small cell lung cancer, induction, followed by surgery, 310–312
other randomized trials of, 312–314
without surgery, 308–310
for AIDS-related primary central nervous system lymphoma, 674
for central nervous system involvement in non-Hodgkin's lymphoma, 604
for mesothelioma, **1099–1115**
for palliation, 1100–1102
potentially curative, 1102–1110
alone, 1102–1103
intensity modulated, 1111–112
target volume distribution, 1109–1110
technique, 1107–1109
three-dimensional conformal, 1110–1111
treatment planning, 1110–1112
with chemotherapy, 1103
with surgery, 1103–1107
for non-small cell lung cancer, stages I and II, **237–261**
altered fractionation, 243–245
accelerated hyperfractionation, 244
acceleration of, 243–244
hypofractionation, 244–245
combined modality therapy, 253–254
dose escalation, 240–243
ongoing trials, 255
other techniques, 253
radiofrequency ablation, 254–255
standard fractionation, 239–240
stereotactic, 245–252
for primary central nervous system lymphoma, 613–614
with high-dose methotrexate, 617–620

normal tissue toxicity, 238–239
postoperative, for resected non-small cell lung cancer, **283–302**
central nervous system relapse, 294–296
general considerations, 283–284
patterns of failure following surgery, 284–286
postoperative chemotherapy and, 292–294
reported results of, 286–291
toxicity and technical considerations, 291–292

Radiofrequency ablation, for non-small cell lung cancer, stages I and II, 254–255

Radiographs, chest, findings in initial evaluation of suspected lung cancer, 220–221
screening for lung cancer with, history of, 211
chest, in management of acute chest syndrome in sickle cell disease, 868–869
of avascular necrosis of femoral head in sickle cell disease patients, 931

Radiology, in measurement of mesothelioma, **1053–1066**
clinical trials of, 1055–1056
computer-assisted, 1062–1064
measuring lesions, 1054–1055
response evaluation criteria in solid tumors and mesothelioma, 1056–1058
variability in, 1058–1062
volumetric measurements, 1064

Ranpirnase, for malignant mesothelioma, 1128–1129

Rapamycin, mammalian target of (mTOR), in lung cancer therapy, 353

Reactive oxygen species, in malignant mesothelioma, 1009–1010

Receptor tyrosine kinases, in lung cancer therapy, 344–352
c-Kit, 351–352
c-Met, 352
epidermal growth factor receptors, 345–350
human epidermal growth factor 2/neu, 350–351
in malignant mesothelioma, 1003

Recombinant plasminogen activator (r-PA), structure, function, and procoagulant effect of, 148–152

Recombinant tissue plasminogen activator (rt-PA), structure, function, and procoagulant effect of, 148–152

Recurrence, after surgical management of gastrointestinal stromal tumors, 550–553
  of primary central nervous system lymphoma, treatment for, 623

Red blood cell sickling, in pregnant women with sickle cell disease, 903–904

Refludan. *See* Lepirudin.

Remodeling agents, pulmonary, in sickle cell patients with pulmonary hypertension, 892–893

Resistance, to antiplatelet drugs, 108

Response, to therapy, imaging evaluation of, in soft tissue sarcomas, **471–487**
  conventional CT and MRI, 472–475
  dynamic contrast-enhanced MRI, 478–481
  gastrointestinal stromal tumors, 482–483
  magnetic resonance spectroscopy, 481
  positron emission tomography, 475–478
  thallium-201 scintigraphy, 482

Reteplase, structure, function, and procoagulant effect of, 148–152

Retinal vasculature, effects of sickle cell disease on, 961

Retinoblastoma tumor suppressor protein pathway, in sarcomagenesis, 433
  Rb-p53-Akt axis, 434

Retinoid signaling pathways, in lung cancer therapy, 354

Retinopathy, proliferative sickle, due to sickle cell disease, 963–966

Reviparin, 5–6
  See also Low molecular weight heparins.

Rhabdomyosarcoma, alveolar, molecular mechanisms of, 439
  in adolescents and young adults, 541–542

Rituximab, for central nervous system involvement in non-Hodgkin's lymphoma, 604–605
  for primary central nervous system lymphoma, phase II trials of, 721–722

S

Salmon patch hemorrhage, due to sickle cell disease, 959

Sandoparin. *See* Certoparin.

Sarcomagenesis, mechanisms of, **427–449**
  cell cycle regulatory proteins and, 431–434
  in specific subtypes, 437–440
    alveolar rhabdomyosarcoma, 439
    Ewing's sarcoma, 439–440
    gastrointestinal stromal tumors, 440
    liposarcoma, 437–438
  karyotype abnormalities and, 434–437
  targeted therapy and, 441–444
    in liposarcomas, 443
    targeting signal transduction cascades, 441
    targeting translocation/fusion gene products, 441–442
    with imatinib mesylate, 443–444

Sarcomas, 427–590
  desmoid tumors and deep fibromatoses, **565–571**
    clinical presentation, 566
    diagnosis, 567
    etiology, 565–566
    genetics, 567
    histology, 566–567
    treatment, 567–569
  Ewing's and primitive neuroectodermal family of tumors, **501–525**
    current clinical trials, 516–517
    epidemiology and clinical features, 502
    genetic and molecular characteristics, 502–503
    localized, treatment of, 503–509
    metastatic, treatment of, 509–511
    progressive and relapsed, 511
    risk for secondary malignancy after curative therapy, 515–516
    stem cell transplantation for, 511–515
  gastrointestinal stromal tumors, **547–564**
    medical management, 552–560
    surgical management, 548–552
  histologic classification, 428–430
  in adolescents and young adults, **527–546**
    demographics of, 527–530
    etiology of, 533–534
    late effects of therapy, 542–544
    management outside clinical trials, 539–542
    presentation of, 534
    psychosocial aspects, 535–536
    treatment issues, 536–539
    tumor biology, 530–533

mechanisms of sarcomagenesis, **427–449**
cell cycle regulatory proteins and,
431–434
in specific subtypes, 437–440
alveolar rhabdomyo-
sarcoma, 439
Ewing's sarcoma, 439–440
gastrointestinal stromal
tumors, 440
liposarcoma, 437–438
karyotype abnormalities and,
434–437
targeted therapy and, 441–444
metastatic, novel therapies for, **573–590**
9-nitrocamptothecin, 585–586
bortezomib, 585
ecteinascidin, 583–585
everolimus, 580
gemcitabine and combinations,
573–578
imatinib, in dermatofibrosarcoma
protuberans, 580–581
in desmoid tumors and other
sarcomas, 581–582
safety and tolerability of,
578–579
oblimersen, 587
paclitaxel, and STA-4783, 583
in angiosarcoma, 582–583
pegylated liposomal doxorubicin,
586–587
SU11248, 579–580
soft tissue, imaging and response in,
471–487
conventional CT and MRI,
472–475
dynamic contrast-enhanced
MRI, 478–481
gastrointestinal stromal
tumors, 482–483
magnetic resonance
spectroscopy, 481
positron emission
tomography, 475–478
thallium-201 scintigra-
phy, 482
of the extremities, **489–500**
adjuvant chemotherapy,
492–495
neoadjuvant chemotherapy,
495–497
prognostic variables,
490–492
surgical management of, **451–470**
biopsy, 453–457
clinical presentation and physical
examination, 451–452
evaluation, 452–453
functional outcome, 466–467
indications for, 457

margins, 461–463
oncologic outcome, 465–466
peri-operative management,
463–465
prior excisional biopsy, 460–461
resectability and limb salvage,
457–460
timing of, 457
Scatter photocoagulation, for treatment of
sickle cell disease affecting the eyes,
967–968
Scintigraphy, thallium-201, in evaluation of
response to therapy in soft tissue
sarcomas, 482
Scleral buckling surgery, for retinal
detachment due to sickle cell disease,
969–970
Screening, for lung cancer, **209–217**
associated studies, 215–216
biases associated with, 210
consensus recommendations, 214
CT-detected nodules, guidelines
for treating, 212–214
current trials of, 212–
reasons for, 209–210
with chest radiographs, history
of, 211
for malignant mesothelioma, 1026–1029
failure of, 1027–1028
for other cancers, 1028–1029
lessons from CA125 and early
detection of ovarian cancer,
1035–1036
mesothelin and soluble mesothelin-
related protein, 1029–1035
use of multiple serum markers
for, 1037
Secondary central nervous system lymphoma.
See Central nervous system
lymphoma, secondary.
Secondary malignancy, after curative therapy
for Ewing's sarcoma family of tumors,
515–516
Seizures, antiepileptic medications for, in
primary central nervous system
lymphoma, 623
Sequestration, acute splenic and hepatic,
transfusion for, in sickle cell disease,
806–807
Shunts, surgical, for priapism in sickle cell
disease, 924
Sickle cell disease, 771–985
acute chest syndrome in, **857–879**
clinical presentation, 860–861
diagnosis, 865–868
epidemiology, 858–860

future directions, 872–873
laboratory features, 863–865
management, 868–872
pathophysiology, 861–863
arterial blood pressure and
  hyperviscosity in, **827–837**
  elevated, 831
  hyperviscosity syndrome, 832–834
  hypotheses on, 830–831
  regulation of, 827–830
  treatment of hypertension,
    831–832
  whole blood viscosity, 832
bone and joint disease in, **929–941**
  bone marrow disturbances,
    937–938
  femoral infarcts, clinical
    identification, 930
  femoral infarcts, 929–934
  growth disturbances,
    930–931
  non-surgical disease,
    931–932
  pathophysiology and risk
    factors, 929–930
  prevalence and incidence, 930
  radiography, 931
  staging, 931
  surgical treatment, 932–934
  humeral infarcts, 934–935
  osteomyelitis, 936–937
  other bony effects, 938
  vertebral infarcts, 935–936
effects on the eye, **957–972**
  clinical features, 957–966
  treatment, 967–970
leg ulceration in, **943–956**
  characteristics of, 947–949
  complications of, 951–952
  history, 943
  incidence and prevalence, 943–944
  risk factors, 944–947
  treatment of, 949–951
new therapies for, **973–985**
  anti-adhesion therapy, prospects
    for, 978–979
  for primary stroke prevention,
    980–981
  for pulmonary hypertension,
    979–980
  Gardos channel blockers, 977–978
  hydroxyurea therapy, 974–976
  omega-3 fatty acids, 976–977
  oral therapy for iron overload, 981
overt and incomplete (silent) cerebral
  infarction in children with,
  839–855
  acute management, 848
  clinical diagnosis, 843–844
  hydroxyurea, 850–851

management algorithm for, 842
neuroimaging, 844–847
neurorehabilitation, 851–852
prevention, 848
risk factors, 840–843
transfusion therapy, 848–850
pain management in, **785–802**
  acute pain syndromes, 786–797
  chronic pain syndromes, 797–799
  classification of painful episodes,
    785–787
  neuropathic pain, 799
  specific recommendations for,
    799–800
pregnancy and, **903–916**
  fetal implications of maternal
    disease, 908–909
  in women with sickle cell trait, 914
  maternal issues, 905–908
  obstetric management
    recommendations, 909–910
  other issues related to, 910–914
    other sickle cell disease
      comorbidities, 913–914
    transfusion therapy in,
      911–913
    treatment of sickle cell pain
      episodes, 910–911
    urinary tract infections, 910
  potential pathophysiologic
    interactions, 903–904
    maternal anemia, 904
    red cell sickling, 903–904
    vascular occlusion, 904
  studies of, 904–905
priapism in, **917–928**
  epidemiology and natural history,
    918–920
  management of acute episodes,
    920–924
  physiology, 917–918
  strategies for secondary prevention
    of, 924–926
pulmonary hypertension in, **881–896**
  diagnosis, 887–889
  hemodynamics and risk factors,
    883–884
  incidence and prevalence,
    884–887
  management, 890–893
  prognosis, 889–890
surgery in, **897–902**
  care measures for, 898–901
  common procedures in patients
    with, 897–898
transfusion management in, **803–826**
  blood product selection, 819–821
  complications of, 816–819
    immunologic, 816–818
    non-immunologic, 818–819

indications for, 805–816
    acute, 806–811
    chronic, 811–814
    controversial, 814–816
  methods, 804–805
  vaso-occlusion in, **771–784**
    as syndrome of chronic vascular
      inflammation, 773–775
    leukocyte adhesion in,
      775–778
    mechanisms of erythrocyte
      adhesion, 772–773
    model of, 780–781
    platelets and plasma coagulative
      factors, 778–779
    sickle hemoglobin
      polymerization, 772
Sickle cell trait, pregnancy in women
  with, 914
Signal pathways, in malignant
  mesothelioma, 1006
Signal transduction, disruption in, in
  sarcomagenesis, 431–433
  Rb-p53-Akt axis, 434
  sarcoma therapy targeting, 441
Sildenafil, for prevention of priapism in sickle
  cell disease, 925
Silent cerebral infarction. *See*
  Cerebral infarction.
Simian virus 40, potential in gene therapy for
  mesothelioma, 1167–1168
Simple transfusion, method for, in sickle cell
  disease, 804
Single-photon emission CT (SPECT), of
  AIDS-related primary nervous system
  lymphoma, 670–671
Skin necrosis, coumarin-induced, 75
  heparin-related, 43–44
Small cell lung cancer, combined
  chemoradiotherapy in, **321–342**
    chemotherapy dosing, 335
    chemotherapy schedules,
      334–335
    choice of chemotherapy agents,
      330–334
    novel approaches to, 335–337
    radiotherapy dosing, 328–329
    radiotherapy volume, 330
    rationale, 322
    sequential *versus* concurrent,
      322–324
    standard *versus* hyperfractionated
      radiation, 325–328
  staging of, 230–231
Social effects, of leg ulcers in sickle cell disease
  patients, 951–952

Soft tissue sarcomas, of the extremities,
  489–500
    adjuvant chemotherapy, 492–495
    neoadjuvant chemotherapy,
      495–497
    prognostic variables, 490–492
  outcomes after surgery for, functional,
    466–467
    oncologic, 465–466
Soluble mesothelin-related protein, in
  detection of malignant mesothelioma,
  1029–1035
Spirometry, incentive, in management of
  acute chest syndrome in sickle cell
  disease, 870
Splenectomy, in patients with sickle cell
  disease, 897–898
Splenic sequestration, acute, transfusion for,
  in sickle cell disease, 806–807
Staging
  non-small cell lung cancer, 225–229
    extrathoracic, 226–227
    intrathoracic, 227–229
  of avascular necrosis of femoral head in
    sickle cell disease patients, 931
  of primary central nervous system
    lymphoma, 699–700
  small cell lung cancer, 230–231
Standard fractionation radiotherapy, for
  non-small cell lung cancer, stages I
  and II, 239–240
Stem cell transplantation, autologous, with
  intensive chemotherapy for primary
  central nervous system lymphoma,
  722–725
  for central nervous system involvement
    in non-Hodgkin's lymphoma,
    605–606
  for Ewing's sarcoma family of tumors,
    511–515
    allogeneic, 514–515
Stereotactic radiotherapy, for non-small cell
  lung cancer, stages I and II, 245–252
Steroids. *See* Corticosteroids.
Streptokinase, structure, function, and
  procoagulant effect of, 148–152
Stroke, acute ischemic, thrombolytic therapy
  for, current clinical practice, 158–162
  in sickle cell disease patients, acute,
    transfusion for, 808–809
    overt and incomplete (silent)
      cerebral infarction in
      children, **839–855**
      acute management, 848
      clinical diagnosis, 843–844
      hydroxyurea, 850–851

management algorithm
    for, 842
  neuroimaging, 844–847
  neurorehabilitation, 851–852
  prevention, 848
  risk factors, 840–843
  transfusion therapy, 848–850
prevention of, chronic transfusions
    for, 812–813
  primary, 812, 980–981
  secondary, 812–813

Stroke prevention, ximelagatran for, in
  patients with atrial fibrillation, 79

Stromal tumors, gastrointestinal. *See* Gastrointestinal stromal tumors (GISTs).

SU11248, for imatinib-resistant gastrointestinal stromal tumors, 558–559, 579–580

SU5416, antiangiogenic therapy for
  mesothelioma with, 1139–1140

Suicide gene therapy, in mesothelioma,
  1148–1150, 1158–1159

Superior vena cava syndrome, in lung cancer
  patients, supportive care for, 376–377

Supportive care, in lung cancer, **369–387**
  for disease-related symptoms,
      369–378
    bony metastases, 375
    cachexia, 377–378
    cough, 375–376
    dyspnea, 369–374
    pain, 374
    superior vena cava
        syndrome, 376–377
  for treatment-related symptoms,
      378–382
    anemia and fatigue, 380–381
    nausea and vomiting,
        378–379
    neutropenia and neutropenic
        fever, 379–380
    oral mucositis, 381–382
  psychosocial issues, 382

Surgery, in sickle cell disease patients,
  897–902
    care measures for, 898–901
      hydration, 900–901
      infection control, 901
      oxygenation, 901
      pain, 900
      preoperative blood transfu-
          sion, 809–811, 898–900
      temperature, 901
    common procedures in, adeno-
        tonsillectomy, 897
      cholecystectomy and
          splenectomy, 897–898
      hip arthroplasty, 898
    for leg ulcers, 951

role in stage IIIA non-small cell lung
  cancer, **303–319**
    chemoradiotherapy without
        surgery in, 308–310
    competing risks of patients with,
        315–316
    heterogeneity of, 304
    induction chemoradiotherapy
        followed by surgery in,
        310–312
    induction chemotherapy followed
        by surgery in, 307–308
    other randomized trials including
        surgery, 312–314
    results of surgery alone in,
        304–305
    toxicity considerations of surgery
        in, 314–315
    trials of adjuvant chemotherapy in,
        305–307
    trimodality including surgery *versus*
        bimodality, 312

Surgical management, of gastrointestinal
  stromal tumors, 548–552
    emerging approaches combining
        imatinib and, 552
    outcomes, 549–550
    preoperative assessment, 548
    primary disease, 548–549
    recurrent or metastatic,
        550–552
  of malignant mesothelioma,
    radiotherapy combined with,
        1103–1107
    predictors of survival in malignant
        mesothelioma patients after,
        1048–1050
  of sarcomas, **451–470**
    biopsy, 453–457
    clinical presentation and physical
        examination, 451–452
    evaluation, 452–453
    functional outcome, 466–467
    indications for, 457
    margins, 461–463
    oncologic outcome, 465–466
    peri-operative management,
        463–465
    prior excisional biopsy, 460–461
    resectability and limb salvage,
        457–460
    timing of, 457

SV40, in malignant mesothelioma,
  1010–1012

Symptomatic treatment, for primary central
  nervous system lymphoma, 623

Synovial sarcoma, in adolescents and young
  adults, 542

T

T-cell primary central nervous system lymphoma, 658–661

Targeted therapies, against Epstein-Barr virus in AIDS-related primary central nervous system lymphoma, 679–681
    disruption of viral functions, 680
    selective drug activation, 680–681
    targeting viral antigens, 679–680

Targeted therapy, for gastrointestinal stromal tumors, 553–560
    role of molecular mechanisms of sarcomagenesis in development of, 441–444
        conceptual approaches, 441–442
            targeting signal transduction cascades, 441
            targeting translocation/fusion gene products, 441–442
        selected examples of, 443–444
            imatinib mesylate, 443–444
            liposarcomas, 443

Tegafur. *See* Uracil-tegafur.

Temozolomide, phase II trials of, for primary central nervous system lymphoma, 719–721

Temperature, body, of patients with sickle cell disease undergoing surgical procedures, 901

Tenecteplase, structure, function, and procoagulant effect of, 148–152

Terathiomolybdate, antiangiogenic therapy for mesothelioma with, 1142

Teratogenic effects, of enoxaparin, 45–46

Thalidomide, antiangiogenic therapy for mesothelioma with, 1140

Thallium-201 scintigraphy, in evaluation of response to therapy in soft tissue sarcomas, 482

Thienopyridines, as antiplatelet agents, 93

Three-dimensional conformal radiation therapy, for malignant mesothelioma, 1110–1111

Thrombin, role in thrombogenesis, 119–124

Thrombocytopenia, heparin-induced, 31–38
        treatment of, 38
        pentasaccharide-induced, 37–38

Thrombogenesis, potential role in sickle cell disease, 778–779
    role of thrombin in, 119–124

Thrombolytic agents, structure, function, and procoagulant effect of, 148–152

Thrombolytic therapy
    current clinical practice, **147–181**
        cerebrovascular thrombosis, 158–162
        complications of, 170–171
        miscellaneous disorders, 170
        myocardial infarction, 152–158
        peripheral arterial thrombosis, 166–169
        venous thromboembolism, 162–166
    See also Antithrombotic therapy.

Thrombosis, pathogenesis of, in research on antiplatelet drugs, 90–91

Thromboxane receptor antagonists, as future antiplatelet agents, 109

Thromboxane synthase inhibitors, as future antiplatelet agents, 109

Ticlopidine, as antiplatelet agent, 93

Tinzaparin, 5–8, 10, 15, 16
    development of generic low molecular weight heparins, **53–68**

Tirofiban, as an antiplatelet agent, 94

Tissue plasminogen activator, recombinant (rt-PA), structure, function, and procoagulant effect of, 148–152

Topoisomerase inhibitors, for malignant mesothelioma, 1121

Topotecan, phase II trials of, for primary central nervous system lymphoma, 719–721

Total hip arthroplasty, for avascular necrosis of femoral head in sickle cell disease patients, 933–934

Toxicity, considerations of surgery in stage IIIA non-small cell lung cancer, 314–315
    to normal tissue in radiation therapy, 238–239
    treatment-related, in primary central nervous system lymphoma, predictors of, 643–645

Toxoplasmosis therapy, empiric, *versus* early biopsy, in AIDS-related primary central nervous system lymphoma, 673–674

Transcranial Doppler ultrasonography, in diagnosis of overt and incomplete (silent) cerebral infarction in children with sickle cell anemia, 844–847

Transcriptional modulation, in targeted sarcoma therapy, 442

Transfusion management, in sickle cell disease, **803–826**
        blood product selection, 819–821
        complications of, 816–819
            immunologic, 816–818
            non-immunologic, 818–819

in pregnancy, 911–913
indications for, acute, 806–811, 848–850, 870–872
chronic, 811–814
controversial, 814–816, 924
preoperative, 898–900
methods, 804–805

Transient red cell aplasia, acute transfusion for, in sickle cell disease, 806

Translocation/fusion gene products, as target of sarcoma therapy, 441–442

Transplantation, of autologous hematopoietic stem cells, for central nervous system involvement in non-Hodgkin's lymphoma, 605–606
with intensive chemotherapy, for primary central nervous system lymphoma, 722–725
of bone marrow, for primary central nervous system lymphoma, 622–623

Transthoracic needle aspiration, in diagnosis and staging of lung cancer, 223–225

Treatment-related neurotoxicity. See Neurotoxicity.

Tricyclic antidepressants, as adjuvants for acute sickle cell pain, 795–796

Tumor vaccines, in lung cancer therapy, 358–360

Tumor-associated antigens, in lung cancer therapy, 357–360
gastrin-releasing peptide, 357–358
neural cell adhesion molecule (CD56), 357–360
tumor vaccines, 358–360

Tunica vaginalis, mesothelioma of, 1080–1081

Tyrosine kinase inhibitors, for imatinib-resistant gastrointestinal stromal tumors, 559–560
for malignant mesothelioma, 1129

Tyrosine kinases, in lung cancer therapy, nonreceptor, 353–354
Akt, 353
angiogenesis and VEGF, 353–354
mammalian target of rapamycin, 353
phosphatidylinositol-3'-kinase, 353
receptor, 344–352
c-Kit, 351–352
c-Met, 352
epidermal growth factor receptors, 345–350
human epidermal growth factor 2/neu, 350–351

U

Ulcers, leg. See Leg ulceration.

Ultrasonography, in diagnosis of overt and incomplete (silent) cerebral infarction in children with sickle cell anemia, 844–847

Unfractionated heparin, mechanism of action, pharmacology, and clinical use, **1–4**

Uracil-tegafur (UFT), adjuvant oral, in lung cancer, Japanese trials with, 273–274

Urinary tract infections, in pregnant women with sickle cell disease, 910

Urokinase, structure, function, and procoagulant effect of, 148–152

V

Vaccines, tumor, in lung cancer therapy, 358–360

Vascular endothelial growth factor, in lung cancer therapy, 353–354

Vascular endothelial growth factor receptor, in malignant mesothelioma, 1005–1006

Vascular inflammation, chronic, sickle cell disease as syndrome of, 773–775

Vaso-occlusion, in sickle cell anemia, **771–784**
as syndrome of chronic vascular inflammation, 773–775
during pregnancy, 904
leukocyte adhesion in, 775–778
mechanisms of erythrocyte adhesion, 772–773
model of, 780–781
platelets and plasma coagulative factors, 778–779
sickle hemoglobin polymerization, 772

Vasoactive agents, for priapism in sickle cell disease, 921–922

Vasodilating agents, for leg ulcers in sickle cell disease patients, 950

Vasodilators, pulmonary, in sickle cell patients with pulmonary hypertension, 892–893

Venous incompetence, role in leg ulceration in sickle cell disease patients, 946–947

Venous thromboembolism, thrombolytic therapy in, 162–166
acute, ximelagatran versus dalteparin for, 78
current clinical practice, 165–166
deep vein thrombosis, 163–164
pulmonary embolism, 164–165

Vertebral infarcts, in sickle cell disease, 935–936

Viscosity, hyperviscosity syndrome, in sickle cell disease, 832–834
of whole blood, 832

Vitamin K antagonists, anticoagulation therapy with, **69–85**
adverse effects of, 74–76
alternatives to, for long-term treatment, 76–80
pharmacology of, 70–74

Vitreous biopsy, in diagnosis of primary intraocular lymphoma, 742

Vomiting, treatment-related, in lung cancer patients, supportive care for, 378–379

W

Warfarin, clinical use as an indirect thrombin inhibitor, 124–126
low-dose, in prevention of central venous catheter-related deep venous thrombosis, 193–194
pharmacokinetics and pharmaco-dynamics of, 71–73
See also Vitamin K antagonists.

White matter abnormalities, and cognitive outcome, with treatment-related neurotoxicity in primary central nervous system lymphoma, 731–732

Wnt pathway, in malignant mesothelioma, 1006–1007

X

X-rays. *See* Radiographs.

Ximelagatran, 77–80
as a direct thrombin inhibitor, 134–139
as an antiplatelet agent, 95–96
for initial and long-term treatment of thrombotic disorders, 77–78
for long-term treatment of venous thromboembolism, 78
for prevention of cardiovascular events after acute coronary syndromes, 79–80
for stroke prevention in patients with atrial fibrillation, 79
for treatment of acute venous thromboembolism, 78

Y

Young adults, sarcomas in adolescents and, **527–546**
demographics of, 527–530
etiology of, 533–534
late effects of therapy, 542–544
management outside clinical trials, 539–542
presentation of, 534
psychosocial aspects, 535–536
treatment issues, 536–539
tumor biology, 530–533

Z

Zinc, for leg ulcers in sickle cell disease patients, 950

Changing Your Address?

Make sure your subscription changes too! When you notify us of your new address, you can help make our job easier by including an exact copy of your Clinics label number with your old address (see illustration below.) This number identifies you to our computer system and will speed the processing of your address change. Please be sure this label number accompanies your old address and your corrected address—you can send an old Clinics label with your number on it or just copy it exactly and send it to the address listed below.

We appreciate your help in our attempt to give you continuous coverage. Thank you.

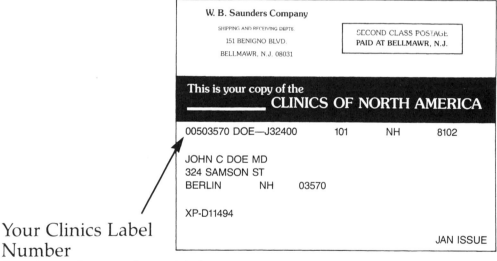

W. B. Saunders Company

SHIPPING AND RECEIVING DEPTS.
151 BENIGNO BLVD.
BELLMAWR, N.J. 08031

SECOND CLASS POSTAGE
PAID AT BELLMAWR, N.J.

This is your copy of the
CLINICS OF NORTH AMERICA

00503570 DOE—J32400   101   NH   8102

JOHN C DOE MD
324 SAMSON ST
BERLIN   NH   03570

XP-D11494

JAN ISSUE

Your Clinics Label Number
Copy it exactly or send your label
along with your address to:
W.B. Saunders Company, Customer Service
Orlando, FL 32887-4800
Call Toll Free 1-800-654-2452

Please allow four to six weeks for delivery of new subscriptions and for processing address changes.

United States Postal Service

Statement of Ownership, Management, and Circulation

1. Publication Title	2. Publication Number	3. Filing Date
Hematology/Oncology Clinics of North America	0 8 8 9 - 8 5 8 8	9/15/05

4. Issue Frequency	5. Number of Issues Published Annually	6. Annual Subscription Price
Feb, Apr, Jun, Aug, Oct, Dec	6	$210.00

7. Complete Mailing Address of Known Office of Publication (Not printer) (Street, city, county, state, and ZIP+4)

Elsevier Inc.
6277 Sea Harbor Drive
Orlando, FL 32887-4800

Contact Person
Gwen C. Campbell

Telephone
215-239-3685

8. Complete Mailing Address of Headquarters or General Business Office of Publisher (Not printer)

Elsevier Inc., 360 Park Avenue South, New York, NY 10010-1710

9. Full Names and Complete Mailing Addresses of Publisher, Editor, and Managing Editor (Do not leave blank)

Publisher (Name and complete mailing address)

Tim Griswold, Elsevier Inc., 1600 John F. Kennedy Blvd., Suite 1800, Philadelphia, PA 19103-2899

Editor (Name and complete mailing address)

Kerry Holland, Elsevier Inc., 1600 John F. Kennedy Blvd., Suite 1800, Philadelphia, PA 19103-2899

Managing Editor (Name and complete mailing address)

Heather Cullen, Elsevier Inc., 1600 John F. Kennedy Blvd., Suite 1800, Philadelphia, PA 19103-2899

10. Owner (Do not leave blank. If the publication is owned by a corporation, give the name and address of the corporation immediately followed by the names and addresses of all stockholders owning or holding 1 percent or more of the total amount of stock. If not owned by a corporation, give the names and addresses of the individual owners. If owned by a partnership or other unincorporated firm, give its name and address as well as those of each individual owner. If the publication is published by a nonprofit organization, give its name and address.)

Full Name	Complete Mailing Address
Wholly owned subsidiary of	4520 East-West Highway
Reed/Elsevier Inc., US holdings	Bethesda, MD 20814

11. Known Bondholders, Mortgagees, and Other Security Holders Owning or Holding 1 Percent or More of Total Amount of Bonds, Mortgages, or Other Securities. If none, check box ▸ ☐ None

Full Name	Complete Mailing Address
N/A	

12. Tax Status (For completion by nonprofit organizations authorized to mail at nonprofit rates) (Check one)
The purpose, function, and nonprofit status of this organization and the exempt status for federal income tax purposes:
☐ Has Not Changed During Preceding 12 Months
☐ Has Changed During Preceding 12 Months (Publisher must submit explanation of change with this statement)

(See Instructions on Reverse)

13. Publication Title		14. Issue Date for Circulation Data Below
Hematology/Oncology Clinics of North America		June 2005

15.	Extent and Nature of Circulation	Average No. Copies Each Issue During Preceding 12 Months	No. Copies of Single Issue Published Nearest to Filing Date
a.	Total Number of Copies (Net press run)	3067	2900
b. Paid and/or Requested Circulation	(1) Paid/Requested Outside-County Mail Subscriptions Stated on Form 3541. (Include advertiser's proof and exchange copies)	1569	1458
	(2) Paid In-County Subscriptions Stated on Form 3541 (Include advertiser's proof and exchange copies)		
	(3) Sales Through Dealers and Carriers, Street Vendors, Counter Sales, and Other Non-USPS Paid Distribution	590	464
	(4) Other Classes Mailed Through the USPS		
c.	Total Paid and/or Requested Circulation [Sum of 15b. (1), (2), (3), and (4)] ▸	2159	1922
d. Free Distribution by Mail (Samples, complimentary, and other free)	(1) Outside-County as Stated on Form 3541	78	121
	(2) In-County as Stated on Form 3541		
	(3) Other Classes Mailed Through the USPS		
e.	Free Distribution Outside the Mail (Carriers or other means)		
f.	Total Free Distribution (Sum of 15d. and 15e.) ▸	78	121
g.	Total Distribution (Sum of 15c. and 15f.) ▸	2237	2043
h.	Copies not Distributed	830	857
i.	Total (Sum of 15g. and h.) ▸	3067	2900
j.	Percent Paid and/or Requested Circulation (15c. divided by 15g. times 100)	97%	94%

16. Publication of Statement of Ownership
☐ Publication required. Will be printed in the **December 2005** issue of this publication.   ☐ Publication not required

17. Signature and Title of Editor, Publisher, Business Manager, or Owner

[signature] Jan M Farucci – Executive Director of Subscription Services   Date 9/15/05

I certify that all information furnished on this form is true and complete. I understand that anyone who furnishes false or misleading information on this form or who omits material or information requested on the form may be subject to criminal sanctions (including fines and imprisonment) and/or civil sanctions (including civil penalties).

Instructions to Publishers

1. Complete and file one copy of this form with your postmaster annually on or before October 1. Keep a copy of the completed form for your records.
2. In cases where the stockholder or security holder is a trustee, include in items 10 and 11 the name of the person or corporation for whom the trustee is acting. Also include the names and addresses of individuals who are stockholders who own or hold 1 percent or more of the total amount of bonds, mortgages, or other securities of the publishing corporation. In item 11, if none, check the box. Use blank sheets if more space is required.
3. Be sure to furnish all circulation information called for in item 15. Free circulation must be shown in items 15d, e, and f.
4. Item 15h., Copies not Distributed, must include (1) newsstand copies originally stated on Form 3541, and returned to the publisher, (2) estimated returns from news agents, and (3), copies for office use, leftovers, spoiled, and all other copies not distributed.
5. If the publication had Periodicals authorization as a general or requester publication, this Statement of Ownership, Management, and Circulation must be published; it must be printed in any issue in October or, if the publication is not published during October, the first issue printed after October.
6. In item 16, indicate the date of the issue in which this Statement of Ownership will be published.
7. Item 17 must be signed.

Failure to file or publish a statement of ownership may lead to suspension of Periodicals authorization.

PS Form **3526**, October 1999 (Reverse)

PS Form **3526**, October 1999